Migraine

T0146107

Migraine

A HISTORY

✳ ✳ ✳

Katherine Foxhall

Johns Hopkins University Press, Baltimore

This book was brought to publication with the generous assistance of the Wellcome Trust.

Johns Hopkins University Press
2715 North Charles Street
Baltimore, Maryland 21218-4363
www.press.jhu.edu

Library of Congress Cataloging-in-Publication Data

Names: Foxhall, Katherine, author.
Title: Migraine : a history / Katherine Foxhall.
Description: Baltimore : Johns Hopkins University Press, 2019. | Includes bibliographical references and index.
Identifiers: LCCN 2018039557 | ISBN 9781421429489 (pbk. : alk. paper) | ISBN 1421429489 (pbk. : alk. paper) | ISBN 9781421429496 (electronic) | ISBN 1421429497 (electronic) | ISBN 9781421429502 (electronic open access) | ISBN 1421429500 (electronic open access)
Subjects: | MESH: Migraine Disorders—history
Classification: LCC RC392 | NLM WL 11.1 | DDC 616.8/4912—dc23
LC record available at https://lccn.loc.gov/2018039557

A catalog record for this book is available from the British Library.

Special discounts are available for bulk purchases of this book. For more information, please contact Special Sales at 410-516-6936 or specialsales@press.jhu.edu.

Johns Hopkins University Press uses environmentally friendly book materials, including recycled text paper that is composed of at least 30 percent post-consumer waste, whenever possible.

CONTENTS

List of Figures   vii
Acknowledgments   ix
Note on Terminology and Names   xiii

1 Introduction: Programmed In?   1

2 The "Beating of Hammers": Classical and Medieval Approaches to
   Hemicrania   22

3 "Take Housleeke, and Garden Wormes": Migraine Medicine in the Early
   Modern Household   42

4 A "Deadly Tormenting Megrym": Expanding Markets and Changing
   Meanings   61

5 "The Pain Was Very Much Relieved and She Slept": Gender and
   Patienthood in the Nineteenth Century   88

6 "As Sharp as If Drawn with Compasses": Victorian Vision, Men of
   Science, and the Making of Modern Migraine   110

7 "A Shower of Phosphenes": Twentieth-Century Stories and the Medical
   Uses of History   135

8 "Happy Hunting Ground": Conceptual Fragmentation and
   Experimentation in the Twentieth Century   155

9 "If I Could Harness Pain": The Migraine Art Competitions,
   1980–1987   184

10 Conclusion   211

Notes   219
Bibliography   243
Index   269

1.1. *Programmed In! (Unwillingly.) Woe Is Me!*, Third Migraine Art Competition, 1985   2

2.1. "Remedies for Healfes Heafdes Ece," from Bald's *Leechbook*, c. 950   23

2.2. "Vein Man" diagram, from "Guild-Book of the Barber-Surgeons of the City of York," c. 1486   36

3.1. "Medecyne for the Megreeme," from Mrs. Corlyon's *Booke of Diuers Medecines*, 1606   51

4.1. "Sainte Anne's Well," from John Speed, *Theatre of the Empire of Great Britaine*, 1611/12   64

4.2. *Monsieur le Médecin*, 1771   86

6.1. Mr. Beck's "Arched Spectrum," from W. R. Gowers, 1895   111

6.2. John Herschel's diary, 22 June 1869   119

6.3. "Diagram of Transient Teichopsia," from Hubert Airy, 1870   121

7.1. "The Heavenly City," Wiesbaden Codex B, from Charles Singer, 1917   136

8.1. "Ordinary Sick Headache," from John R. Graham, 1956   159

8.2. *"Migril" Masters Migraine!*, 1961   172

8.3. "Mrs. Janice Everett, age 41," 1969   173

8.4. *Migraine Is Two Headaches*, undated   173

9.1. Untitled artwork, Third Migraine Art Competition, 1981   185

9.2. Untitled artwork, First Migraine Art Competition, 1981   193

9.3. Untitled artwork, Second Migraine Art Competition, 1982   194

9.4. Untitled artwork, unspecified Migraine Art Competition, undated   197

9.5. Untitled artwork, Second Migraine Art Competition, 1983   198

9.6. Untitled artwork, Second Migraine Art Competition, 1983   198

9.7. Untitled artwork, First Migraine Art Competition, 1981   200

9.8. *The Power of Pain*, Third Migraine Art Competition, 1985   200

9.9. *The Onset of Migraine*, Third Migraine Art Competition, 1985   202

9.10. Untitled artwork, Third Migraine Art Competition, 1985   203

9.11. Untitled artwork, Third Migraine Art Competition, 1985   204

9.12. *The Five Ages of My Migraine*, First Migraine Art Competition, 1981   205

My early ideas for a history of migraine were formed at the Centre for the History of Science, Technology, and Medicine at the University of Manchester. I thank Michael Worboys and the late John Pickstone for giving me the opportunity to take up a research fellowship; Michael Brown, Emma Jones, Victoria Long, Rob Kirk, Neil Pemberton, Carsten Timmermann, Elizabeth Toon, and Duncan Wilson shared ideas, commented on my project proposals and early papers, and were an invaluable source of support, friendship, and sensible advice. Brigitte Soltau, Kate Smith, Melissa Bentley, and Leo Tavakoli were wonderful company and a source of solidarity, food, and wine during my weeknight stays in Manchester and London.

Generous funding from the Wellcome Trust (grant no. 091650/Z/10/Z) for a Medical Humanities Research Fellowship (2011–2014) made this whole thing possible. Thanks are due to the Medical Humanities Committee for their faith in the project, and to the three anonymous reviewers who provided insightful feedback on the initial proposal. At the Wellcome Trust, Lauren Couch fought in my corner at a difficult time, for which I am immensely grateful. More recently, Hannah Hope and Diego Baptista on the Open Access team have helped navigate this aspect of the publication process.

The majority of the research for this book was undertaken during my Wellcome-funded three-year fellowship in history at Kings College London (KCL), a time I remember principally for wonderful conversations over books and images (and a few underground cocktails) with Bonnie Evans, Florence Grant, Keren Hammerschlag, Ludmilla Jordanova, Anna Maerker, Sophie Mann, Richard A. McKay, Ann Poulson, Dionysios Stathakopoulous, and Rosemary Wall. At KCL, I also thank Brian Hurwitz, Paul Readman, Adam Sutcliffe, and the scholars in the Menzies Centre for Australian Studies for their support and welcome.

At KCL, it was a privilege to work with, learn from, and be mentored by Ludmilla Jordanova, who enthusiastically saw the potential for this project from my first vague and speculative email. Since 2013, at Leicester, Clare Anderson has supported me through the enormous challenge of juggling my first lecturing post and young children. I cannot stress enough how valuable the intellect, advice, and encouragement of these two remarkable women and role models has been and continues to be. Thank you.

In late 2013, I joined the School of History (now HyPIR) at the University of Leicester, where I have worked and taught with some wonderful colleagues, including Bernard Attard, Andy Hopper, Sally Horrocks, Zoe Knox, George Lewis, Toby Lincoln, Prashant Kidambi, Jo Story, Roey Sweet, Deborah Toner, Lynne Wakefield, and Sarah Whitmore. A special mention must also go to the fabulous BSWs: Eureka Henrich, Emma Battell-Lowman, Kellie Moss, Katy Roscoe, and Maeve Ryan.

As I have developed this project, I have had countless conversations about migraine with friends, family members, colleagues, and strangers—on trains and buses; in elevators and on the school playground; over emails and cups of tea; and on Twitter and Facebook. A huge number of people have given helpful feedback, shared personal experiences, and asked pertinent questions that have all made positive contributions to this book. This includes seminar audiences at the London School of Hygiene and Tropical Medicine; the History of Medicine Unit at the University of Birmingham; the Late Modern History Seminar at St. Andrews; the University of Leicester Centre for Medical Humanities, and the Durham Centre for Visual Arts and Cultures. Attendees at conferences and workshops include the Case Studies of Medical Portraiture Workshop (KCL, 2011), the American Association for the History of Medicine Conference (Baltimore, 2012); the Social History Society Conference (Leeds, 2013); the European Association for the History of Medicine and Health (Cologne, 2015); the Society for the Social History of Medicine Conferences (Queen Mary University of London, 2012; Kent, 2016; and Liverpool, 2018); and the International Congress of History of Science, Technology, and Medicine (Manchester, 2013). In 2012, I organized the Illness Histories and Approaches Workshop at KCL, and I thank all the speakers and attendees at that event who, through their engagement, made me think hard about how to approach the history of illness and disease.

Some of the research for chapter 9 was carried out with additional support from the University of Leicester Research Impact Development Fund in 2016. At the head office of Migraine Action, Rebekah Aitchison and Simon Evans politely humored my repeated inquiries about the art collection and were a pleasure to work with as we put together the Migraine Art Collection website. I am indebted to Steve Ling for his infectious enthusiasm for the artworks and the care with which he approached the cataloging and research for that project, and delighted that our work has played a part in securing a permanent home for the artworks at the Wellcome Library.

An early version of some of the material on Hildegard of Bingen in chapter 7 was published as "Making Modern Migraine Medieval: Men of Science, Hildegard of Bingen, and the Life of a Retrospective Diagnosis," *Medical His-*

tory 58 (2014): 354–374. This work is available through Open Access, online at https://doi.org/10.1017/mdh.2014.28/. Other paragraphs have been revised from the research included in "Digital Narratives: Four 'Hits' in the History of Migraine," in *The Routledge History of Disease*, ed. Mark Jackson (London: Routledge, 2017), 512–528. My thanks to the editors and anonymous reviewers for their constructive engagement with these pieces.

The Wellcome Library in London is one of the great repositories of human knowledge, and it has a brilliant team of archivists and librarians who make visiting and working there a joy, including Elma Brenner, Phoebe Harkins, and Ross Macfarlane. At the Queen Square Archives and Library at the UCL Institute of Neurology, Sarah Lawson and colleagues have been unfailingly helpful and welcoming in retrieving books and documents from the dauntingly long list I handed over. I would also like to thank archivists at the Royal Society of London, the Alan Mason Chesney Medical Archives in Baltimore, the Neurological Institute at Columbia University, the East Sussex Record Office, the Leicestershire County Record Office, and the British Library. For help with images, I thank Arike Oke and Holly Peel (Wellcome Library), Fazila Patel (Migraine Action), Domniki Papadimitriou (Cambridge University Library), Katherine Marshall (Royal Society), and the British Library Licensing Team.

I have received heartening encouragement and helpful leads from people who have responded to my posts on the Remedia blog, the Recipes Project, the Wellcome Library blog, and my own research blog, as well as for pieces in The Conversation website. Thanks to Jenni Nuttall for allowing me to use her translation of William Dunbar's poem, to Lauren Kassell for helping me read the Napier casenotes, and to Anne MacGregor and Mark Weatherall for responding to my queries about aspects of migraine medicine.

A number of people have read and given feedback on earlier drafts and full chapters: my gratitude to Sarah Easterby-Smith, Keren Hammerschlag, Mark Jackson, Ludmilla Jordanova, Rich McKay, Molly Rogers, Trish Skinner, Kate Smith, and Matthew Smith. In addition to all her practical and emotional support and advice, Sally Foxhall's knowledge of grammar, and her ability to spot repetition at a hundred paces, has improved my writing considerably.

It has been a pleasure to work with the team at Johns Hopkins University Press. I am grateful to Jacqueline C. Wehmueller for making the initial contact, and to the anonymous reviewers for their critical engagement and positive report on my initial proposal. Matthew R. McAdam and William Krause have smoothly guided the book through reviews and into production. In particular, I want to thank Matthew Smith and Joanna Kempner for their critical, generous engagement and extremely helpful suggestions for revision of the manuscript. Kathleen M. Capels has provided meticulous copyediting and made that process a real pleasure. Any errors of interpretation or fact in this book, of course, remain entirely mine.

This project first began to take shape in 2010. The process of researching and writing it has spanned three house moves, three fixed-term employment contracts, marriage, and the birth of two children. I therefore dedicate this book to Andrew Creese, who is still my superstar, and to Toby and Elin, who have changed my ideas about everything.

If we are to avoid undermining, belittling, or stigmatizing migraine and the people affected by it, then the words we choose matter. Throughout this book, many of the words I use reflect historical ideas about migraine, but, as accepted conventions for the appropriate terms are constantly in flux, it is important to be clear about the rationale I have followed when selecting my terminology. Since 2016, the American Headache Society has accepted and described migraine as a "neurological disease." In Britain, the website of the National Migraine Centre also uses "disease," while the main advocacy charity Migraine Trust describes migraine as a "complex neurological condition." In this book I use the terms "disease," "condition," and "disorder." The authors of historical sources often talked of migraine as a disease, while I use the terms "syndrome" and "illness" when historically appropriate. In particular, I understand illness as denoting the presence of a subjective sense of unwellness, to differentiate it from the notion of disease as an underlying condition that may not manifest in tangible symptoms. I use "migraine" to refer to the underlying condition and "attack" to describe individual episodes.

It is also important to consider how we speak about people. Unless used by my sources, I refer to a "person with migraine" or a "person who experiences migraine," rather than "migraineur." Although many people with migraine, including migraine scholars, have actively adopted the term migraineur to describe themselves and their identity (as well as using migraine as a verb, as in "I'm migraining"), others find the label unhelpful. To talk of someone as a migraineur implies that they are defined by their migraine. As Joanna Kempner has suggested, these kinds of words can imply that migraine is something that people *do*, and, therefore, have control over—so their use (or not) should be a personal choice. I try to avoid words related to "suffer," "sufferer," or "complaint" altogether, except when necessary in quotes or when paraphrasing historical material. In so doing, I follow the lead of neurologist William B. Young, who has done a great deal to raise awareness of the effect of terminology in migraine and who has provided clear guidance for talking about migraine.[1]

As published work becomes ever more visible online, we must consider carefully how we reproduce the details of personal medical records. For this reason, in chapter 5 the patients from London's National Hospital for the Paralysed and Epileptic are referred to only by their first name and the initial of their surname, as requested by the archivists at the University College London Institute of Neurology, Queen Square Library.

The artists who submitted their work to the Migraine Art competitions in the 1980s have not been named, either on the website that now makes the entire collection available or in the discussion in this book. While, at the moment of submitting their pieces, entrants freely gave their names and agreed that their artwork could be used, this was in a period before the internet. Particularly because many of the artists were children at that time, it would have been wrong for us to have a person's name digitally available in a way that would make elements of their medical history visible without their knowledge.

Migraine

CHAPTER ONE

Introduction

Programmed In?

Nature's Rotten Tricks, 1985

A woman's head with neatly bobbed hair stares out of the picture (fig. 1.1). At least, it would do so if the arcade games machine did not obscure her face. A strange black-and-white crescent shape—a spiky, glowing zigzag—fills the screen of the migraine computer where the woman's eyes should be. The shape emanates outward from a small dot in the jaws of the arc on the right hand side of the screen. The artist has entitled the painting *Programmed In!*, and, in much smaller writing to the side, an easily missed subtitle: *(Unwillingly.) Woe Is Me!* The arcade machine—generously supplied by Nature's Rotten Tricks—offers a list of animated games, all for free, that the player can choose. Some of these, such as Rainbow or Expanding Angular, suggest the special effects that might be encountered while playing, while others are more cryptic. Does Mobile Stellate involve intergalactic travel, perhaps, or Fortification some kind of siege? In fact, the game titles on the arcade machine are all types of migraine aura, taken from a lecture given by the renowned Victorian neurologist William Gowers in 1895. The zigzag arc on the screen is a rendering of a well-known diagram of a "scintillating scotoma," drawn by Dr. Hubert Airy, physician son of the famous astronomer George Biddell Airy, and first published in 1870. In this artist's imagination, Airy's scotoma has been reimagined as Pac-Man, the main character of a coin-operated arcade game released by the Japanese company Namco Ltd. in 1980.[1] In the original game, the yellow Pac-Man gobbled a trail of white dots, all the while being chased by four multicolored ghosts. Here, we might imagine chasing a never-ending supply of little white pills in a constant search for relief from an incurable disorder.

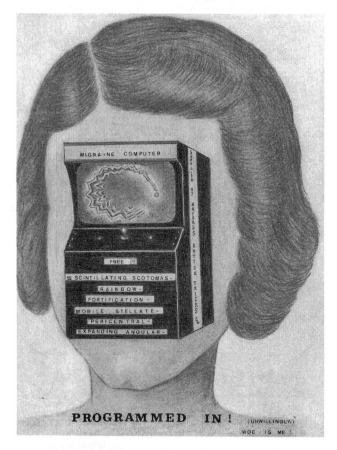

Fig. 1.1. *Programmed In! (Unwillingly.) Woe Is Me!*, submitted to the Third Migraine Art Competition, unnamed artist, 1985, image 449. Courtesy of Migraine Action via the Wellcome Collection, licensed under CC-BY

This revealing image is from 1985, and it was submitted to the third of four Migraine Art competitions held between 1980 and 1987. The electronic machine and the reference to programming illustrate the contemporary emergence of a modern neurological framework for describing migraine, yet the nineteenth-century language and imagery overlaying the face seem to define what migraine is and how it can be talked about. It is not just the illness, but the cultural and historical frames of reference available to speak about it that are programmed into the unwilling woman's head.[2] The machine effaces the woman's identity and prevents her from communicating and experiencing migraine on her own terms. The artist's lament at migraine being programmed in attests to the significance of heredity in determining who gets migraine. At the same time, we might read this title as a defiant rejection of a modern tendency to attribute migraine to some kind of personal failing or weakness, a disorder primarily associated with women that could be avoided if only they would eat better, sleep more regularly, and avoid stress. While women are overwhelmingly represented in the ranks of those who experience migraine, as *Programmed In!* implies, it is their voices, and their experiences, that are often marginalized.

The blending of modern and historical references in *Programmed In!* neatly illustrates the central argument of this book: a modern neurological framework that defines our current understanding of migraine as a neurobiological disorder located in the brain has determined a narrow set of boundaries with which to understand and talk about migraine. This process, I argue, has had a profound effect not only on our understanding of migraine's history, but also on our ability to account for, and take seriously, the huge range of experiences that people with migraine encounter in the present. In this study, I propose a way to think afresh about migraine's past; to reveal the ways people have described, explained, and treated migraine since the Middle Ages; and to show how and why that long history has shaped our modern knowledge of, and approach to, this extremely common condition and the people who have it. While there are certain continuities in a cluster of symptoms that have been called migraine over hundreds of years, our understanding of migraine's causes and symptoms, the therapeutic practices we use to deal with it, and our cultural and social attitudes toward the people who have migraine all have long histories that warrant investigation. Changing ideas about the role of humors and blood circulation in the body, the physiology and function of the brain, gender, the relationship between various acute and chronic illnesses, national medical cultures, institutional specialization, and the weight we give to particular symptoms have all contributed. We cannot understand modern migraine without a knowledge of its fascinating and varied history.

What Is Migraine?

For nearly two thousand years, people have known of a disorder called migraine. The origins of our modern term can be traced to the second century, when Roman physician, surgeon, and philosopher Galen coined the term "hemicrania." The essence of Galen's hemicrania was a symptom: a pain that affected half the head. This symptom (and the related disturbance of the stomach that he also identified) has remained important to concepts of migraine ever since, although migraine is now often, though not always, considered to include such one-sided pain.[3] Through translation and use, Galen's term spread. It became *emigranea* in Latin and Middle English. In medieval Welsh we find *migran*. The fifteenth-century Scots poet William Dunbar used "magryme." The early modern period saw a wide variety of variations on the English vernacular "megrim" or "meagrim." For example, within Jane Jackson's recipe book, we find "migrim," "migrims," "migrime," "mygrime," and "mygrim." In printed works, common since the sixteenth century, the letters *i* and *y* were often considered interchangeable, depending on the typesetter's preference. Examples include "migrime" or "mygryme."[4] Galen's term provides the common root (*m*, *c/g*, and *r*) for the German *migräne*, the Spanish *migraña*, and the French *migraine*. In Swedish, we find *migrän*. Czech and Hungarian have *migréna*; modern Greek, *imikranía*. Today *migrena* would be recognized in Croatia, Azerbaijan, and Poland. And so on.

Over time, other symptoms besides head pain and gastric disturbance have been added, or became important to, developing concepts of migraine. In the early medieval period, sensory symptoms were often included in discussions of migraine, before slipping out of common use until late eighteenth-century European writers incorporated them once more. The significance of gastric disturbances has waxed and waned, depending on the changing medical frameworks that best seem to explain migraine at any particular time. By the turn of the nineteenth century, English-language speakers often used "sick headache" or "bilious headache" to reemphasize the relationship between the key symptoms of head pain and nausea, apparently in response to an evolution of the meaning of megrim toward an association with nervous disorder over the preceding century. Nineteenth-century authors spilt much ink explaining which words denoted particular kinds of headache. In the 1870s, Cambridge physician Edward Liveing used the English term in his influential text *On Megrim*, but by then the majority of his contemporaries preferred the French term *migraine*.[5] Migraine has also been allied with many other disorders, from the humoral concept of rheum in the seventeenth century; to vertigo in the eighteenth; epilepsy and hysteria in the nineteenth; and chronic daily headache, cluster headache, and trigeminal autonomic cephalalgia in our own time.[6] These discussions have all played an important role in shaping migraine's history.

What is migraine in the twenty-first century? For writer and broadcaster AL Kennedy, it's "a ghost, it's a gaoler, it's a thief, a semi-perpetual dark companion."[7] Rudyard Kipling, on the other hand, thought his hemicrania was "a lovely thing," though it literally divided him in two: "One half of my head in a mathematical line from the top of my skull to the cleft of my jaw, throbs and hammers and sizzles and bangs and swears while the other half—calm and collected—takes notes of the agonies next door."[8] Around the world, migraine affects approximately a billion people, or one in seven, of whom two-thirds are women. This means that virtually everyone will live with, work with, be related to, or be friends with someone who has migraine. Globally, it is the most common, and the most economically burdensome, of all the neurological disorders, as well as the third leading cause of disability among the under-fifty age group. It is more prevalent than diabetes, epilepsy, and asthma combined.[9]

Migraine is a spectrum disease, usually manifesting as an episodic or chronic primary headache disorder, characterized by attacks that can last from a few hours to up to three days. It is two to three times more prevalent among women than men, and women experience higher levels of pain, longer lasting attacks, and greater disability than men.[10] For much of the twentieth century, migraine's causes were considered to be vascular, and the pain a result of dilation of the cranial blood vessels. Since the 1970s, the emphasis has shifted, and it is now defined as a disorder involving nerve pathways and chemicals in the brain, to which people are often genetically predisposed. While migraine is still understood to affect the neurovascular system, it seems likely that the headache pain comes from neurogenic inflammation, rather than vasodilation. This is a problem of brain function, rather than structure. As the website for the National Migraine Centre in London explains, "if the brain is a computer, migraine is a software not a hardware problem."[11] Nevertheless, a huge amount remains unknown, including the role of the hypothalamus (the part of the brain that controls the endocrine system and has a role in the menstrual cycle, pain modulation, and governance of the body's circadian rhythms), the cause of premonitory symptoms, the extent to which antimigraine drugs can access the brain, and the role of the blood-brain barrier.[12]

Migraine headaches pulsate, are frequently one sided, can be extremely painful, and often are aggravated by normal physical activity. Other well-known symptoms include nausea and vomiting, as well as visual or sensory disturbances, known as aura, that usually take from five to twenty minutes to develop and can last for up to an hour before resolving completely. Before and during a migraine attack, many people encounter various symptoms, such as tiredness, emotional disturbance, poor concentration, sensitivity to light or sound, blurred vision, nausea, and yawning. On average, migraine sufferers experience one or two attacks a month. For more than two-thirds of women with migraine, and just under half of men, these attacks last longer than a day. In addition to the pain and discomfort felt during each attack, the cumulative effect of migraine can bear on all aspects of daily life, affecting relationships with family, partners, friends, and work.[13]

There are two major types of migraine. Migraine *without* aura (previously known as common migraine), is experienced most frequently, is usually more disabling, and is often related to the menstrual cycle in women. Migraine *with* aura (known since the late nineteenth century as classic, or classical, migraine), is characterized by recurrent neurological disturbance, particularly of vision, which precedes the onset of headache. The word "aura" comes from the Greek for "breeze," and visual aura is the most common sensory symptom. A visual aura, usually lasting between five and thirty minutes, is often characterized by zigzag patterns that develop from a central originating point into a C shape that spreads outward across the field of vision, but they can also take the form of a corona, stars, or loss of sight in some of the visual field. Aura can affect any of the human senses, appearing as pins and needles, whistling sounds, numbness, or speech disturbance.[14] In 2011, Serene Branson, a reporter for CBS in Los Angeles, famously was unable to make herself understood when she experienced migraine on air while reporting from the Grammy Awards ceremony, leading many to assume that she was either drunk, on drugs, or having a stroke.[15] Aura can also take the form of vertigo, tinnitus, reduced hearing, difficulties balancing or walking, or even decreased consciousness. For some people, an occasional visual aura may be the only symptom of migraine they ever experience. For others, the aura is a signal, announcing the imminent onset of a debilitating migraine headache, with all its associated symptoms.

As Dawn C. Buse and her colleagues observe, the striking difference in migraine prevalence among women and men in our own time is one of migraine's hallmarks.[16] Yet, as this book demonstrates, a gendered ratio is not an inherent characteristic of a timeless disorder, but a result of evolving ideas about the kinds of people who are most likely to get migraine, and of key decisions about which symptoms should, and should not, be included in the category of migraine. It is only since the global acceptance of the *International Classification of Headache Disorders* (*ICHD*) criteria from 1988 that this gender ratio has become widely accepted, a remarkably recent development. We also now know that men and women experience migraine differently. By comparing women with women, and developing clear criteria for menstrual and menstrual-related migraine, British specialist Anne MacGregor and her colleagues have demonstrated that menstrual attacks (which account for more than half of migraine in women) are "clinically different" from nonmenstrual attacks: they "last longer, are more severe, are more likely to relapse, are less responsive to treatment, and are associated with greater disability." Significantly, migraine attacks that are directly associated with menstruation tend not to include symptoms of aura, even if those women develop attacks of migraine with aura at other times. Only around one in eight women experience visual aura, compared with around a third of men. In short, for women overall, it seems that migraine is a less visual, but distinctly more painful thing to reckon with.[17]

Other factors beyond gender determine the likelihood of experiencing migraine. Migraine is common in children, affecting between 6 and 8 percent (9.7% for girls and 6.0% for boys). Often, recurrent, severe abdominal pain in childhood can be a precursor for the development of migraine later on. For girls, prevalence increases after puberty, rising from 7 percent under the age of fourteen to nearly 10 percent by the age of twenty.[18] Migraine tends to increase in severity until around age forty before declining, particularly in women.

As socioeconomic status decreases, chronic migraine prevalence seems to increase.[19] The question of whether lower socioeconomic status is a cause of migraine (for example, because of the increased likelihood of factors such as poor nutrition, high stress, and limited healthcare) or whether it is a result of the disease affecting education and employment prospects, is a thorny question. Advocates and headache professionals alike are wary of suggesting that socioeconomic factors can directly cause migraine, emphasizing instead that they most likely trigger or exacerbate an underlying neurological condition.[20] Yet important questions about the extent to which migraine prevalence and experience varies by race and ethnicity, and how this intersects with other social and economic factors remain greatly underexamined, a blind spot reflected in the historical sources on which this study is based. Much more research is needed to understand how the collection of epidemiological data regarding self-reported pain, disparities in access to healthcare, and the quality of healthcare received are factors in differing migraine burdens across social groups. This situation for migraine reflects a broader state of persistent gender, racial, and socioeconomic bias and discrimination when it comes to developing and prescribing treatments for pain in general.[21] Discussions about the significance of social status, heredity, and gender all have an important part to play in this history and have fundamentally shaped the interpretation of migraine's modern biological reality.

Themes

The idea to write a history of migraine came from a chance conversation with some medical historian friends in a bar one evening. We were contemplating how strange it was that a pain so intense could appear to be devoid of any real bodily purpose or reason. I began to wonder how people had explained and dealt with such a pain historically. This question remains a central preoccupation of this book. In sources that span hundreds of years, I have been repeatedly struck by how vividly people have found ways to describe the quality and severity of the pain they have associated with a disorder named migraine, and how precisely they have been able to account for migraine's force in the body, using the explanatory frameworks available to them in their era.

Understanding how people in the past have rationalized migraine pain does more than simply bear witness to its existence. Looking at the ways in which the causal frameworks people have used to explain migraine change over time helps us identify how different groups of people, as well as individual lifestyles and choices, come to be associated with migraine, as well as draws our attention to how people rationalize illness within their own life narratives—what we might term the "Why me?" question. This book draws from, and contributes to, a wider body of literature that emphasizes pain as an embodied and highly gendered historical phenomenon.[22] Since the Middle Ages, the consistency of descriptions of migraine pain as arrows and hammers, drilling and boring, or a vise that grips is striking, but it is important for us not to lose sight of how the experience of pain is affected by changing cultural, social, and political contexts. As a methodological approach, *paying attention* to how and when pain is discussed or becomes significant reveals its political as well as its phenomenological role in this history.[23]

Practical attempts to manage, cope with, and relieve pain on a day-to-day basis run through the long social and cultural history of migraine. From classical times, pain was at the heart of humoral ideas about hemicrania and its treatment. Since the late seventeenth century, this book argues, there has been a gradual erosion of the conceptual centrality of pain to medical discussions of migraine. This begins almost imperceptibly with linguistic shifts that saw megrim become associated with dizziness, vertigo, and nerves. In the late nineteenth century, the marginalization of pain became explicit, as men of science denied that subjective experiences of pain had troubled the reliability of their accounts of visual disturbance. Hubert Airy's image, in particular, shaped not only how neurologists understood migraine's biological reality, but also its history. As physicians conferred diagnostic primacy on aura, the field of migraine research fragmented under the weight of competing theories. Most recently, as vascular theories have fallen out of fashion, words that denote sensations—such as pumping, throbbing, and dilating—have given way to an altogether gentler neurological lexicon: pathways, transmission, irritation, and blocking. I am not suggesting that physicians have forgotten, or don't realize, that migraine is painful; of course they do. But even as pain remains the prime target of pharmaceutical developments, a particular framing of migraine as *more than* just a headache has paradoxically served to undervalue the serious pain that does define a migraine experience for the majority of people, particularly women and minorities.

In her memoir about a decade with an "unrelenting, totally unreasonable headache," Paula Kamen concludes that while she could still find "absolutely no meaning in the pain itself," pain has been crucial to determining the relationships between female patients and the predominantly male physicians and neurologists she has encountered. Kamen's identification of the continuing influence of historical prejudices about women's pain in particular confirm the necessity for an historical analysis that examines the cultural and social subtexts that underlie our modern-day practices and assumptions.[24] Despite increased understanding of the pathological mechanisms and factors relating to its prevalence, and clear evidence of its substantial global burden, migraine, along with other headache disorders, has a credibility problem. It remains underfunded, underdiagnosed, and undertreated, with an estimated 50 percent of people with the disorder never consulting a doctor about it.[25] A 2007 study of headache research support in Europe found that although migraine attracted relatively strong pharmaceutical investment, it was the least publicly funded of all brain disorders, relative to societal and economic impact.[26] In 2017, America's National Institutes of Health allocated only $19 million to migraine, compared with $51 million for smallpox (declared globally eradicated in 1980), and just 11 percent of its total $161 million budget for epilepsy research.[27]

In *Not Tonight*, an excellent study of the relationship between gender and biomedicine in contemporary knowledge about migraine, sociologist Joanna Kempner describes this situation as migraine's "legitimacy deficit," a status exacerbated for individuals by many neurologists' lack of interest, as well as their skepticism and reluctance to persist with patients who are seen as being time consuming, emotionally challenging, and difficult to treat. "Delegitimation," Kempner explains, is "a fundamental component of the migraine experience."[28] In researching this book, I have been fascinated by the historical development of this notion of legitimacy. If migraine has existed as a medical diagnosis for hundreds if not thousands of years, Kempner asks, then why have medical advances "so far not been sufficient to validate the experiences of those with migraine, nor to bring resources to [its] study and treatment?" For Kempner, who focuses on the period since the late nineteenth century, the answer lies in the persistence of gendered images, metaphors, and stereotypes that continue to define how migraine is perceived culturally—affecting people who are weak, feminized, oversensitive, and unable to cope—even as medicine, advocacy groups, and patients alike claim migraine for the gender-neutral brain.[29]

In this book, I propose that we need to think slightly differently about this problem of legitimacy, because much evidence suggests migraine had been taken seriously in both medical and lay literature throughout the classical, medieval, and early modern (c. 1500–1800) periods as a serious disorder requiring prompt and sustained treatment. This only began to change in the eighteenth century, as migraine became associated with a range of nervous disorders, and then came to be seen as characteristic of sensitivity, femininity, overwork, and moral and personal failure. While gender plays an important role in this development, other factors are also significant and often intersect with it, including national cultures of medical knowledge, the social status of patients, changes in vernacular terminology, the social and cultural contexts in which people obtained medical advice and treatment, and attitudes toward bodily experiences of pain. While a lack of proof is not confirmation that migraine's belittlement was absent in earlier centuries, I argue that there is a clear, identifiable point in the eighteenth century when migraine began to attract less than serious attention.

Taking a long historical view suggests that the current state of affairs in which migraine's legitimacy is diminished is only a relatively recent one. In this light, the wealth of evidence from the medieval and early modern periods that does take migraine seriously provides an exciting opportunity. It allows us to write a rich new history that emphasizes the historical contingency of legitimacy, rather than its permanence, and allows us to bear positive witness to the attempts, over hundreds of years, people have made to care for, treat, and provide explanations for people with migraine. This is a history that validates a wide variety of experiences and explanatory models beyond our own gendered neurological paradigm, at the same time as it situates our current understandings within a much longer trajectory that emphasizes the inevitability of change.

The varied history of attempts to treat migraine is important, because it makes us confront a contemporary situation in which millions of people still do not have access to sufficiently cheap and effective treatments. For centuries, people have attempted to find methods and remedies to manage and treat migraine, including phlebotomy, herbal remedies, surgical procedures, and pharmaceutical preparations. We might be tempted to ridicule seventeenth-century recipes that recommend the application of earthworms, to condemn the extent to which people in the (not so distant) past accepted bloodletting, or to be profoundly unsettled by relatively recent experiments with cranial surgery. We might find it easy to reassure ourselves that such practices have been consigned to the past. Yet there is still no cure for migraine. We have drugs that can abort or reduce the symptoms of individual migraine attacks once they have begun, but these do not work for everyone, and for those who do experience benefits, this relief is by no means total. Beyond the effort it takes to convince physicians, employers, family, and friends of the severity of the disease, managing migraine on a day-to-day basis takes a huge commitment to avoid triggers, juggle medications, negotiate side effects, and regulate stress, sleep, and exertion. In addition, the long-term effects of frequent medication use, and the growing prevalence and burden of chronic migraine—defined as migraine attacks on fifteen or more days per month—are attracting growing concern. We may no longer make use of sedative substances such as valerian, luminal, and hydrocyanic acid, but the prescription of opioid medications remains both a political and a medical problem. Future generations may not be very complimentary about our own distinctly inadequate therapeutic offerings.

A history of therapeutics does more than simply ask whether a medicine worked. As medical historian Jack Pressman has argued in the context of frontal lobotomy: "A therapy's usefulness is contingent upon a particular historical era. To ignore this is to overlook what was at stake in a given treatment —for the individual patient, the medical profession, or society."[30] The long history of migraine medicine reveals more than a list of substances people have taken for migraine. Remedies from early modern recipe collections reveal something of the personal, intellectual, and social networks on which people with migraine from across the social spectrum could draw for support, advice, knowledge, and relief. The stories that people have told illuminate the effects of illness on lives, and methods for mixing recipes suggest something of how migraine was understood both as an acute and a chronic condition. On the other hand, examining the ways in which nineteenth-century physicians developed pharmaceutical products in institutions reminds us that medical power and authority is not achieved without human cost.

Blood has always been a part of the migraine story, whether conceptually or therapeutically. Yet the often explicit rejection of vascular theories since the late 1970s, and a language of reclaiming migraine for the brain and neurology, has had a profound influence on how neurologists have represented migraine and its history. In particular, blood has been noticeably sidelined in this endeavor, a circumstance this book seeks to rectify.[31] Even as scientists have come to regard vasodilation and vasoconstriction as epiphenomenal to migraine's causal mechanisms, blood continues to shape neuroscientific research into migraine, particularly in efforts to understand whether disruption or inflammation of the blood-brain barrier plays a role in migraine, and the extent to which drugs must penetrate it to act centrally in the brain. While it seems likely that existing migraine drugs must be able to cross the blood-brain barrier to enough of an extent to have a therapeutic effect, the quite recent development of anti-CGRP antibodies (very large molecules that would be unable to penetrate the blood-brain barrier) suggests that they are acting peripherally. This has led researchers to focus on the trigeminal ganglion in this hunt for a possible migraine generator.[32] Neither the meaning nor the role of blood in relation to migraine has remained stable or continuous over time, and we should not try to make direct links between the phlebotomy practices of the medieval period and the late twentieth century's fascination with serotonin and blood platelets. But whether the emphasis has been humoral, menstrual, surgical, neurochemical, or genetic, blood's flows, pulses, sensations, and functions have been consistently evoked to describe, observe, conceptualize, and treat migraine since at least the Middle Ages.

Another important theme is the concept of patienthood—who has or has not been a patient—and what it means for people with migraine to become visible as such in particular contexts. In medieval and early modern sources, the experiences of individuals generally remained inferred or abstract. During the seventeenth century, personal correspondence and casebooks began to provide substantial evidence about how people with migraine interacted with physicians.[33] In the nineteenth century, migraine started to appear in institutional settings, a development that had implications not only for those seeking help, but also for clinicians, who used them to advance their own theories, and therapeutic development. In hospitals and asylums, the presence of poor, working-class patients prompted investigation into migraine's causes, as well as experiments with how to treat it. This book continues scholars' efforts to take account of the history of subjectivity, as well as the impact of illness on patients' economic and domestic lives.[34]

Finally, the story of migraine is a very visual history. From diagrams of vein men, which taught medieval physicians the rules of phlebotomy, to twenty-first-century MRI scans showing brain abnormalities in migraine patients, the visual imagery of migraine has been a powerful tool for attempting to communicate migraine's pathological processes in the body. Here, I consider images not just as illustrations, but as meaningful historical evidence in their own right.[35] A significant reason for migraine's visually rich history is the experience of aura, as well as the central role aura has played in modern conceptualizations of migraine. As we have already begun to see in the image that opened this introduction, one of the most important single images in this history has been Hubert Airy's 1870 diagram of his aura (see fig. 6.3), which rapidly became a shorthand for authentic, accurate migraine experience from the late nineteenth century on. Then there is the staggering collection of artwork submitted to the four Migraine Art competitions in Britain in the 1980s, which powerfully attest to the violent disruption of a life lived with migraine. These are the subject of chapter 9. In this book, I argue that visual imagery does much more than illustrate migraine's history. It shows us how a particular way of seeing migraine has come to dominate the neurological framework. This also has shaped medical research and the way in which doctors approach migraine.

In his memoir, Andrew Levy makes an important historical point about the visibility of people with migraine. He notes that in recent times, "we have tended to treat migraine as a private affair, between a migraineur and a migraineur's head in a dark room," that is, as something to be hidden when one is out in public. People in the past, Levy observes, had a different idea: with bands, plasters, and caps, sufferers (including Charles Darwin) literally wore their treatment on their heads.[36] It is also important to think about the moments in which migraine becomes visible on the human body. The signs have often been subtle: the characteristic facial pallor of the migraine attack, or the young servant whose shaking left hand was the only outward hint of the condition she sought help for in 1895. In the Middle Ages, the scars of repeated bloodletting in the temporal veins would have left a distinct corporeal reminder of measures taken to calm humoral turmoil.

Bringing together questions of gender, pain, legitimacy, treatment, patienthood, and visibility requires us to take seriously not just how medical knowledge has changed over time, but how contexts of power and authority have shaped migraine's cultural and social history, as well as its present form. What counts as evidence? Whose voices are amplified when they claim to know migraine either subjectively or objectively? How do ingrained assumptions determine whose words seem to transcend the messy business of pain, fatigue, confusion, and nausea, and whose testimonies are ignored, or considered unreliable? The content of this book is driven by the conviction that while medical practitioners and theorists are an important part of the history of migraine, their ideas are not its *only* history. As well as taking account of changing scientific and medical frameworks, as a social and cultural historian I am interested in a history of migraine from below, that is, one that includes the lives and experiences of men and women with migraine and how they have talked about, understood, and treated this extremely common, but still incurable, disorder.[37]

Writing a History of a Disease

When I've talked about this project with others, a common response has been to ask how far back people have *known* what a migraine was. This is a difficult question to answer, and it is, in large part, the subject of this book. It depends on what you think these individuals should have known about, and whether we want to understand those ideas in their own terms. The question "Did they know?" gets to the heart of an issue that historians, and clinicians interested in history, have long debated: what is it that we are looking for when we write histories of disease, illness, or medicine?[38] Do works that apply our modern biomedical categories to the past tell us anything about history?[39] If not, then how do we respect and contextualize this knowledge on its own terms, however distant, inaccurate, or strange those contemporaneous disease categories might now seem to our modern gaze?[40]

This volume contributes to an important and growing body of literature addressing the histories of a range of medically elusive, noncommunicable disorders—such as allergy, fibromyalgia, autoimmunity, multiple sclerosis, and some mental disorders—that straddle the boundaries of acute, episodic, and chronic disease. Like many of these afflictions, migraine can often be characterized by periods of disability and pain, followed by remission, a situation that medical historian Catharine Coleborne has aptly termed "unpredictable illness trajectory."[41] While technological and pharmacological interventions have transformed diseases such as AIDS, diabetes, or kidney failure into manageable chronic disorders, modern migraine drugs that abort acute attacks when used frequently seem increasingly liable to exacerbate a very unwelcome transition to chronicity. Migraine is thus an important case for studying how pharmacological interventions can shape the ongoing character of an illness, rather than effecting its cure.[42]

Even as historians have carefully analyzed social, cultural, and political contexts that have shaped our ideas about individual diseases, they have often assumed the disease entities have an essential transhistorical identity that either has been discovered, or could be.[43] This is not just the case for diseases caused by an infectious pathogen. For instance, one recent history presents depression as a "comparatively consistent disease phenomenon," and older terms—such as vapors, spleen, and melancholia—as simply different words for the symptoms of "what we would now call depression."[44] Siddhartha Mukherjee considers cancer to be an "ancient disease," which has existed with its fundamental feature of "the abnormal growth of cells intact for four thousand years."[45] In some cases, as for migraine, we can see that a particular word *has* consistently signified one or more symptoms over many centuries. An example is the history of asthma. The word asthma has existed since classical times and has had the idea of "shortness of breath" at its conceptual heart. Nevertheless, medical theories about asthma's place in the body, as well as social interpretations of it, have changed substantially over that time.[46]

Concepts of disease, as historian Adrian Wilson explains in an influential article in 2000, "are human and social products which have changed and developed historically." In the case of pleurisy, Wilson shows that while the concept of what pleurisy is has altered over time, it has nevertheless always been seen as "a strictly bodily ailment."[47] Others have suggested that studying the act of diagnosis itself can illuminate past mentalities in relation to disease at very specific moments.[48] This approach is particularly useful in the case of migraine, because it forces us to consider what significance migraine words themselves held when used either in relation to a particular person or in a more general theoretical sense.

I should stress that while I do not assume that our own neurological basis for migraine is timeless, I certainly do not deny the neurological, biological, and genetic realities of migraine in the twenty-first century. Rather, I work on the basis that the biological actuality of a disease can only ever be understood (and, to some extent, experienced) in light of the medical, social, and cultural concepts and technologies that are available to any one person at any particular time. Put simply, if your conceptual framework is humoral, your migraine cannot be neurological. Here, I investigate both what people in the past have believed to be the physiological (and at times psychological) reality of their, and their patients', migraine, and the contemporary meaning and effects of that socially and culturally constructed reality.[49] As I have suggested at the beginning of this introduction, I am interested in seeing how supposedly outdated concepts and ideas become layered into new ways of thinking about migraine.

My approach to migraine's history is somewhat different from studies that already exist, of which Mervyn Eadie's *Headache through the Centuries* is the most substantial contribution. Eadie, a professor of clinical neurology and neuropharmacology at the University of Queensland from 1977 to 1997, scrupulously applies modern headache definitions to descriptions of headaches found in historical sources.[50] Individual thinkers—always men—waymark medicine's progress toward modern neurological ideas, breaking the shackles of outdated thought as they go. Eadie is not interested in wider social or historical contexts, despite his comments that lay writers in the sixteenth and seventeenth centuries regarded migraine as an important entity, well before formal medicine did, a tantalizing observation he pursues no further.[51] While Eadie is careful to acknowledge that centuries of thought have yet to produce a satisfactory understanding of migraine and headaches, he nevertheless assumes the historical validity of his own neurological viewpoint.[52] Such an approach marginalizes even quite recent theories that don't accord with a neurological model. Thus endocrine therapies are hardly mentioned, menstruation—so central to how a majority of women experience migraine—receives only one paragraph, and women feature in his history only when they can be retrospectively diagnosed as sufferers. Psychological and allergic theories, so important to discussions between the 1920s and 1950s, are absent.

My approach insists that we must give as much respect to past concepts of, and treatments for, disease as we give to our own. This is particularly important for a disease such as migraine, where so much still remains to be discovered.[53] Recognizing that concepts of migraine have constantly been redefined in dynamic interaction with social, cultural, and medical conditions necessarily makes us accept that this process will continue in the future. Our own ideas, too, will seem painfully out of date sooner than we might care to admit.

Sources

A wealth of previously unexamined evidence contributes to the history of migraine presented here. Sources include medieval manuscripts, household recipe books, medical journals, printed manuals, physicians' casenotes, newspaper advertisements, pharmaceutical advertising, private diaries and letters, art, poetry, songs, and YouTube videos. My research for this book has been profoundly shaped by an explosion of digitized material available online, the possibilities of which we are only just beginning to appreciate.[54] Digitized searching enables us to explore bodies of material that would previously have been beyond the reasonable scope of a research project. Comparing recipe ingredients in early modern manuscripts with those that appear in printed books, for example, reveals how recipes were adapted to local conditions and then recycled for later generations. Mentions of migraine in nineteenth-century criminal trial transcripts give a sense of how theoretical discussions in medical journals of the time played out in the lives of ordinary people. But we also need to take care. Finding words is not the same as finding history, and, as Lauren Kassell astutely observes, "seeing is not knowing or understanding."[55] It is incumbent on us to continue to pay critical attention to the contexts, narratives, and influences that surround the words we can find and the physical sources in which they exist.

Digitization has changed the way we write history, and it is tempting to believe that any history can be written from the comfort of a good chair, with access to the internet. But this remains far from the case. The vast majority of historical material is still *not* digitized. In general, modern casenotes are one class of material that remains beyond the scope of digitization, not least because of issues of patient confidentiality.[56] Furthermore, as Tim Hitchcock has observed, "the very process of digitization is effectively reproducing a kind of Western cultural hegemony that would not be acceptable if it was a product of self-conscious policy."[57] These circumstances shape which words about illness gain authority, as well as how different kinds of knowledge or valid viewpoints can be rendered invisible by technology.[58] Online content is continually in flux, and the internet is not a democratic space. Socioeconomic status, gender, geographical location, and disability all play major roles in controlling who can find, access, consume, and create online material. In many ways, the limitations of the sources available mirror the blind spots modern medicine has in relation to migraine's global prevalence, an issue to which I return in chapter 10, the conclusion. I acknowledge that limits of time, funding, and linguistic ability (not to mention space) mean the history I have written here is based primarily on English-language translations and sources. I am also aware that in attempting to chart a course through a thousand years of history, I may tread clumsily at times in historical periods where others are far more expert than I. This book leaves open the very real possibility that a history of migraine might look completely different if written from the perspective of French, Chinese, or Arabic material, and I hope these possibilities will spur further research.

Chapter Outline

Each chapter in this volume begins with a single source, as a platform from which to examine what people in the past have meant by migraine, and what migraine has meant to them. Chapter 2, on classical and medieval approaches to migraine, begins with Bald's *Leechbook* (c. 950), which contained four remedies for a half head ache, or "healfes heafdes ece" in Old English. The chapter considers how classical ideas about the humoral causes of hemicrania were interpreted, and how knowledge of symptoms, mechanisms, and therapeutics—including herbal remedies and phlebotomy—spread and evolved through learned and vernacular medical cultures in manuscript, print, and imagery up to the fifteenth century. Descriptions of fumes, burning, boiling, and hammering evoked the seriousness of a disorder understood as the result of "evil humours flowing."

Chapter 3, taking Mrs. Corlyon's recipe book from 1606 as its basis, reveals the extent of vernacular knowledge about treating migraine in the early modern period. It traces how individual recipes in manuscript and printed remedy collections from the sixteenth and seventeenth centuries were shared and adapted over time. In addition, it considers the variety of ways in which ordinary people understood and dealt with migraine, including evidence that migraine could be thought of as both an acute and a chronic disorder.

Chapter 4 moves away from domestic medicine and into the medical marketplace, examining the variety of treatment options and professional advice available to the paying public from the sixteenth to the eighteenth centuries. Starting with Francis Thomson's desire to travel to the warm springs bubbling up in the Derbyshire hills, it moves to the chaotic streets and back alleys of eighteenth-century London, and then to the genteel drawing rooms of fashionable Bath, to show how reputable medical practitioners and itinerant gone-tomorrow salesmen and -women alike dispensed advice, promises, waters, and pills to those in search of relief. By examining the way migraine was discussed in a variety of contexts—including astrological casebooks, advertisements for cheap preparations, correspondence between physicians and patients, and the reports of charitable establishments for the poor—this chapter demonstrates how the meaning of the vernacular English word megrim began to diverge from the classical sense of hemicrania by the eighteenth century, particularly under the influence of continental ideas about migraine. It is in this change, I argue, that we can begin to see when migraine started to become something of a joke. The shift matters, because it is in the late eighteenth century's failure to take migraine seriously that we can find the seeds of our own highly gendered way of understanding—and dismissing—this disease.

Chapters 5 and 6 explore two parallel nineteenth-century histories that, together, are crucial to ushering in migraine's modern profile, as well as our assumptions about gender. Chapter 5 examines how nineteenth-century medical writers discussed the relationships between illnesses, including sick headache, megrim, and hemicrania. As they revised the classical categories of head pain, physicians formulated new theories about head disorders in medical journals, texts, and everyday use. Ideas about nervousness, hysteria, and the sympathetic relationship between head and stomach cemented a tendency to assert particular types of individuals (i.e., young women) tended to suffer from headache disorders, including migraine. In asylums and specialist institutions, such as London's National Hospital for the Paralysed and Epileptic, people with migraine were transformed into inpatients who would become the ideal subjects for theoretical observation and pharmacological experimentation.

Even as medical writers and researchers firmly began to associate migraine with women, Chapter 6 traces the emergence of a parallel, but very different, cultural profile for migraine. In the 1860s, a group of astronomers, photographers, and physicians began openly talking about their experiences of visual disturbance. At first, these men rarely acknowledged feeling any pain; these were strictly scientific discussions about vision, light, and the brain. It was through these commentaries that visual aura became an important symptom of migraine, and then began to define the modern formulation of migraine we recognize today. The chapter explores how, as a consequence of texts such as Edward Liveing's classic *On Megrim*, a very particular visual representation of migraine—Hubert Airy's diagrams of his migraine aura—came to define authentic, accurate, and, most important, *trustworthy* migraine experiences. This has profound implications for contemporary understandings of how migraine intersected with gender, class, and heredity. Together, chapters 5 and 6 explain how, by the twentieth century, doctors could simultaneously be enthralled by the neurological implications of migraine's visual characteristics (associated with male intellect), while the pain of the patients whom they regularly attended to in their clinics became invisible, hidden behind simple assertions of pharmaceutical efficacy.

Chapter 7 examines three historical stories about migraine that have oft been repeated since their emergence in the first decades of the twentieth century. It first considers the case of the celebrated St. Rupertsberg abbess, Hildegard of Bingen (1098–1179), and how she came to be diagnosed with migraine by a young historian of science, Charles Singer, in 1913. Although Singer's diagnosis took little account of Hildegard's own ideas about illness, his theory became a commonly accepted fact. I suggest it is no coincidence that Hildegard's diagnosis occurred around the same time as two other migraine stories (which would prove to be similarly tenacious) were created: the idea of trepanning as one of migraine's most ancient treatments, and the retrospective diagnosis of seventeenth-century noblewoman Anne Conway. Rather than either accepting or rejecting the truth of these three historical stories, the chapter examines why ideas such as a post facto analysis of Hildegard's migraine have become so attractive both for neurologists, who seized opportunities to anchor neurological ideas in a millennium of history, and the people who have seen their own experiences of migraine reflected in Hildegard's diagnosis.

Despite the emphasis on aura in the early twentieth century, the ascendance of a neurological framework for understanding migraine was by no means assured. Beginning with the case of a young woman treated for allergy in the early 1930s, chapter 8 explores how, in the early twentieth century, competing medical theories from the fields of psychology, allergy, endocrinology, surgery, and neurology reconfigured and fractured medical understanding of migraine. Migraine became, in the words of influential British neurologist Macdonald Critchley, a theoretical "hunting ground," despite pharmaceutical breakthroughs that had begun to promise genuine relief. From the late 1930s, the verifiable and obvious efficacy of ergotamine-based medicines validated the physiological concept of migraine as a vascular disorder, even as ideas about the existence of a "migraine personality" took hold. As this chapter makes clear, none of these competing theories were able to provide an answer to the ongoing fundamental issue of whether migraine was one disorder, or many.

Between 1980 and 1987, in the context of patient advocacy, art therapy, the idea of migraine as an essential part of a migraineur's identity, and the founding of specialist patient clinics, the Boehringer Ingelheim company and the British Migraine Association charity ran four international competitions in which they invited people with migraine to represent their aura and their experiences of life with migraine. What the organizers did not expect was the deluge of responses that focused on pain. The submissions for the competitions form an extraordinary archive of nearly six hundred images. An analysis of this collection forms the basis for chapter 9, examining how ordinary people found ways to creatively express their daily experience of migraine and its impact on their lives. Most significantly, it argues, the Migraine Art Collection is a profound witness to the realities of poorly treated and inadequately acknowledged pain.

Chapter 10, the conclusion, looks at very recent advances in migraine treatment, which offer hope of a radically improved quality of life. It also describes the acceptance of an internationally recognized classification that has transformed epidemiologists' ability to calculate migraine prevalence on a global scale. Nevertheless, I argue, it is as important as ever that we continue to ask, who speaks for and about migraine and those who live with it? Whose knowledge gets taken seriously, whose experiences are silenced, whose pain is minimized or left untreated, while others are privileged?

CHAPTER TWO

The "Beating of Hammers"

Classical and Medieval Approaches to Hemicrania

Bald's *Leechbook*, c. 950

A medical text from the tenth century contains six herbal remedies for the "healfes heafdes ece," or half headache, as well as revealing the causes—known as "tokens"—of the disease:

> For ache of half the head. Take the red nettle of one stalk, bruise it, mingle with vinegar and the white of an egg, put all together, anoint therewith. For a half heads ache, bruise in vinegar with oil the clusters of the laurus, smear the cheek with that. For the same, take juice of rue, wring on the nostril which is on the sore side. For a half heads ache, take dust of the clusters of laurel, and mustard, mingle them together, pour vinegar upon them, smear with that the sore side. Or mix with wine the clusters of laurel. Or rub fine in vinegar the seed of rue, put equal quantities of both, rub the back of the neck with that.[1]

The "healfes heafdes ece" was the result of either "evil humour flowing" or "evil vapour," or both. In order to counteract the dangerous effects of such internal bodily disturbances, the patient must first have blood let from a vein early on in the disease. This was to be followed by a wort drink, and then, the author promised, "the sore places shall be cured."[2]

Bald's *Leechbook*, the remarkable Anglo-Saxon collection of recipes, remedies, charms, and diagnostic and surgical guides in which these revealing instructions can be found, is the oldest near-complete medical text surviving in Old English, and the oldest remaining text in Europe that is not written in Latin or Greek (fig. 2.1).[3] The *Leechbook* seems to be the collection of a knowledgeable medical practitioner. It is a textbook for practical use, perhaps either as a general reference manual or for training, at a time when medical practice

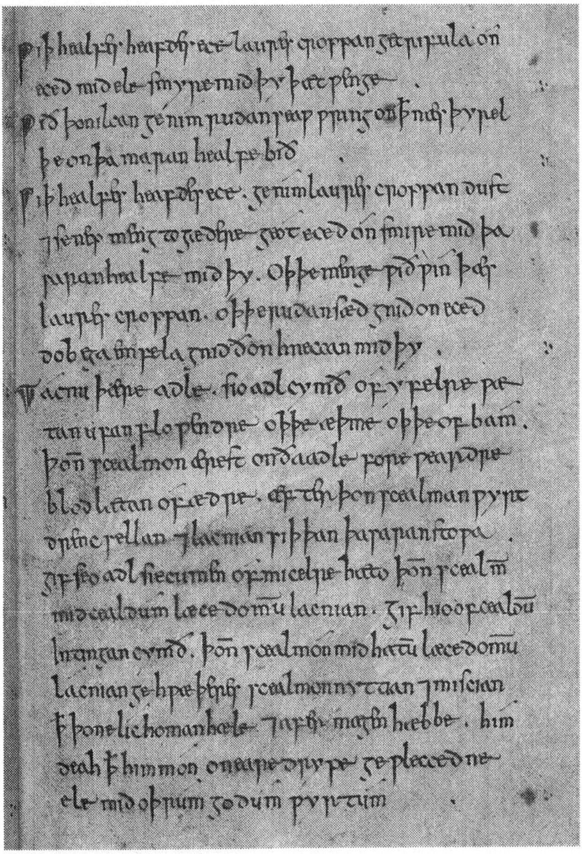

Fig. 2.1. "Remedies for Healfes Heafdes Ece [half headache]," from Bald's *Leechbook*, f. 8r, c. 950. © The British Library Board

brought together herbal remedies, minor surgery, urinary inspection, blood-letting, charms, amulets, and healing rituals in a mix of local traditions with the echoes of classical Mediterranean teaching.[4] As historian Marilyn Deegan has explained, the *Leechbook* represents the "mainstream of the intellectual life" of its day. It provides important evidence of the theory and practice of medicine at the turn of the first millennium and is a compelling and valuable source with which to begin our journey through migraine's history.[5]

As this chapter shows, there is a great deal of evidence from the Middle Ages in which practitioners took seriously a painful disorder that affected approximately half the head. It had initially been named hemicrania in the second century CE by Galen, the most famous philosopher and physician in the Roman Empire. From this basis, people developed a range of strategies and treatments for migraine, including herbal preparations and phlebotomy. Some of these individual remedies can be traced across centuries, showing how approaches that had first been developed in the classical period persisted through Arabic translation and practice and came back to Europe in the medieval period. Though interpretations of hemicrania's, or emigranea's, humoral causes differed over time and place, manuscript evidence shows that medieval writers widely accepted it as a powerful, painful illness, and this knowledge traveled far and wide.

Most important, texts from the classical and medieval periods answer an important question that I have frequently been asked as I have researched this long history of migraine: did people that far back *know what a migraine was?* The answer, quite emphatically, is yes, in their own terms. This chapter examines a wealth of evidence showing how migraine was identified and treated in the classical and medieval periods, but, most tellingly, it also reveals the sophisticated interpretations of humoral theory that explained its causes, symptoms, and effects on the body.

Bald's *Leechbook*

Life expectancy in Anglo-Saxon England at the time when Bald's *Leechbook* was compiled would not have been much more than thirty years, particularly for young men in societies frequently at war or under Viking attack, and for women, who often died in childbirth. Archaeological and textual evidence reveals that diseases such as fever, eye infections, tuberculosis, arthritis, and rickets were common. It is likely that women performed the majority of healing work in these mainly rural, agricultural societies, as women's burial sites have been found to contain small canisters for herbs that would have been attached to belts.[6] For ordinary people, herbal remedies would have formed the basis of most medical treatments, while learned medicine was concentrated in religious establishments. Although we have little information about who Bald was or his intentions for the *Leechbook*, we do know that he was the manuscript's owner, and that he had instructed another person, Cild, to compile it, possibly at the priory scriptorium attached to the cathedral in Winchester, the most important city in the Kingdom of Wessex, in southern England.

The *Leechbook* followed standard classical practice by considering diseases affecting specific places from head to toe before moving on to diseases of the whole body, then those caused by worms or parasites, and, finally, paralysis, fevers, and madness.[7] Examining Bald's *Leechbook*, historian Michael Cameron imagines "an experienced physician at work . . . picking out what he had found to be useful in his practice and arranging it in a manner convenient for others to use, leaving out everything that he thought did not contribute to the subject of his chapter or which might confuse others less skilled than himself."[8] One striking passage instructs the practitioner to treat his patients as individuals, considering their strength and condition, such as whether they were strong and vigorous, or delicate and frail. The practitioner must remember the "great difference" between the bodies of men, women, and children and the varying strengths of the daily laborer, the leisured, the old, and the young, as well as those used to hardship and those who were not.[9]

Thanks to the work of Marilyn Deegan, whose research reveals how the compiler selected, adapted, and rearranged items from a range of different classical sources, we can trace the origin of the remedies for the "healfes heafdes ece" back further. They came from the *Physica Plinii*, a compilation derived from several versions of the work of Roman naturalist, philosopher, and author Gaius Plinius Secundus—more commonly known as Pliny the Elder—dating from the fifth century.[10] Pliny, described elsewhere in the *Leechbook* as the "great physician," was one of its most significant sources.[11] The *Leechbook* identifies evil humors and vapors within the body as the cause of half headache. The idea of humors originated in the Hippocratic corpus, the first substantial body of Western medical texts from the Greek city-states, dating from the late fifth and early fourth centuries BCE. Hippocratic physicians contended that the four humors were central to the body's condition, explaining a person's physical and emotional character, their health, and their behavior. Humoral theory conceived of the body as an envelope containing and nourished by four essential fluids that could move, or flow, around the body: phlegm, yellow bile (choler), black bile (melancholy), and blood. Galen synthesized the Hippocratic writings, developing a comprehensive explanatory system emphasizing the constitution, temperament, and responsibility of the individual in governing health and wellness. Galen explicitly attributed the cause of hemicrania as the ascent of vapors that were either excessive in amount, too hot, or too cold.[12] In particular, Galen attributed head pain to bilious humors arising in the stomach. This humoral theory of hemicrania, particularly its association with bile and the notion of a sympathetic relationship between the stomach and the head, would persist in understandings of migraine well into the nineteenth century.

The humoral system was a holistic approach to health, in which a person's body was intimately connected to the world around them and was a micro-cosm of the universe. The four humors equated with the four basic elements. Thus choler was hot and dry, as fire; phlegm was cold and wet, like water; black bile was cold and dry, corresponding to earth, and blood was hot and wet, associated with air. The humors were also connected to the four seasons. As the humoral balance changed during a person's life cycle, old people tended to be drier than children, while women were perceived as colder and moister than men. A person's internal humoral balance explained their temperament. For instance, melancholic people were said to have an excess of black bile, while too much blood could make a person prone to anger. A person's humoral balance could also make them susceptible to particular disorders, so correcting that imbalance through a practice such as phlebotomy aimed to restore health, either by evacuating humors or preventing problems from aris-ing.[13] Among the bodily organs, the brain was considered cold and moist.

The idea that substances derived from animal, vegetable, or mineral sources had certain qualities that could be used to either counteract or enhance a person's bodily makeup was integral to a system of knowledge that under-stood humors, bodies, and diseases in terms of heat and cold, moisture and dryness. In particular, plants were assigned one of four qualities (hot, cold, dry, and moist) on a scale of four degrees, with one being the mildest and four the most intense, even poisonous. The most famous classical authority on the subject was Greek physician Dioscorides's *Materia Medica*, from the first cen-tury CE, whose wisdom was later reproduced in popular herbals. Plants could have further sensory qualities—they could be sweet, bitter, sharp, or have a pleasant or unpleasant smell—which could help identify whether they were poisonous or safe.[14] We will consider the importance of this system as a ratio-nale for migraine remedies more fully in the following chapter, but it is worth realizing here how Bald's ingredients would have been understood in his time. All four of the herbal ingredients in the *Leechbook*—nettles, laurel, rue, and mustard—were thought of as hot and dry. Thus, even though the *Leech-book* explained that hot humors or vapors could be a cause of the ailment, this suggests that in practice, hemicrania was primarily considered to be the re-sult of cold and moisture within the body. As we will see, this understanding persisted throughout the early modern period.

The quantities of the ingredients required for the *Leechbook*'s remedies for half headache were mostly left up to the practitioner to determine, but these were relatively simple preparations that could be mixed up quickly with no equipment required, besides a mortar and pestle, and easily committed to memory. Plants such as laurel, rue, and nettles that were named in the *Leech-book* as being good for half headache would have been readily available in gardens or households, while vinegar, eggs, mustard, and wine were common, inexpensive staples.[15] Having several remedies to choose from gave the practitioner flexibility in selecting an appropriate medicine, based on the idiosyncratic constitution of the person to whom they were prescribing a treatment or, perhaps, on the seasonal availability of items. For example, a recipe requiring evergreen laurel would be better suited to winter than one requiring flowering plants, such as nettle or rue.

Humoral Hemicrania

Bald's *Leechbook* is remarkable, but other sources give further rich insight into how widely, and for how long, coherent concepts of migraine have existed. If Galen can be credited with coining the term "hemicrania," he was not the first physician to talk of a pain occupying only one side of the skull. The famous Ebers papyrus is commonly given as the earliest written evidence of this ailment. Dating from circa 1550 BCE, the text mentions a "disease of one half of the head." But the treatment given is not conclusively aimed at a disorder that can be firmly identified as migraine. The instruction to anoint the head with the skull of catfish, fried in oil or fat for four days, was the same as was indicated for a thorn in the side, in order to draw the thorn out of the wound. The Ebers papyrus offers other remedies for removing pain from the head, including ingredients such as terebinth resin, cumin, and juniper berries.[16]

For many neurologists, a passage from the Hippocratic *Epidemics*, dating from the fifth century BCE, seems to be the first clear description of the symptoms of migraine with aura in the historical literature.[17] It described a young man, Phoenix, with

> flashes like lightning in his eye, usually the right. And when he had suffered that a short time a terrible pain developed towards his right temple, then in the whole head, and then into the part of the neck where the head is attached behind the vertebra behind, and there was stretching and hardness around the teeth. He kept trying to open them, straining . . . vomits, whenever they occurred, averted the pains I have described, and made them more gentle. Phlebotomy helped.[18]

Greek physician Aretaeus of Cappadocia, believed to have lived in the first century CE, first classified headaches into three types. "Cephalalgia" was an acute pain, while "cephalaea" was more chronic. Of most interest to us is the category of "heterocrania." This was a one-sided headache that brought about "horrible and terrifying things," including glassy eyes, painful sinews, nausea, and misery (if not death). The patient would feel slow, be offended by odors, and be averse to light. Aretaeus identified the cause as "cooling, along with drying out."[19]

At the same time as Arataeus and Galen were formulating ideas that would come to dominate an understanding of hemicrania in the West for nearly two thousand years, there is evidence of migraine treatments from China during this period. Gwei-Djen Lu and Joseph Needham suggest the Chinese were using acupuncture for treating migraine in the second century. A famous physician of the Han dynasty, Hua Tho, treated Emperor Tshao Tshao (Wei Thai Tsu) for his migraine headaches, mental disturbance, and dizziness. Dynastic history records that Hua Tho immediately cured the emperor by giving him acupuncture at "a point in the sole of the foot and the general was immediately cured."[20] This practice was also followed at the Thang imperial court, including by royal physician Chin Ming-Hao, using the acupuncture point known as *pai-hui* to cure Emperor Thang Kao Tsung of "an eye affection with migraine and dizziness" in 683.[21]

In European medicine, one of the clearest early examples of the adoption of a humoral theory of migraine comes from a sixth-century text known as *The Wisdom of the Art of Medicine*, which gave brief summaries of ideas about the body, its illnesses, and treatments.[22] It divided the body into four parts (head, stomach, belly, and bladder), discussed the humors and sinews, and gave instructions for seasonal bleeding and purging to maintain humoral balance and prevent unhealthy conditions. Unusually, the *Wisdom* assigned the four humors to particular parts of the body, which classical medical practitioners had not done.[23] Migraine was associated with red bile (choler), which predominated on the right-hand side of the body, under the liver. Faith Wallis's translation of the *Wisdom* tells us: "These things are hot and sharp and cause bodies to be depleted in summer time, but plump and phlegmatic in the winter. Their fumes rise up to the human brain and cause heat in the head, earache, and migraine." The fumes of black bile could ascend through the body to the brain, but these caused subtly different disorders, namely, headache and dizziness in the head. The *Wisdom* explained how humors changed over one's life cycle. At fifteen years old, "the heat of the blood comes upon him and there surges up in him red bile; and now it behoves to let blood. Red bile will dominate in him until he is twenty-five."[24]

Humors were an extremely strong bodily force determining a person's well-being. The twelfth-century text *Causae et Curae*, created by the celebrated St. Rupertsberg abbess, Hildegard of Bingen (1098–1179), presented a compelling rationale for emigranea's one-sided nature. Rather than blaming yellow or red bile (choler) for the ailment, *Causae et Curae* identified emigranea as a disorder stemming from melancholy (black bile) and "all bad humours present in a person."[25] The text leaves us in no doubt as to the power of these humors. Emigranea seizes only half the brain at a time, because "its strength is such that if it seized the whole head, a person would not be able to endure it." *Causae et Curae* gave clear instructions for a remedy that was supposed to sedate the pain and enrich the brain. Aloe and myrrh should be reduced to a fine powder, mixed with wheat flour and poppy oil to make a dough, and then the whole head should be covered with the paste. The patient placed a cap on top and kept it on the head for three days and nights.[26]

More examples of medieval treatments survive in other manuscripts. A recipe from eleventh-century Chartres gave instructions to stroke peony root frequently over the site of the pain, take a bath with sweet-smelling herbs boiled in vinegar, or use a cap made with well-boiled hot abrotano (artemisia).[27] In thirteenth-century Wales, patients were instructed to eat a baked or roasted hare's brain stuffed with rosemary flowers, followed by sleep, to treat the migran.[28] An influential thirteenth-century medical compendium, the *Antidotarium Nicolai*, from the famous medical school in Salerno indicated the compound known as theriac could be used for a multitude of diseases and chronic illnesses, including epilepsy, apoplexy, headache, migraine, bronchitis, spitting of blood, asthma, leprosy, smallpox, and chills. Theriac (from which we derive the modern word treacle) was one of the best-known medical preparations in medieval Europe. This was a complicated preparation, often containing up to eighty different ingredients, and was one of the most important Galenic medicines. Originally used as an antidote for poisons and snakebite, theriac became something of a universal cure-all. By the fourteenth century, it was commonly used against the Black Death.[29]

These remedies and explanations span over a thousand years and cover a huge geographical area. Yet they all share one important characteristic: while medieval treatments for some medical conditions incorporated elements of magic or religion, this consistently appears not to have been the case for migraine.[30] Rather, the remedies proposed and the ideas about hemicrania's causes contained within early texts offered practical suggestions based on secular traditions of healing and bodily knowledge. In particular, natural ingredients with specific qualities or physical interventions (including phlebotomy) were designed to remedy an illness that could be convincingly explained as the result of imbalanced or bad humors.

Old Knowledge for New Audiences

It is difficult to imagine a more precise evocation of the burning, throbbing, internal turmoil of a migraine attack than one we find in the thirteenth-century encyclopedia *De Proprietatibus Rerum* ("On the Properties of Things"), compiled by Franciscan monk Bartholomaeus Anglicus (Bartholomew the Englishman). Emigranea was a "most grievous" ache that, for the patient, felt like "there were beating hammers in his head." One would be unable to tolerate noise, voices, or light. The head pain seemed to pierce and prick, burn and ring, its cause identified as "choleric smoke, with hot wind and windiness."[31]

Classical sources for *On the Properties of Things* included the Bible, Augustinian theology, Aristotle, and Pliny.[32] Bartholomaeus's ideas about emigranea came—as he acknowledged—from Constantine the African's succinct medical handbook *Viaticum*, dating from the late eleventh century, itself a translation from the Arabic of a tenth-century medical work by physician Ibn al-Jazzar. Constantine had composed *Viaticum* at the Benedictine monastery of Monte Cassino in southern Italy. This was one of the most important centers of new medical learning and translations in medieval Europe, and it sponsored Constantine's rendering of more than thirty texts from Arabic into Latin.[33] *Viaticum* would come to be broadly disseminated throughout Europe within a larger compilation of medical texts known as *Articella*, which formed the basis of the medical curriculum at Salerno. It appears to have been widely used by monks and commented on in universities.[34]

Bartholomaeus's discussion of emigranea came in the seventh of the nineteen books that made up his encyclopedia.[35] It followed the customary *a capite ad calcem*, or head to toe, format of medical handbooks, beginning at the top of the body, with a discussion of general head pain. Bartholomaeus explained that headache (*cephelea*) had two types of causes: internal and external. External ones included a blow to the head, or they could be of climatic origin, such as from the effects of warm or cold air. If the headache came from within, it could be because of a defect in quality, such as the body being too hot or too cold, or from humoral imbalance. The kind of head pain a person felt helped to identify the causal factor. Citing Galen, Bartholomaeus explained that intermittent pains could come from sharp humors oppressing the stomach, while a continuous pain was the direct result of a problem with the humors. The likely cause could be narrowed down by paying attention to the location of the pain. If it came from choleric fumes (yellow bile), "heat will be felt in the nostrils, dryness in the tongue; there will be wakefulness and thirst, the pain will be greater on the right side than on the left, because that is where the seat of choler is." Phlegm produced a "heavy" pain. The head could also be divided into four sections, helping to explain why some parts could hurt more than others. Blood dominated the forehead, while choler was on the right side, melancholy on the left, and phlegm at the back. So if melancholy (black bile) was the cause, then the pain would be felt more intensely on the left.[36]

Having outlined these general rules in relation to the head, Bartholomaeus next turned more specifically to emigranea, providing an explanation that would aid a diagnosis and outlining a plan for treatment. Reassuring his readers that the affliction could be quickly taken care of, Bartholomaeus indicated a number of procedures that should be followed. First, the practitioner must withdraw blood according to the position of the pain within the head. So, for pain in the back of the head, the vein in the forehead must be opened. If the pain was at the front of the head, a nosebleed should be induced. Alternatively, Bartholomaeus recommended scarifying—making a series of shallow cuts, often using a mechanical instrument—in the shins, in order to draw the humors, fumes, and spirits away from the site of pain in the head and transfer it to the lower parts of the body. After bleeding, the patient should be purged, using "appropriate" medicines, and then lukewarm water should be poured over the head, hands, and feet to open the pores and let the fumes evaporate. Understanding the location of pain in relation to the humors guided the next step. The offending humor in emigranea was "hot and choleric," so it required the use of cold medications in order to restore balance. "We anoint the temples, nostrils, and pulsating veins with rose water, together with the milk of a woman who is nursing a male child, and we induce sleep," Bartholomaeus explained.[37] Should these treatments fail, Bartholomaeus was reluctant to take responsibility for anyone considering alternative, more drastic measures and referred his readers back to his sources. "If you wish to use stronger medications," he advised, "consult the Viaticum of Constantine."[38]

On the Properties of Things, originally composed for the friars at Magdeburg, where Bartholomaeus taught theology, became perhaps the most popular of the medieval encyclopedias, and it was widely circulated throughout Europe as a comprehensive source of both theoretical and practical knowledge. It was translated from Latin into French, German, and Italian during the fourteenth century. John Trevisa, a Gloucestershire vicar, translator, and writer, rendered this encyclopedia into English in 1398, before London printer and publisher Wynkyn de Worde produced the first printed version in English almost a century later. Thomas Berthelet printed a second edition in 1535, and Stephen Batman "corrected, enlarged, and amended" the text in 1582.[39] Although Bartholomaeus's encyclopedia continued to be reprinted and disseminated into the early modern period, it seems that some of the classical ideas about migraine he repeated were becoming less influential. In particular, the notion that migraine could result from either hot or cold causes seems to have given way to a general acceptance that cold ones were the most usual culprit, for which hot and dry ingredients were the best remedy.

The emerging preference for warming treatments is reflected in a mid-fifteenth-century manuscript collection, written in English, of over a thousand remedies for treating diseases and injuries. The collection contains at least eight ways to relieve mygreyne, or mygrayn. This includes three kinds of plasters to be laid on the head, two simple mixtures to be chewed in the mouth, a thick medicine that could be stored in a bladder pouch, a powder to be eaten, and a thick egg-based mixture to be applied to the forehead. One recipe for a powder stands out as being a particular favorite of the manuscript's compiler. Attributed to Galen, "the gode philosophir," it was also used by "my Lord John, the Duke of Somerset, in the Lent-time when he went over the sea." The compound should be eaten "first and last byside [other] receytis." The recipe was not simple, but it would certainly have been aromatic and sweet, requiring ginger, nutmeg, cloves, spikenard, anise, elecampane, licorice, and sugar, all beaten together into a powder. Mixed into pottage or a drink, or taken straight from a spoon, the text promised that the patient would be better within four days.[40]

Spikenard is the most significant of the ingredients in this preparation. Also known as muskroot, and often as Indian spikenard, or just nard, it is a member of the valerian family (to which we will return in chapter 4), native to the Himalayas. The plant, mentioned in the Bible, had been used medically by Pliny and Dioscorides, including for "cold" diseases and against headaches, and it was often a component of incense.[41] In addition to spikenard itself, this fifteenth-century remedy contained a number of the aromatic ingredients that had been required for nard oil. This substance was described in the ninth-century dispensatory of Nestorian physician and pharmacologist Sābūr ibn Sahl, from southwestern Iran, which is one of the earliest pharmacopeia written in Arabic. Nard oil most likely would have had sedative properties and was indicated for the treatment of hemicrania, among other things. It was an expensive recipe, requiring over twenty herbal ingredients, including cyprus, laurel, elecampane, citronella, myrtle leaves, wild caraway, forget-me-not, sweet marjoram, stalkless roses, fresh myrtle-water, myrrh, and grape ivy. These had to be prepared with different liquids, in three stages, over a period of several days. The third stage took Indian spikenard (the ingredient that gave nard oil its name); pounded it together with cloves, storax, and nutmeg; and added this mixture to fresh water, balm oil, and the strained oil from the previous two stages. Then the whole concoction was boiled until the water had disappeared, before being bottled, stored, and used as required. Two other recipes in the fifteenth-century manuscript also contained spikenard as a key ingredient, and both mixed the plant with vinegar, mustard, and honey. These concoctions would have been aromatic (if not distinctly pungent) and warming. One remedy produced a thick mixture to be held in the mouth for as long as it took to say two *Agnus Dei*, and before bed one should drink a draft in God's name.[42]

These examples from the thirteenth and fifteenth centuries provide important evidence of how medical information, derived from a corpus of classical knowledge—in this case, in the form of recipes for treatments of a particular disease—had been reintroduced to Europe via Arabic texts and then spread through learned centers, such as universities and monasteries, and, later, in print. These ideas, however, were not reproduced uncritically. Recipes could be adapted, so if the original classical ingredients were not available, they could be replaced by herbs that grew more locally, a theme we will see again in the early modern period.

Lay Understandings

One of the issues that comes from having to rely on medieval manuscript texts is that these sources tend not to reveal a great deal—Bartholomaeus's wonderfully evocative account of beating hammers is an exception—about the extent to which this knowledge was passed on to or reflected understandings within the wider population. Nonetheless, two examples from the fifteenth century—a poem, and the banns of an itinerant leech—do provide glimpses of how migraine might have been understood more broadly.

"My head did ache last night," Scottish poet William Dunbar wrote, as he addressed his patron, King James IV of Scotland (1488–1513), the morning after a migraine, in a three-verse poem called "On His Heid-Ake":

so much that I cannot write today
So painfully the migraine does disable me

piercing my brow just like any arrow
that I can scarcely look at the light.[43]

We might imagine Dunbar seeking refuge from the bustle of the court, hiding from the narrow rays of sun that pierced the dusty gloom of his lodgings. In the second and third verses, the poet captured a sense of the migraine aftermath: of being "dulled in dullness and distress" as the "postdrome" came with the arrival of the new morning. Although he was relieved of pain, when he sat down to write he could find no words. His head dulled, his body unrefreshed, his spirit sleeping, he found himself unable to rouse for mirth and minstrelsy, revelry and dancing.

Dunbar's migraine poem is something quite different from his usual representations of the Scottish court and society.[44] It is a personal and reflective piece, a petition to the king to ask for forgiveness for the poet's temporary failure to entertain. The poem is a rare and important historical document, because, rather than being the instructions for a treatment, as most other sources from the Middle Ages are, it so clearly evokes what Dunbar and his contemporaries understood a migraine attack and its aftermath to *feel* like. It is particularly significant that Dunbar talked of his "magryme" as being accompanied by sensory symptoms—an aversion to light, an inability to think—combined with a severe headache.

Another piece of evidence from the fifteenth century indicates how learned medicine might have become accessible to a wider audience. Peripatetic practitioners, known by the term "leech," advertised their whereabouts, the services they offered, and their prices through documents called "banns," which were designed to be read out loud in public. In one surviving English example, the leech offered his services to "any man or woman that is diseased in any divers sickness." Charging a penny for urine analysis, and another penny for a written prescription, the leech promised (with the Grace of God) to cure wounds, bruises, aching or broken bones, cankers, worms, flux, deafness, and all manner of scabs and gouts, as well as "mygreyn." This, the bann explained, was a malady that affected half a man's head and lessened the sight in his eye.[45] It is noteworthy that the bann enumerated these symptoms to potential customers. While broken bones, deafness, bleeding, burns and scalds, sores, and boils were obvious enough to require little explanation, the leech also did not feel the need to describe the symptoms of gouts and cankers. He only elaborated on three of the diseases he promised to be able to cure. As well as explaining mygreyn, he stated that a "whistle in a man's jaw" was a hole that was always running, while "morphew" made a person faint and "greatly discoloured in his visage."[46] The extra information in the case of these three illnesses suggests either that people would not have had the knowledge to be able to diagnose themselves, or that the leech was aware of different definitions of (or words for) these diseases and was describing his own understanding of them. As in Dunbar's poem, the leech conceived of mygreyn as involving pain in one side of the head and affecting vision, setting it apart from other headaches. The leech's clarification on these points suggests that these medical banns had an educational as well as a promotional purpose. As he traveled around, an itinerant physician provided geographically dispersed communities with a common terminology for a particular set of symptoms.

Blood

Bald's *Leechbook* and Bartholomaeus's *On the Properties of Things* both recommended bleeding as a first resort for hemicrania. This is not surprising. With new translations of classical texts, bloodletting became common practice for dealing with both physical and mental illnesses within a context in which blood played a hugely significant cultural role in religion, law, and medicine. Blood was believed to reveal the truth; it held body and soul together, determined emotions, and transported the humors around the body. In the second century, Galen considered bloodletting appropriate for any disorder, if a physician knew when, where, and how much to bleed and made sure to take the patient's constitution into account. The practice of phlebotomy became a standard way to remove excess humor.[47] The thirteenth-century surgeon Lanfranc of Milan explained that there were three types of bloodletting: to preserve health, to protect one from sickness, and to remove illness. Lanfranc recommended bleeding for those who ate meat, drank good wine, and took little exercise. It could be used against strong pains in the head without fever, quinsy, pleurisy, pneumonia, or illnesses that came from an overabundance of blood. In such cases, phlebotomy could remove either an incipient or an established illness.[48] Bleeding would have been particularly appropriate for a localized pain disorder like migraine, which was understood so clearly, in humoral terms, as the product of excess or bad humor.

In the fifteenth-century "Guild-Book of the Barber-Surgeons of the City of York," a slim, white, longhaired, naked man stares out at us from the page (fig. 2.2). Twenty red lines emanate from points around the man's body: from the forehead, face, and neck, down the arms to the elbows and hands, and then to the penis and feet. Each line represents a bleeding point on a vein, showing

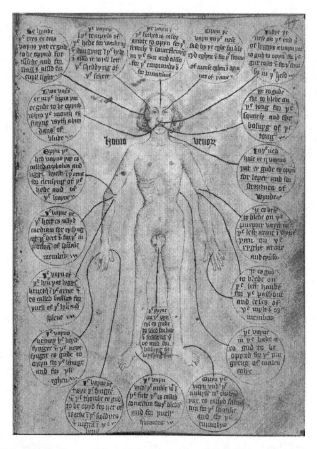

Fig. 2.2. "Vein Man" diagram, from "Guild-Book of the Barber-Surgeons of the City of York," f. 50r, c. 1486. © The British Library Board

the range of illnesses that could be treated by taking blood from these places. Each line leads to a circle, which contains a concise instruction giving the position and name of the vein and recommending which diseases might benefit from an opening to release blood at this point. Some of the instructions dealt with particular humors: bloodletting in the back, for instance, purged melancholy, while opening the vein under the ankle and inside the foot drained "yvelle humors" in general. Other instructions mentioned particular illnesses, including quinsy, "leper," a "boiling or bruising" penis, and "evils" of the heart, liver, and spleen. Several of the veins were suitable for being opened to treat disorders of the head. If you wished to cleanse the head and brain, you could open the cephalic vein, lying high in the right arm above the elbow. For "evyll sight," bleed the two veins behind the ears.

Follow the line connected to the point between the thumb and first finger of the man's right hand. It leads to a circle in the bottom left-hand corner of the image, which contains directions for opening the vein between the fingers and thumbs in order to treat pain in the shoulders and "migram" in the head.[49] Beyond the specific identification of the correct vein, however, much knowledge is assumed on the part of the practitioner, including how to diagnose a migram, how much blood to take, or whether there were rules about bleeding at particular times or seasons. Tellingly, this bleeding point between the thumb and forefinger is also used now in some modern migraine treatments. Paula Kamen describes having a transcutaneous electrical nerve stimulation machine attached to a pressure point between the thumb and forefinger on her right hand, and this is also a recognized acupuncture point for headaches.[50] While it would be wrong to infer any direct continuity, the similarity is certainly striking.

During the fourteenth and fifteenth centuries, images of *homo venorum,* or vein man, such as this one in the York guild book, began to appear more widely.[51] These diagrams gave physicians simple, practical instructions about when and where to undertake bloodletting and showed the points on the body from which blood could be drawn. The images themselves range from basic sketches of the male human form, marked with bleeding points, to detailed illuminated manuscripts naming individual veins, giving clear instructions, and specifying the disorders that could be treated by opening each vein. Historians have suggested that the diagrams and charts in documents such as these may have been used to train apprentices, or that the York volume contained the knowledge required of professional practitioners with a guild background.[52]

Drawing vital blood from a body—any body—whether suffering from migraine, mania, leprosy, or quinsy, was not to be taken lightly. As Bettina Bildhauer observes, even normal or harmless bleeding, such as menstruation, was considered with suspicion and "circumscribed as a moment of crisis."[53] A range of evidence from across the period suggests some of the factors a person with migraine would have needed to take into account when deciding whether, and how, to bleed. We have already seen how careful Bartholomaeus was to outline the location of bleeding in the head, depending on where the pain was felt, or to note that a patient could be scarified in the shins to draw the humors away from the site of the problem. Phlebotomy could be performed gently, using leeches, or, more commonly, by venesection with a lancet or scarificating tool. The patient should be comfortable. A ninth-century ground plan of a Benedictine monastery shows a bloodletting facility complete with beds, privy, and four chimneys, so the recipients of bloodletting could be kept warm before the procedure.[54] There were seasonal considerations, too, and springtime was widely accepted as the best time to bleed patients prophylactically.[55] Bald's *Leechbook* advised that the optimum moment for bloodletting was early on during Lent (specifically, April), which was when evil humors that had been "drunken in" during winter could be "gathered" and taken from the body.[56] Several centuries later, William Clowes, one of the best known of the late-sixteenth-century surgeons, advised that phlebotomy should be avoided in extremes of temperature; thus spring and autumn were the most convenient times. Clowes explained that blood should be let on the right-hand side in spring, and on the left during autumn and winter, which might well have had implications for relieving one-sided headaches. During summer, phlebotomy should be undertaken at eight o'clock in the morning; in winter, at noon. The patient should exercise before bloodletting, while the sick and old should be encouraged to fortify themselves beforehand by taking bread and "stipticke wine" to help with clotting.[57] Few authors gave instructions regarding the quantity of blood that should be taken from each point, though the famous French surgeon Ambroise Paré, whose work was widely translated into English, urged bloodletters to consider the strength of the patient and the "greatness" of the disease. He warned that blood should not be drawn from "ancient people" unless immediately necessary.[58]

There were two theoretical approaches to bleeding, both based on the understanding that humors flowed around the body and could be brought back into balance by taking blood. "Revulsive" bleeding aimed to draw bad humors to a distant part of the body before they had a chance to settle (as in the York guild book), while "derivative" bleeding withdrew blood at, or close to, the affected part of the body, in order to draw bad humors out directly.[59] In the thirteenth century, Bartholomaeus's instructions regarding migraine incorporated both approaches by recommending bleeding either from the head or from the shins. Lanfranc of Milan preferred to let blood from the vein of the thumb for head ailments, because it weakened the patient less than taking it from the head. Perhaps more importantly, fewer serious mistakes could be made when bloodletting from the hand. Before bleeding a patient at the extremities, Lanfranc advised that their hands or feet should be put in hot water for an hour, with the blood flow then constricted above the wrist or ankle.[60] By contrast, the *Regimen Sanitatis Salerni*—an aide-memoire in poetic form, possibly originating in the thirteenth century, and one of the most widely disseminated and translated medical texts into the early modern period— recommended opening either the veins in the temples at the side of the head or the cephalic vein (running from the shoulder down the arm) on the left-hand side for diseases of the head, including megrim.[61] In the sixteenth century, Nicholas Gyer's *English Phlebotomy* recommended cutting the cephalic vein in the middle of the arm for any disease above the head or neck, including "passions of the heade," as such as hemicrania, mygrame, and mania. Gyer explained that it was safe to open this vein in the arm, because "there is no sinew or artery under it." Even if a cut missed the vein in the first attempt, "he may be bold to strike it again: for there is I say, no ieoperdy [danger] to cut any muskle."[62] William Bullein's popular *Newe Booke Entituled the Gouernement of Healthe* recommended opening the middle vein of the forehead against "megrim, forgetfulnes, and passions of the head," though only after purging the head.[63] Jacques Guillemeau's *Frenche Chirurgerie* also specified the temporal vein, bleeding it on the side corresponding to the pain of the hemicrania, as Galen had recommended so many centuries before.[64] These examples reveal that, over time, the practice of bleeding from the head for migraine (the derivative technique) seems to have become more popular, a trend reflecting a more widespread rejection of the revulsion method since the Renaissance.

Although the fifteenth-century writer Jacques Despars largely dismissed astrological judgments as being "uncertain, unstable, ambiguous, and often deceptive," medieval phlebotomists paid much greater attention to astrological calendars than their classical forebears had done.[65] The phases of the moon, positions of the planets, and season of the year were all relevant to determining bleeding practices.[66] Around the turn of the seventeenth century, another striking image of a man, this time showing twenty-one bleeding points, began to appear in printed almanacs. These were common across Europe in the early modern period and, for much of the population, were perhaps the only secular literature they would come across. They contained information about the seasons, religious events, signs of the zodiac, and diet, reinforcing understandings that a strong connection existed between the weather, the environment, and a person's health.[67] Elisheva Carlebach has argued that these folk, or shepherds, calendars were probably not intended to be purchased by the herders themselves, but by "those who read to them, instructed them, or employed them" in order to correct their "superstitious" ways.[68]

At least seven editions of the *Shepheards Kalendar*, published between 1595 and 1656, contained the same woodcut image. Each point on the vein man was labeled with a letter from A to U, beginning in the middle of the forehead and working down the left-hand side of the body, before returning to the right eye and then down the right arm. For sufferers of megrim, two veins in the head were of interest. The point marked A, the vein in the middle of the forehead, should be bled to relieve aches and pains of the head, as well as for fevers, lethargy, and megrim. Point C represented two veins in the temples "called the Arteries, for that they pant." Opening these, it was noted, was a more drastic procedure, to be used when the patient suffered from gout or megrim or wished to take away a "great repletion and abundance of bloud that is in the brain" affecting the head and eyes. The vein man diagram in the *Shepheards Kalendar* emphasized the astrological as well as the humoral requirements of the procedure. Precise instructions about the timing of bloodletting according to astrological rules ran vertically down the margin of the page. "Natural" days for bloodletting were when the moon was neither new, nor full, nor in the quarter. In addition, the moon must be in a sign that was considered good for bleeding, unless that sign was the one dominating the part of the body where blood was to be let, in which case "it ought not for to be touched." In general, days when the moon entered Aries, Libra, and Sagittarius "be right good" for bleeding, while Taurus, Gemini, Leo, and Capricorn "be evill for bleeding." In the case of megrim, bleeding should be avoided when the moon was in Aries, since this sign governed the head and face.[69] Writers had long noted the dangers of bloodletting in the head when the moon was in Aries. One fifteenth-century folded almanac instructed its reader not to make an incision in the head or face, or in the great vein of the head, when the moon was in Aries.[70] Another almanac went even further, warning that at the beginning of Aries, it is "full p[eri]lous" to let blood for headaches, and doing so was likely to cause "longe endurynge" of the disease, or even death.[71]

Conclusion

This chapter has revealed the range of humoral interpretations for hemicrania that existed between the classical and medieval periods. In particular, a consistent association of hemicrania with bile tells us something very important about the kinds of people expected to experience it. Yellow/red bile (choler) was associated with the fire of youth, while black bile (melancholy) was more likely to dominate during adulthood. Humoral theory, like present-day ones, seems to have presented migraine as a disorder that would often have become apparent during childhood or the teenage years and would last through adulthood.

Almanacs provided a source of practical information for the lay population, allowing a knowledge of phlebotomy—and thus an important strategy for treating migraine—to spread beyond learned practitioners, such as those in the York guild or in monasteries. Even if a person would most often go to a barber surgeon for the procedure itself, an almanac could arm the patient with important information about when to seek out a phlebotomist and ensure that they were bled correctly. The popularity of phlebotomy suggests that, in the medieval period, a person with migraine might have become visible in a very particular, if subtle, way. If, for many people, bloodletting was a seasonal fixture in an annual routine of maintaining bodily balance, for a person with migraine, it might have been a much more regular occurrence that could be performed quickly, and relatively cheaply, when the need arose. It is worth considering the cumulative scarring effect that frequent, deliberate cuts—particularly when your practitioner favored letting blood from the temples—might have had on a person's body.[72] Migraine, so often considered an invisible disease in our own time, may well have previously been quite visible through the marks that were left by frequent attempts to remove evil humors from the head.

As printers started to reproduce manuscript texts in greater numbers by the late fifteenth century, medical works gained a wide circulation throughout Europe. Within these, emigranea and megrim continued to find a prominent place, just as they had during the medieval period. But ideas about what migraine was, and how to deal with it, had changed over time. While early writers—including Galen, the unspecified author(s) of the *Wisdom of the Art of Medicine*, and Bartholomaeus Anglicus—attributed hemicrania to either hot or cold bodily causes, by the fifteenth century, the remedies that seem to have been absorbed most often into vernacular practice were the ones that used hot and dry ingredients to counteract a disease understood to have cold and moist causes. Though we have no way of knowing whether the experience of migraine in ancient Rome, or Anglo-Saxon England, or twelfth-century Rhineland was the same as ours, early explanations of the pain, discomfort, and sensory symptoms that characterized migraine appear, in many ways, to be remarkably familiar. Early medical approaches to hemicrania reveal a rich culture for dealing with a well-known and extremely painful disease.

CHAPTER THREE

"Take Housleeke, and Garden Wormes"

Migraine Medicine in the Early Modern Household

Mrs. Corlyon's *Booke*, 1606

A noblewoman's recipe book, dated 1606, explains that "you shall know the Megreeme by this it lyeth in the Browes, or in the Noddell [the back of the head], or in the one side of your heade."[1] The book belonged to Alathea Talbot, Countess of Arundel and Surrey, well known for her interest in physic, but its authorship was attributed to a woman named Mrs. Corlyon. One of the principal factors in head pain, Corlyon explained, was a physical process she described as "the opening of the heade," for which she identified three common causes: too much moisture about the brain, a sudden jump or fall, or the shaking of "vehement riding or such like." In order to recognize when your head had opened, Mrs. Corlyon gave a relatively straightforward and quick diagnostic test that could be undertaken by anyone. First, you must "bowe downe the end of your thombe." Then you should attempt to fit the half of the thumb between the two knuckles into the space between the upper and lower teeth of the fully opened mouth, with the upper joint pointing toward your upper teeth and the lower joint to your lower teeth. If you cannot fit the portion of the thumb between the two joints into the space between your teeth, "then your heade is opened," she explained.

Corlyon's simple thumb test provided a quick way—which could also be used preemptively—to determine whether further action was needed to treat a head that was opened. She also provided a simple physical method for, quite literally, forcing the two sides of the head back together. Leaning over a table on your elbows, put your face in your hands with your thumbs under the two sides of the skull bone behind the ears, with the fingers facing toward the top of the head. Gathering your face into your hands, squeeze the face and temples together, so the fingers met at the top of the head. This hold should be continued for half an hour at a time and repeated as often as necessary. To be sure of success, Corlyon recommended that the sufferer also anoint their temples near the ears and the back of their head with either her ointment for palsy or one made of lavender; recipes for both were provided later in her book. The ointments should be taken in a drink of cow's milk mixed with green or dried balm, rosemary, and nutmeg. Every day, the patient should drink a quart of this concoction, as hot as possible, so the perfumed air "may ascende into your heade."[2]

Mrs. Corlyon included detailed instructions for the preparation of three herbal remedies for megreeme. The first, a remedy "to staye the humours from fallinge to the Eyes, and goode for the meegreeme," came in the first chapter, for diseases of the eyes, in a section that also included preparations to take away redness and soreness in eyes, clear the sight, remove growths, and prevent cataracts. Two more migraine remedies came in the chapter on diseases of the head: a "gargas" (gargle) to be held in the mouth, and a plaster to be applied to the forehead and temples after using the gargle. Other remedies in her chapter included concoctions to "stay the rhewms," procure sleep, and clear the head of corrupt air or wind.[3]

Mrs. Corlyon's directions for diagnosing and treating migraine through both physical and herbal means take us beyond learned physicians and formal texts. Her book provides a unique and invaluable insight into how migraine in the early modern period might have been understood by ordinary people, and how it was treated within the home. In the present chapter, Mrs. Corlyon's collection forms the basis for tracing a path through early modern ideas about the symptoms, causes, and treatment of migraine, its relationship to other conditions, and the rich variety of medicaments that could be made up and applied. During my research, I collected nearly a hundred separate recipes from manuscript remedy collections and printed books from the sixteenth and seventeenth centuries. There are different kinds of treatments, including plasters and caps to be placed on the head, drinks, powders, gargles, and aromatic preparations to be held in the mouth.[4] These remedies incorporate nearly sixty separate herbs and plants, in addition to spices or strongly flavored ingredients such as nutmeg, cumin, cinnamon, ginger, and mustard, as well as twenty different oil, resin, and liquid bases, including wine, ale, olive oil, frankincense, and turpentine. Egg white, honey, and bread helped bind other elements together into pastes that could stick to linen or leather patches. A number of recipes called for earthworms, the rationale for which we will discuss later in this chapter. While many of the collections did contain instructions for minor surgical operations, the practice of bloodletting appears to have remained beyond the purview of domestic approaches to megrim, which were concerned almost entirely with the production of medicines using ingredients derived from plants and animals.[5]

Although recipes and instructions such as Mrs. Corlyon's tell us little firsthand about the lives of individual sufferers, and although, in many cases, we do not have much information about the owners of the books, the instructions about the qualities of the ingredients required, and the manner in which these concoctions must be made and followed, do reveal a lot about the kinds of diseases these writers anticipated. In the previous chapter, we saw that medieval writers often identified both hot and cold causes for migraine, while here we find that most "receipts" called for "hot" and "dry" herbs (as in Mrs. Corlyon's one for "Megreeme in the heade"), revealing that by the early modern period, migraine was widely understood in everyday practice to be brought on by excess moisture and cold humors in the head. When they are assembled and analyzed together, recipes and remedies provide a rich picture of the ways in which people dealt with migraine and their ideas for managing a disease that could be both acute and chronic. They also give important insight into the ways in which medical information circulated between print and pen among householders in the early modern period.

Early Modern Household Recipe Books

Mrs. Corlyon's *Booke of Diuers Medecines, Broothes, Salues, Waters, Syroppes, and Oyntementes* is modestly sized and bound in its original calf leather cover. The initials stamped in gold leaf on the cover and the inscription on the first page reveal that the book was owned by Alathea Talbot, but a note inside the front cover explains that most of the recipes "have been experienced and tried by the special practize of . . . Mrs. Corlyon." The date suggests that the blank volume may have been a gift on the occasion of Alathea's marriage to Thomas Howard, the second Earl of Arundel (1586–1646), into which Alathea transcribed the contents, perhaps from Mrs. Corlyon's own book.[6] Recent research by historians has revealed that the Wellcome Library's manuscript is identical to another in the Folger Shakespeare Library, suggesting that Mrs. Corlyon belonged to a well-known family of Cornish gentry.[7]

Mrs. Corlyon's *Booke* is one of the best preserved in the Wellcome Trust's archive of early modern manuscripts containing domestic recipe collections.[8] These were both practical household manuals and highly prized family heirlooms. Because of their importance, a great number of similar manuscripts have been carefully maintained over time and can be found in major libraries and archives.[9] Elaine Leong has described them as "treasure stores of practical knowledge," filled with information to be used "just in case."[10] Recipe books contained a wealth of shared, collected, and inherited knowledge to aid in the running of a household, including instructions on how to concoct medicines and salves, clean a gunshot wound, make basic pies for everyday meals and elaborate puddings for special occasions, preserve gluts of seasonal produce, and administer veterinary treatments to maintain the health of precious livestock. These volumes are a revelatory window into the goings-on of early modern lives, and they allow us to combine the history of household medicine with the broader culture of scientific knowledge, the commercial economy of the medical marketplace, and the reception of early printed material.[11] While Alisha Rankin's work on networks of respected noblewomen healers in Germany has used recipe books to showcase these women as integral to mainstream cultures of pharmacy, scientific experiment, patronage, and exchange, other historians have emphasized that such books are not just indicative of women's knowledge, but also are illustrations of how generations of men and women contributed to the compilation of family books.[12] More recently, attention has shifted to how these collections—particularly exemplars such as Mrs. Corlyon's, which was devoted to the everyday practice of medicine—can help us understand the history of particular disorders and states of health, often by examining the contents of the recipes themselves.[13]

Although many manuscript recipe books are written in several hands and bear the marks of being added to and passed on over generations, Alathea Talbot's version of Mrs. Corlyon's *Booke* is a "best copy," written in the same handwriting throughout and meticulously set within carefully ruled borders. Each remedy is titled in red ink, with the rest of the writing in black, a common way of laying out medieval and early modern manuscripts. We might best understand this manuscript as a personal treasure, rather than a practical manual that Alathea used on a regular basis. A few supplemental remedies that appear on the spare pages at the end of chapters and in the back of the volume seem to have been added later. Nearly all of these are credited to named individuals, suggesting that Alathea chose to supplement her collection with just a few trusted recipes, in addition to the majority that initially came from Mrs. Corlyon. Individual recipes deemed particularly valuable are accompanied by terms such as "soveraign," "*probatum est*," "experienced," or "these drinks do help."

Corlyon's collection is organized in twenty-five thematic chapters. As had been standard practice for medical handbooks during the medieval period, it follows a head-to-toe organization, starting with the eyes, then progressing downward through the body in chapters dedicated to the head, ears, face, teeth and mouth, throat, lungs, and stomach, until reaching disorders of the digestive system. Five additional chapters deal with preparations for less localized disorders, including jaundice, bleeding, sweat, plague, and gout. One chapter lists "generall medecines for particular effectes," and the final five chapters deal with different types of medicine: broths, waters, syrups, salves, and ointments. There are remedies for ailments as diverse as deafness, toothache, sciatica, consumption, kidney stones, and the expulsion of wind, as well as a number of preparations for general, less diagnosable weaknesses. Together, the recipes cover a huge number of different problems. This is a highly personal early modern encyclopedia of bodily and medical knowledge.

Between Print and Pen

While some elements of Mrs. Corlyon's approach, such as the diagnosis of an open head, are distinctive, in general her ideas are representative of the humoral and herbal knowledge contained in manuscript and printed collections of the period. Corlyon's identification of excessive moisture, or the dangers of too much shaking, reflected widely held ideas that the sources of head pain could either be internal (humoral) or external, the latter for reasons such as the temperature being too hot or cold, or individuals eating the wrong foods (though, in the early sixteenth century, Sir Thomas Elyot's *Castel of Helth* suggested that vehement shaking might usefully serve to cure, rather than provoke, "mygrimes").[14] It is not clear, however, where Mrs. Corlyon obtained her theory about the dangers of an open head as the cause of headache. Neither her rationale for head pain, nor her description of such a physical treatment, appear in any of the manuscript or printed sources that I have been able to find from the early modern period.

Mrs. Corlyon defined megreeme by the location of the pain (in the brows, the nape of the neck, or one side of the head), which reflected an ongoing influence of the classical division of headaches into three types. What is unusual is that she included this information in her recipe book, when she, like her contemporaries, rarely gave details about the character or symptoms of diseases for which she offered treatments. In fact, Corlyon included diagnostic information with only two recipes in the book: how to tell what was a megreeme, and how to distinguish between a stitch and a more serious pleurisy.[15]

For many gentlewomen, printed medical books would have been an important addition to their collection, particularly in the case of those for whom providing physic within the local community, as well as the household, was an important aspect of their social role.[16] By the sixteenth century, the diagnostic information for individual ailments that is missing from recipe collections could commonly be found in printed medical books. Andrew Boorde's *Breuiary of Helthe*, published in 1547, is one of the earliest medical texts in vernacular English, rather than the Latin of learned authors.[17] It, too, offered a great deal of information about megrim. Boorde's *Breuiary* was arranged alphabetically by the Latin terms for ailments, with English-language descriptions in the margins alongside for easy reference. Each entry also gave the Greek names for the illness, as well as its characteristic symptoms and causes, before offering a remedy. The *Breuiary* placed a heavy emphasis on diet, both as a cause of sickness and in its treatment. This approach certainly reflected the continuing importance of ideas about balancing humors and regimens, but it also conveniently led Boorde's readers to his companion book, *A Compendyous Regyment or a Dyetary of Helthe*.

We might usefully think of Boorde's *Breuiary* as a handbook that aimed to help an ordinary person understand the terminology their physicians might use. Boorde explained that he did not want to exasperate genuine doctors and masters of the science of physic with his publication, nor did he expect it to allow people to cure themselves. He kept his entries brief, so he did not reveal the science of physic to all, which might lessen public regard for physicians and allow "every bungler" to practice it. Instead, Boorde provided enough information for patients to diagnose their disorders, arming readers with the ability and confidence to make a more informed judgment about the credibility of those who offered cures.[18]

Boorde began his entry for hemicrania by explaining to readers unfamiliar with Latin that it was a compound of the terms "hemi," meaning "the mydle," and "craneum, which is to say the skulle." "Megryme," to use its English word, would thus be felt in the middle part of the head, with pain descending to the temples, "and doth fetch a compas lyke a rayne bowe." At different times the pain might lie more to one side of the head than the other.[19] Boorde's use of the term "compas," meaning to range over the head, can be traced directly back to Bartholomaeus's thirteenth-century *On the Properties of Things*, which had been much reproduced since. It is important to note that Boorde's reference to a rainbow was not a description of the kind of visual experiences of aura that artists and scientists would come to depict in the nineteenth century, but of the *shape* of the pain, as an arc around the top of the head. Nevertheless, the fading nature of rainbows, and their tendency to appear brighter on one side in the sky, made this a particularly telling analogy. Boorde explained that megryme was caused by a "reume" (a flow or flux of humors, particularly one originating in the head) that was "intrused" (projected inward) in the head and could not be removed other than by using medicine.[20] Rheums could be either hot or cold, and they were often described as "thin" or "sharp." Rheums became a problem, and caused disease, when they moved, or "flowed," usually downward into the nose, eyes, or neck. This idea is apparent in the first of Mrs. Corlyon's recipes, which was supposed both to prevent humors from falling to the eyes and to be good for meegreeme.

Roughly forty years later, Philip Barrough's *Method of Phisicke* defined hemicrania as "a painefull evill remaining in the one halfe of the head, either on the right halfe or on the left, and is distinguished by the seame that runneth along in the skull ... this griefe in Englishe is called the migrime."[21] Barrough gave a number of different explanations for the effects of humors in causing headaches, and he dedicated several pages to apprising readers of the best ways to treat headaches resulting from heat and cold, dryness and moisture, and the humors of blood, choler, and phlegm. He also offered remedies for pains from "windynes" (an echo of Bartholomaeus again), the stomach, fevers, or a simple hangover. Barrough's ideas about the causes of different kinds of headache were complex, but he showed how the quality and severity of the pain could give clues as to what created it and help identify appropriate treatments. For example, a dry cause might produce a moderate pain, but if the abundant humors had a "sharpe and byting qualitie," the pain would prick and shoot accordingly. Inflammation of the head caused a beating, pulsing headache.[22] For migrime, Barrough identified the source as "the ascending and flowing of many vapours or humours eyther hote or cold, eyther by the vaines, or by the arteries, or by bothe," an explanation that had changed little since Galen. Sometimes the eruption of pain could emanate from the brain thrusting out its "excrementes and superfluityes."[23] The dangers of vapors were not necessarily just internal. Ambroise Paré identified goldsmiths and metal gilders as particularly at risk from megrim, because they routinely breathed "noysome vapour or smoake," such as that given off by antimony or quicksilver.[24] In 1615, London physician Helkiah Crooke made an early connection between migraine and vomiting, commenting: "Seeing the stomack hath obtayned so many sinewes, it is no wonder if when the braine bee stroken or affected, the stomacke also bee disturbed, and vomitings caused, especially in the Hemicrania or Meigrame."[25] Crooke's discussion of vomiting was unusual at this point in time, as the association of megrim with nausea or sickness only became more common from the eighteenth century on.

Although Boorde and Barrough had different ideas about migraine, due either to the effects of trapped rheums or rising vapors, both men acknowledged, as had been common since the classical period, that pain could result from either hot or cold causes, and that the disease was characterized by an excess of humors or moisture in the head. For Boorde, the key to successfully alleviate all head pains was to determine their humoral characteristics and then treat them accordingly, either by bleeding, purging, heating, or cooling. These remedies were designed to draw out the offending stuck rheum, rather than to moderate the sufferer's temperature. Boorde recommended purging the head with "gargaryces and sternutacions" (gargles and sneezes), and then anointing the temples with oils or applying a mustard plaster to the temples. Above all, the sufferer should avoid becoming constipated and protect their head against extremes of temperature, whether hot or cold.[26] Barrough also recommended purges to remove humors, again chosen to either cool or heat the affected area, depending on the cause of the migrime. An ointment consisting of oil made from the herb dill and powder from the pulverized root of the "ireos" lily (which could be imported from Florence) treated a distemper produced by cold. If hot humors or vapors were the culprit, a sufferer could take remedies based on mildly cooling ingredients, such as oils of roses or chamomile. This course of action was particularly recommended for women, children, and eunuchs, all of whom, by virtue of already being cold, should not be cooled too much further. For more drastic cooling, juices made from houseleek, purslain, knotgrass, unripe grapes, nightshade, and lettuce were useful ingredients. The juices of poppies or mandrake, on the other hand, should be avoided.[27]

It is notoriously difficult to find the extent to which information printed in books was either read or used in practice, or what the sources of that information were in the first place. In some cases, there is direct evidence of a knowledge exchange between manuscript and printed recipe collections. One example is a "singuler remedy for all diseases in the head" in John Partridge's *Widowes Treasure*. This required a handful each of chamomile, betony, and vervain leaves, pounded together and steeped in ale wort, then mixed with cumin seeds, hartshorn powder, vinegar, egg yolk, and saffron to form a hot plaster to be laid on the head. Seventy years later, Thomas Collins reproduced two versions of this recipe in his *Choice and Rare Experiments*.[28] The recipe appears again in Miss Shaw's manuscript collection of recipes, probably dating to the second half of the seventeenth century.[29] But it is also true that even the most well-circulated printed recipes were not necessarily incorporated into manuscript collections. Thomas Moulton first published his *Myrour or Glasse of Helth* in 1531, and, over the remainder of the sixteenth century, the volume went through at least seventeen editions.[30] Moulton included one recipe "for the migrym" that required four handfuls of red rose flowers and three handfuls each of chamomile and vervain. These herbs should be boiled together in white wine, then put into a linen bag and placed on the head "as hote as the sicke may suffer." Although relatively easy to prepare, Moulton's recipe seems not to have caught the attention of compilers of household collections, perhaps on the simple grounds of practicality. As well as relying on the seasonality of a particular color of roses, it required constant reapplication of the hot plaster for a day and a night, or longer if need be.[31] Recipes involving more obscure ingredients, derived from the medieval and Mediterranean traditions of classical medicine, also appear not to have translated well, such as one from Thomas Cartwright requiring "Bole Armoniack, Sanguinis Dragonis, and Terra Sigillat."[32]

While published books often contained details of and uses for single herbal ingredients, known as simples, compilers of manuscript recipe collections rarely stuck with one item when several would do. Yet, as we have already seen, these were not just randomly thrown together concoctions of whatever leaves and roots could be found in the back garden. Their combination reflected a distinct rationale, informed by centuries of accumulated knowledge regarding the natural properties of plants. During the early modern period, printed herbals—such as those published by William Bullein, William Copland, and Rembert Dodoens in the sixteenth century and, most famously, by Nicholas Culpeper in the seventeenth century—reproduced the classical knowledge of Greek physician Dioscorides, thus widely disseminating the information needed to mix together different ingredients that would either complement or moderate each other.

Using this system, we can begin to understand the mentality behind Mrs. Corlyon's recipes. "A Gargas or Medecine for the Megreeme in the heade" advised (fig. 3.1):

> Take Sage Rosemary and of Pellitory of Spaine, the rootes of eche of these a like
> quantity, and boil them in a pinte of Vineger, uppon a chafing dish of coales,
> untill halfe be consumed, then putt therein two good spoonefulles of Mustard

beyng made with good Vineger, and so lett it boile a while, And then take a litle of it, as hott as you can suffer and holde it in your mouthe, as you shall feele occasion and then spitt it out, and take more and this doe five or six tymes euery morninge so long as you shall fynde occasion or feele your selfe greeved.

Mrs. Corlyon's recipe for a gargle required the roots of three different herbs. Rosemary was widely considered to be beneficial for head pain. An anonymous early seventeenth-century pamphlet extolled the virtues of the "quintessence of rosemary flowers." It recommended those "that are subject to Melancholy, Lethargie, Megrim, Lunacie, Vertigo, Apoplexie, and any other

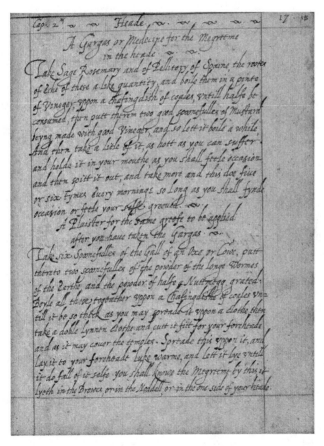

Fig. 3.1. "Medecyne for the Megreeme," from Mrs. Corlyon's *Booke of Diuers Medecines, Broothes, Salues, Waters, Syroppes, and Oyntementes*, 1606. Courtesy of the Wellcome Library, London, licensed under CC-BY

infirmities that come to the head by reason of humiditie and coldnes" to take one or two drops in broth or good wine.[33]

According to Copland's *Herbal*, sage was hot in the first degree and dry in the second. Rosemary, too, was hot and dry, and both herbs were characterized by a strong (and not unpleasant) savory aroma that might have seemed to enhance the effect of the remedy infusing through the head when chewed or inhaled. Pellitory of Spain (also called Spanish chamomile), a small perennial with feathery leaves and a daisylike flower, had similar qualities, although to a greater degree.[34] Accordingly, it was well known for its use in remedying head complaints. Thomas Cogan's *Hauen of Health*, a manual first published in 1584 and reprinted in several editions through the first decades of the seventeenth century, described pellitory of Spain as "hot in the third degree fully, and dry in the second," its chief use being to purge the head of rheums and other grief. Cogan recommended chewing a little piece of the dried root to draw out an abundance of "flegmaticke and waterish humours."[35] Gerard's *Herball* described pellitory root as "very hot and burning," useful against "the megrim or continuall paine of the head . . . the apoplexie, the falling sickness . . . a similar good and effectuall remedy for all cold and continuall infirmities of the head and sinewes."[36]

Hot and dry herbs like these appear in a number of manuscript recipe collections for plasters, drinks, and preparations to be gargled, or held in the mouth. Mixing these aromatic hot and dry herbs with pungent items from the kitchen, such as vinegar and mustard, would further enhance the effect of the herbs, whether they were designed to penetrate or warm through the skin, or create vapors that would ascend through the head from the nose or mouth.

In 1526, a very similar remedy for migraine, "postume," and dropsy in the head appeared in the anonymously published *New Boke of Medecynes*. It required "iiii penyweyght of the rote of Pyllatory of Spayne / a half peny weyght of Spygnarde [spikenard]." These should be ground together and boiled in vinegar, mixed with a spoonful of honey and a saucer of mustard, and held in the mouth a spoonful at a time.[37] This same recipe can also be found in a fifteenth-century manuscript recipe collection.[38] Thomas Vicary's *English Man's Treasure*, the first textbook of anatomy to be published in English, contained an herbal remedy to purge the head. The recipe consisted of, among other things, "Pelitorie of Spaine," "Stavisacre," ginger, and cinnamon, placed in a linen bag soaked in vinegar and held in the mouth.[39] Vicary's recipe bears more than a passing resemblance to Corlyon's remedy, but we can trace this combination back further. A fourteenth-century collection of medical recipes from the British Library has one for "mygrenen" requiring "peletir of spane and stafsacre in a litil poke," which should be held for a long time between the teeth on the sore side and chewed.

If we replace the requirement for spikenard and stavesacre (in the delphinium family) with the similarly hot and dry sage and rosemary in Mrs. Corlyon's recipe, we can see that Corlyon and her contemporaries were adapting long-established and trusted remedies, substituting plants with similar qualities that could be more easily obtained or grown in a northern European garden in place of the more exotic herbs. Versions of this medicament were still being widely circulated in the mid-seventeenth century. The Townshend family's collection of medical and cookery recipes noted the mixture's suitability for toothache and headache as well as megrim, recording that they had received the recipe from a Mr. Bamfield.[40] Other common herbs in remedies for megrim include vervain, betony, chamomile, fennel, and marjoram. These, too, were all considered to be hot and dry in various degrees.

At this point, it is worth noting a somewhat surprising absence from these early modern recipe collections. Feverfew has a regular place in today's herbal remedies and is commonly understood as having been used for centuries. It was certainly known in earlier periods. In the seventeenth century, Nicholas Culpeper's *English Physitian* explained that "featherfew" was very effective against all pains in the head that had a cold cause, and John Pechey's *Compleat Herbal* instructed readers to warm a handful of feverfew in a frying pan before applying it hot. Feverfew is easy to grow—its delicate leaves and clusters of pretty, white, daisylike flowers show up yearly in my own garden—but it seems to have rarely, if ever, appeared in early modern domestic practice.[41] A likely explanation for this is that feverfew was native to the Balkan region of Europe and, although it was known, it was not commonly available in northern and western Europe until introduced more widely in later centuries.[42]

The principle of using warming, drying ingredients applied to a range of disorders. Rheums of different sorts are mentioned in several places in Mrs. Corlyon's *Booke*. A recipe to "stay rheums" in the chapter for disorders of the head also made use of sage, as well as the dry ingredients salt and bran, which would draw excess moisture outward from the brain. Her medicine to cleanse the brain used rosemary, with the explanation that chewing the leaves would allow the fragrant air to ascend into the head, and the offending humors would then be voided from the mouth. Recipes for toothache again used rosemary to draw out rheum, while Corlyon noted that if the cause of a sore throat was a cold rheum, then the reader could simply add a little sage to her gargle recipe.

She also recommended adding hot and drying herbs—including sage, rosemary, and thyme—to a bath for treating legs swollen with cold.

If a number of different disorders appeared to be manifestations of the same humoral cause, they might all be treated by a single medicine. For example, William Langham's *Garden of Health* recommended the ashes of ash bark for both megrim and toothache, while the anonymously authored *Here Begynneth a New Boke of Medecynes* contained two recipes "for the Mygrayme in the heed, for the dropsy in the heed, for yᵉ fevour in the heed & for all aches in the heed."[43] The collection of Johanna St. John (an English gentlewoman who employed a team of herb gatherers and distillers to run the productive gardens at Lydiard Park, her country house in Wiltshire), contained one recipe "for the megrim convulsions fitts or falling sickness" and another for a seasonal purging ale to be taken in April and September against "dropsys palsys megrime fowlnes of the lungs pains of the stomach."[44] Dr. Stephen's water— a staple cure-all in both printed and manuscript collections—was, Mrs. Corlyon noted, particularly useful "for all diseases that come of rheume." The recipe for Dr. Stephen's water contained rosemary, thyme, sage, "pelitory of the wall," and chamomile, as well as warming spices such as cinnamon, aniseed, nutmeg, and coriander seed. If a person with migraine in the early modern period found they were unable to make or procure a specific remedy, it is likely that they would have turned to the ubiquitous Dr. Stephen's water in the same way that we might take a general painkiller in the absence of a more targeted drug. Other recipes treated migraine together with giddiness, dizziness, or falling sickness, an important association we will return to in the following chapter.

Earthworms

"A Plaister for the same greefe to be applied after you have taken the Gargas" (see fig. 3.1) recommended:

> Take six Spoonfulles of the Gall of an Oxe or Cowe, putt thereto two Spoonfulles of the powder of the longe Wormes of the Earthe, and the powder of halfe a Nuttmeg grated: Boyle all these togeather uppon a Chafing dishe of coales untill it be so thick as you may sproade it uppon a clothe then take a doble lynnen clothe and cut it fitt for your foreheade and as it may couer the temples. Spreade this uppon it, and lay it to your foreheade luke warme, and lett it lye untill it do fall of it selfe. you shall know the Megreeme by this, it lyeth in the Browes, or in the Noddell, or in the one side of your heade.

The first part of Mrs. Corlyon's remedy, the "gargas" discussed earlier, was relatively simple to make, only required readily available ingredients, and was easy to prepare in large batches. It could have been included without difficulty into the daily morning routine of, or made for, a person with frequent attacks. It was not, however, designed to be used on its own, and the second part of her recipe required some distinctly less appealing ingredients to make a plaster that could be stuck to the head and left there until it fell off of its own accord. Corlyon undoubtedly considered the pairing of the recipes to be important, as elsewhere in the book she warned that "there is no helpe in any medicine unless it be carefully ministred, according to the trewe prescription thereof."[45]

Nutmeg was a common ingredient in migraine remedies. One of Jane Jackson's recipes from her collection simply required the sufferer to grate a nutmeg onto a cloth, wet it with wine and rosewater, and bind it to the temples and forehead overnight. Johanna St. John's remedy warmed more aggressively, calling for celandine (considered hot and dry in the third degree), and as much ginger and nutmeg "as will lye on a Groat." In Lady Ayscough's recipe, dating from 1692, nutmeg was one of several spices—including frankincense, mastic, cloves, and cinnamon—to be combined with a number of hot herbs.[46]

The two main elements in this part of Mrs. Corlyon's medicament were ox gall and earthworms. Animal parts had been a common ingredient in remedies since the ancient Egyptians, and particularly so after the first century, when Greek physician Dioscorides had singled out specific parts of animals and humans for their general medical value. We have already seen that a thirteenth-century Welsh remedy for migraine involved the skinned and boiled or roasted head of a hare.[47] In a fifteenth-century leechbook, a recipe for "mygreyne" required the gall of an ass mixed with powder from the stavesacre plant, which should be beaten, skimmed, and then applied on the head like a plaster.[48] Mrs. Corlyon made use of animal ingredients in several recipes. Those who needed to strengthen their backs or take away aches were offered an ointment of earthworms.[49] She used slugs against a "pyn or webb" in the eye and snail shells for colic, while "an especiall & good medicine" for falling sickness instructed the reader to take an ounce of "the Skull of a Man's heade."[50] This was by no means an outdated practice. The Royal College of Physicians of London's *Pharmacopeia* discussed the medical virtues of the different parts of various creatures, including vipers, swallows, and scorpions. William Salmon believed earthworms, in particular, to be beneficial for many complaints, including consumption, jaundice, hectic fevers, and diseases of the head and brain.[51] Other publications from this period mentioned using earth-worms, including Pope John XXI's *Treasury of Healthe* (1553), which told suf-ferers to take a dead earthworm and make a plaster to be laid on the back of the head for "the palsey."[52] Thomas Collins's *Choice and Rare Experiments* used a handful of earthworms in a remedy for general head pain.[53]

Why use earthworms? We can find a valuable explanation for this in Eliz-abeth Sleigh and Felicia Whitfield's collection of medical receipts from the late seventeenth century. They explained that nature's remedies had "extreme subtile parts," which were able to "undermine that which is hard, open that which is stopped & shut," and gently expel offensive matter. They singled out creatures "bred of putrefaction," such as earthworms, "timber sowes" (earwigs), snails, and the flesh of snakes—though admitting these might be "loathsome to take"—as particularly useful.[54] The rationale behind Corlyon's use of earth-worms in a plaster for "megreeme" is thus revealed as being quite straight-forward. It worked on the principle that creatures such as earthworms, which in life existed on rotting and putrefying matter, could counteract similar pro-cesses in the human body.

Another migraine medicament containing garden worms appears in at least three places in the seventeenth century, including in an anonymous pub-lication, the popular *Closet for Ladies and Gentlewomen*. The recipe is short and simple, and the ingredients easily obtainable: "Take Housleeke, and Gar-den wormes, the greater part being Housleeke, stampe them together and thereto fine flower, and make a playster in a fine cloth and lay it the forehead and temples."[55] Unlike the warming sage and rosemary used by Mrs. Corlyon, however, houseleek was known as a cold herb, as were plants such as prim-rose, red rose, yarrow, and blessed thistle. While dry and hot herbs seem to have been most often used in household manuscript collections, suggesting that, in practice, migraine was most often understood as being the result of cold and moisture, ingredients with cold properties became a commonsense approach to treat a pain with a sensation of heat or burning.

Houseleek often appears in migraine remedies. In 1642, Jane Jackson re-produced two versions of the earthworm recipe in her manuscript collection, as well as a third worm-based preparation that omitted houseleek and simply mixed worms with bread. In 1655, the original recipe of houseleek and worms was republished in a book called *Natura Exenterata*, recycling the mixture for a new generation of medical readers.[56] The persistence of the earthworm rec-ipe across several decades, in both manuscripts and print formats, reinforces a point made by Paul Slack: many of the printed medical works that proliferated in the Tudor period did not attempt to change the attitudes or practices of their readers, or introduce fashionable practices or innovations, but instead were conventional and conservative, with the aim of reinforcing other sources of medical knowledge, rather than promulgating new ideas.[57] Whether or not readers of *Natura Exenterata* were aware that this recipe had been around a long time, it remained authoritative as long as it seemed relevant.

Worms were again a key ingredient in the third of Mrs. Corlyon's migraine remedies, "A Medecine to staye the humours from fallinge to the Eyes, and goode for the meegreeme," which appeared in her chapter for diseases of the eyes:

Take one handfull of wilde Dasye rootes and washe and dry them in a cleane clothe, then shredd them and take a dozen greate earthwormes, and stampe them well together: Putt to all this as much as a pretty A[p]ple of sharpe Leaven Beate all well togeather and mingle all with the white of an egge and spredd it uppon a doble lynnen clothe so large as the foreheade is, that it may come even to the browes and cover the temples: Let the party lye uppon his backe one hower after the Medecine is laid on, after binde it with a kercher [kerchief], and so lett it lye till it be all loose of it selfe. When you use this Medecine make a bagg of dryed sage, so large as will cover from the moulde of the heade to the napp of the neck, and take a pretty quantity of Greeke Pitche and melte it alone in a litle earthenn pott, and spredd it with a flatt stick upon the flesh side of the best Glovers Leather, and cutt your plaister so large as it may lye betweene the shoulders and upp towards the napp of the neck and lett it lye so long as it cleaveth. It is very good for the patient to forbeare much butter or any thinge wherein Garlicke, Onions, or any Leekes be used.[58]

This third remedy again contains two parts: the first instructions are for a plaster to be applied to the brows and temples, with a second plaster for the neck to be made out of sage and placed in a linen cloth. Here, Corlyon combined earthworms with daisies, another herb with a well-established reputation for treating migraine. John Gerard's influential *Herball* (first published in 1597) mentioned using daisies as a cure for megrim, explaining that sniffing the juice of the leaves and roots up into the nostrils would purge the head of "foule and filthy slimie humors" and help the megrim.[59] Corlyon's final advice to the patient—to make sure that they avoided particular foods—also has a long provenance that we can trace. As Luke Demaitre has observed, medieval authors believed that leeks, onions, cabbages, and nuts were "smoky" foods and therefore could cause headaches.[60] Accordingly, Boorde's and Barrough's books both recommended that people with migraine should refrain from eating garlic, "ramsons," and onions, as well as avoiding wine, strong or new ale or beer, and new bread.[61] Barrough added mustard and radish roots to this list, explaining that such ingredients send "sharpe vapours up to the head."[62]

The Temporality of Disease

Recognizing that there is a strong rationale behind the combinations of ingredients in these remedies takes us a long way toward understanding early modern perceptions of migraine's causes and its effects on the body. Moreover, details about the preparation and administration of medicines can provide further valuable glimpses in this regard. The recipe in Corlyon's *Booke* that required both one plaster applied to the head and another, spread on the "best Glovers leather," for the shoulders and neck, called for a significant commitment from both the supplier of the medicine and the patient if it was to work. As well as necessitating a substantial collection of ingredients, processes, and materials, it required the patient to avoid certain foods, wear two different plasters, lie down for an hour, and then keep the plasters on for as long as it took for them to fall off. This was not a remedy that could be swigged down, with the rest of the day continuing normally. Then, as now, experiencing and managing migraine affected how people lived their lives.

Jane Jackson's recipe book is one of the most revealing collections for contemplating what kind of disease early modern people thought megrim to be. Jackson included no fewer than six separate entries for "Migrim in the Head." The first recipe was for the houseleek and garden worms remedy we have already considered, one that was quick, cheap, and simple. Jackson instructed her reader to pound the two elements together, mix them with fine flour, and then spread the paste onto a fine cloth, to be laid "to the forehead temples and all." Assuming that houseleek was readily available, the recipe would take a few minutes at most to prepare. The second remedy replaced the flour with vinegar, to make a plaster to be laid on the nape of the neck.[63] The simplicity of these medicaments, as well as the speed and ease with which they could be prepared from readily available ingredients, suggests that they were designed to be made up quickly and used as and when they were needed, perhaps frequently. The later recipes in Jackson's book became more complex. One required using "knoted wormes," but this time the instructions for their collection were quite specific: the worms must be gathered in the morning and left to stand until four or five o'clock in the afternoon. Then they had to be taken out of their pot one by one, cast into a second vessel with a good piece of rye bread, and finely pounded together. Before going to bed, the paste should be wrapped in a linen cloth and bound to the temples all night. Moreover, the remedy was not expected to cure straight away; it would perhaps need to be applied four or five times before the head would "be whole." This was a time-consuming remedy to produce, suitable for an illness expected to last for several days.[64]

The fifth recipe required equal portions of frankincense resin, mastic, turpentine, galbanum, olive oil, linseed powder, laurel, anise powder, and cumin, all mixed together and laid into a cap of leather, bound tightly round with a linen cloth.[65] It took planning and financial outlay to source so many unusual ingredients. We might understand the making or purchase of such a medicine as an investment. Moreover, while linen was commonly specified as the fabric for a plaster, this recipe required a leather cap. Such a commitment, however, would pay off, as Jackson promised the reader that once made, the medicine would last for twenty years. Jackson's recipe book illustrates a progression from everyday remedies that could be easily memorized and made up in minutes to a more sophisticated medicine that would give service for decades. It suggests that seventeenth-century notions of migraine, just as in our own time, appreciated that it could occur as an occasional acute attack, or as a chronic disease that could last for several days at a time, requiring vigilance and management over a significant part of a life cycle. Another interpretation is that the simplest, quickest recipes would also have been the ones a person without the means to buy medicine could either make at home or have someone, such as Jackson, provide the mixture as a philanthropic gesture, perhaps to a neighbor or a servant.

Conclusion

Tracing the provenance of recipes and their ingredients reveals a great deal about everyday knowledge of migraine—its causes, character, and treatments—in the early modern period. Most remedies followed a humoral framework that emphasized the virtues of hot, dry, aromatic ingredients in treating a disorder most often understood as caused by trapped cold and moisture. Understanding the degrees to which herbs such as sage and rosemary were hot and dry meant that older recipes, derived from a Mediterranean classical tradition, could be adapted and updated to better reflect the local availability of ingredients. While some mixtures were quick, simple, and cheap to make, others involved many ingredients, including imported spices and substances that would have to be purchased from an apothecary. Comparing printed remedy collections with those in manuscripts also reveals that just because a recipe appeared again and again in print, it did not mean it necessarily translated into everyday practice, while others remained in current knowledge over centuries. Perhaps most important, these recipes suggest people understood that there were different types of migraine. The available treatments providing a flexible, varied—and, especially, practical—treasure trove of knowledge, allowing practitioners of domestic medicine to provide individual therapies that corresponded both to the quality and the temporality of a common, well-recognized illness.

CHAPTER FOUR

A "Deadly Tormenting Megrym"

Expanding Markets and Changing Meanings

Francis Thomson's Letter, c. 1590

It is difficult to say for certain exactly when, and in what town, Francis Thomson, hiding in his pigeon house, was composing a letter, but it was certainly a Monday morning, in England, around the last decade of the sixteenth century. It was an urgent request for help from Sir Michael Hickes, the secretary to Lord Burghley, Queen Elizabeth I's lord treasurer. Hickes was certainly a powerful man. As a central figure in the practical administration of the queen's business, Hickes greatly influenced the distribution of royal favors, and in the 1590s he was at the height of his powers. Thomson's letter might have found its way to Hickes's desk among requests from mayors needing assistance against their enemies, petitioners requesting grants and sales of land, and churchmen asking for ecclesiastical appointments.[1]

Written on a single page, in the formal secretary hand common to the Tudor period, Thomson's letter is an unusual one among the petitions and obsequious pleadings now bound in a thick, leather-cased volume in the British Library. After several lines of the usual flattering formalities in which he begged the secretary's "diligence & assistance of frendshipe," Thomson got to the point: a Mr. Toplyff "intendeth shortly to bringe me in truble." Thomson pleaded with Hickes and Lord Burghley to take pity on a man in his "old dayes," so he might live without Mr. Toplyff troubling him. In return for protection, Thomson promised Hickes a gelding, purchased from his brother at considerable cost. He signed his letter, but then added a further note at the bottom, emphasizing his difficult situation: "I am much troubled so by the mygrame & sciatica in my hypp." Thomson had planned to go to Buxton for his ailments, "but now I know not what to doe for feare of Mr. Toplyff."[2] Although it contains only the briefest of references, Thomson's letter gives us a sudden insight to his world. He suffered from two long-term, perhaps chronic conditions, and his belief that his infirmities would continue had shaped his travel plans for the summer ahead, but the religious and political atmosphere of post-Reformation England made a rude intrusion into his chances of getting treatment. In writing to the representatives of the very highest authority in the land, Thomson hoped his plight would be taken seriously. Unfortunately, we have no further information about Thomson, whether he received a response from Hickes, or whether he did, in the end, make it to Buxton.

Thomson's letter takes us out of the domestic setting and into the public sphere. While the continued availability of herbal remedies and phlebotomy attest to continuities and adaptations from earlier eras, there were always new things to try in an increasingly commercialized medical marketplace. From the hills of Derbyshire to the chaotic streets of central London and the drawing rooms of fashionable Bath, from the most reputable of society physicians to astrologers and itinerant, gone-tomorrow street corner salesmen and -women, we have a great deal of evidence about the variety of treatments available to the pained—and paying—early modern customer. Thomson's letter is just one of many sources from the early modern period that give a real sense of migraine as a chronic debilitating disorder affecting people from across the social spectrum, disrupting their ability to work, earn, and contribute. As well as providing rich evidence of the treatment options, including bathing and astrological medicine, available to those seeking a cure for migraine, this chapter examines sources from the early modern period that reveal significant shifts in the understanding of what migraine was. In 1661, we get the first sense that a person's identity might be defined by the chronic condition of having migraine. Thomas Blount's *Glossographia* introduced the term "hemicranick" to describe a person "subject to the sickness called Megrim or Hemicrania."[3]

While humoral theories certainly remained relevant, by the seventeenth century, migraine was increasingly being allied to various disorders, including the vapors, apoplexy, vertigo, epilepsy, and hysteria. It is not until the eighteenth century, however, that we begin to see migraine being discussed in the context of wider concerns about nervous diseases as the product of luxurious urban living, rich diets, and sedentary lifestyles. At that point, migraine had begun to be perceived as the disorder of a particular kind of person, someone who was sensitive, effeminate, and nervous.

Taking the Waters

Francis Thomson's wish to go to the isolated town of Buxton, nestled among the hills of Derbyshire, is explained by the presence of St. Anne's Well, which had long been held to have holy and medicinal properties. Many wells and springs had gained a reputation for miraculous healing during the Middle Ages, reflecting what Alexandra Walsham has called a "sacralised landscape" of traditional piety. Wells offered a resource for people who could not afford to pay for medical care, or whose ailments seemed otherwise incurable.[4] Archaeological evidence suggests that there had been a bath at Buxton ever since the Romans had called the place Aquae Arnematiae. By the twelfth century, there was a chapel dedicated to St. Anne.[5] In 1460, William Worcester wrote of a well and "many miracles making the infirm healthy," noting that even in winter, the water was warm.[6] During the Reformation, Buxton was one of multiple sites associated with miraculous healing and Catholic worship coming under attack from religious reformers. In 1538, Sir William Bassett, working for Thomas Cromwell, removed the images of St. Anne at Buxton, defaced the tabernacles, and took away the crutches, shirts, and sheets that "yngnorantt pepull" had left as offerings. Although Bassett locked up the baths and wells, within decades the visitors had returned.[7]

In 1569, the Earl of Shrewsbury's physician recommended that his wealthy patient visit Buxton to relieve an attack of gout. The earl was so impressed he bought the well, chapel, and surrounding grounds.[8] Next to where the Buxton springs flowed into a brook, the earl built "a very goodly house," square, solid, and four stories high, capable of lodging thirty visitors to the spring at one time. Seats, protected from the cold air, surrounded the baths, and fires aired clothing.[9] The significance of Buxton as a place of medical pilgrimage is shown in John Speed's famous *Theatre of the Empire of Great Britaine*, the first printed volume to comprehensively map all the English and Welsh counties. In the bottom right-hand corner of his early seventeenth-century map of Derbyshire, Speed depicted the Earl of Shrewsbury's lodgings at St. Anne's Well (fig. 4.1), one of two only bathing places portrayed among the university colleges, ancient monuments, great castles, historic battles, and sea monsters. The other was St. Winifred's Well in Flintshire, which, like Buxton, had received royal patronage. In 1416, Henry V visited St. Winifred's Well after his victory at Agincourt. Though Speed mocked the "zealous, but blind devotion" of the pilgrims who traveled to the Welsh holy well, his prominent inclusion of these

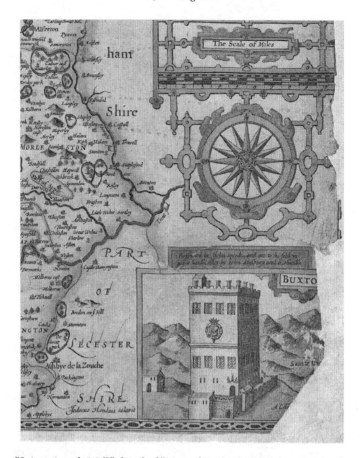

Fig. 4.1. "Sainte Anne's Well," detail of "Map of Derbyshire," Atlas 2.61.1/21, from John Speed, *Theatre of the Empire of Great Britaine*, 1611/12. Reproduced by kind permission of the Syndics of Cambridge University Library

two bathing places, and his mention of reports that the waters of St. Anne's Well had effected "great cures," nevertheless witness their importance as sites of healing. Speed acknowledged that "daily experience sheweth that they are good for the stomacke, and sinewes, and very pleasant to bathe the body in."[10]

Visitors to the Buxton baths paid a local poll tax for their use: a registration fee of 4d (around half a day's pay for a laborer), with an additional levy, dependent on a person's rank, increasing from 1s for a yeoman, to £3 10s for a duke. The influx of wealthy visitors attracted beggars, and the Poor Law of 1572 contained a clause forbidding any "dyseased or ympotent poore person living on Almes" to come to Buxton unless they had received permission from two justices of the peace and an understanding that their own parish would provide the necessary funds.[11] By the end of the 1570s, Buxton boasted two inns and eight alehouses to cater to visitors.[12] Although its water was cooler than at Bath, physician John Jones—author of the first popular guide to the baths, published in 1572—stated travelers to Buxton did not have "halfe so many greevouse accidentes" as at the more well-known destination.[13]

Buxton's most famous visitor was Mary Queen of Scots, seeking relief from her ailments. She first came there in 1573, staying for five weeks, and returned a further eight times, until 1584. These trips caused great consternation for Queen Elizabeth I, who constantly feared Mary's involvement in plots. Lord Burghley, the recipient of Thomson's letter, was the man charged with Mary's strict surveillance. In 1587, Mary Queen of Scots was executed after being found guilty of involvement in the Babington Plot, the seeds of which, some historians have speculated, may have been sown during meetings in Buxton.[14] The town's popularity with Catholics attracted considerable attention and suspicion, for "much intrigue went on under the cover of taking the waters."[15] It is clear that Francis Thomson's fears for his safety were he to undertake a journey to Buxton were well founded. In 1578, Richard Topcliffe had warned the Earl of Shrewsbury of the "sundry lewde Popish beasts" who congregated at his well.[16] During the 1580s and 1590s, Topcliffe was notorious as a hunter of recusants, like Thomson, who refused to attend Protestant church services. Describing himself as a "Discoverer and Taker Up of Papists," Topcliffe interrogated and tortured Catholics imprisoned by the government.[17] Thomson's letter, his experience of migraine and sciatica, and his desire to go to Buxton for treatment can only be fully understood within the religious and political contexts of the time. Going to Buxton was more than a journey of healing, it was also an act of political resistance.

John Jones's promotion of the Buxton baths sheds further light on its attraction for someone like Thomson. Downplaying the potential for miracles, Jones instead explained the medicinal effects of the "Buckstones Bathes" through its chemical properties. They strengthened weak members, promoted respiration, and "wypeth awaye fylth." Because the water was temperate, rather than hot (as at Bath), it moderated "overheated members" and dried those that were too moist. Thus the Buxton baths helped alleviate diseases caused by too much heat, as well as those resulting from too much cold and moisture. Jones's list of disorders that could be cured by the waters was long, including rheums, fevers, headaches, "weak sinews," ulcers, cramps, itching, vomiting, ringworm, consumption, inflammation, obstructions of the liver, and burning urine. The baths benefited those who were "short of wind," as well as re-lieved green sickness and "stone." He recommended the waters for various sexual difficulties, such as for women who had trouble conceiving or "weake men that be unfrutefull." A visitor should bathe for up to two or three hours, both morning and evening, after exercise and purging, but before eating meat. The best time of year was when the sun was high (between early May and late September), but pestilential seasons should be avoided. Jones had reinterpreted the source of Buxton's curative powers for a post-Reformation audience, but he did not entirely dispense with religion. He beseeched those persons who came away uncured "not to exclaim upon God and good men," for some in-firmities became deeply rooted over time, so no remedy would be effective. He included a prayer, to be recited before bathing, that called on God to provide relief, comfort, and ease, as well as to "strengthen these baths."[18]

If Jones presented Buxton as some kind of balneological cure-all, other healing wells and springs were known to cure specific ailments. Robert Storye of Leicester traveled twenty miles to the new King's Newnham bath in War-wickshire for his migraine.[19] Pilgrims traveled to Loch Siant in Skye, an island off the northwestern coast of Scotland, to cure headaches, kidney and bladder stones, and consumption.[20] Had Francis Thomson been looking for a cure for migraine and sciatica in the 1720s, he might well have been tempted to visit the "English Spaw" in the forest outside Knaresborough, which physician and alchemist Edmund Deane recommended for inveterate headaches, "migrims," "turnings and swimmings of the head and braine," dizziness, epilepsy (or fall-ing sickness), and the like, such as "cold and moist diseases of the head."[21] Deane explained that the chemical virtues of the spring came from its quali-ties of "vitrioll," a classical term denoting the ability "to heate and dry, to bind, to resist putrefaction, to give strength and vigour to the interiour parts," as well as to cleanse and purify the blood. Thus "vitrioline waters," as at Knares-borough, could heal diseases that seemed without hope of recovery by drying the "over moist braine"; cutting, loosening, and purging the body of "vicious and clammy humours"; and comforting the stomach.[22]

Consulting the Cosmos

If Thomson did decide that the trip to Buxton was dangerous, he might well have been tempted to try another contemporary treatment option: a consulta-tion with an astrologer, such as Richard Napier or Simon Forman. Napier, an alchemist, physician, and Anglican minister, had been tutored by astrologer-physician Forman, whom he first consulted in 1597. Forman had established his reputation during the plague of 1592, but, without formal education, he made a lifelong enemy of the College of Physicians, who believed him (ironically) to be ignorant of astrology.[23] Napier and Forman met in London and Buckinghamshire, and they would become the most famous astrologer-physicians of the time. Most remarkably, between them, the two men left a staggering 80,000 case records.[24] Between 1597 and 1634, thousands of patients, from all social backgrounds, consulted Napier, who has been described by historian Michael MacDonald as "the last Renaissance magi," at his home in Great Linford, Buckinghamshire. Napier saw up to fifteen patients a day, a number in line with other astrologers, who recorded seeing between one and two thousand patients a year.[25] As MacDonald notes, Napier was no quack, but rather a physician who "presumed that the maladies of mind and body could be studied as systematically as the movements of the planets."[26] Napier's casenotes follow a standard format, recording the patient's name, whether he saw them in person, their age, their occupation, where they lived, and the exact time and date of the consultation. On a "horary chart"—a grid drawn on the page—Napier could then map the heavens at a specific point in time. By locating the patient (and the problem) relative to the cosmos at the precise moment they asked their question, the astrologer placed them "at the vortex of the natural forces that impelled the universe."[27] Below this grid, Napier could record details of the patient's description of their ailment, his observations of their symptoms, information from the stars (and whether this tallied with the account he had been given), and his prescription for any treatment.

Napier's casebooks contain at least eighteen instances in which megrim was the topic of the question asked of the astrologer. These cases included slightly more men than women, the patients ranging in age from their early twenties to an anonymous "old woman," aged sixty-five. Although it is perhaps surprising that there are not more examples of megrim in the casebooks, the records nevertheless provide important first-hand evidence—rare from this period—of how the experience of megrim was understood at the turn of the seventeenth century. For instance, Thomas Norman described a pain that was "hot."[28] Other cases suggest a chronic illness, which perhaps explains the decision to consult the astrologer. Goody (a title denoting a married woman of lowly station) Joan Markham came to Forman with a "continuall megrim" in May 1598. Although not recording if he offered her a prescription, Napier judged that the woman's illness had been the result of her taking "a great grief" after the death of her son.[29] In 1603, when Francis Dale consulted Napier's assistant, Gerence James, he described a megrim and pain in his head of "long continuance."[30] Jonas Tanner had suffered a megrim in his head and eyes for twelve years, but he consulted Napier when the megrim gave him more trouble than before.[31]

Goodman John Roughead was a frequent visitor to the astrologers, appearing around twenty times in Napier's casebooks, and once each in Forman's and James's. Napier described Roughead several times as a neighbor, or "of our towne." Proximity partly explains why he consulted Napier so often, but it is also clear that Roughead had a longstanding problem with megrim. He first appears to have consulted Napier in May 1601 for a "hot megrim" that a blow with a "flale" had helped. In 1602, Roughead visited three times: in March, "payned in his head"; in May, for hemicrania; and in June, for megrym. In January 1607, he would return for his "deadly tormenting megrym in his head," and again in 1609, for his "great extreeme payne" in his head.[32] On several of these occasions, Napier prescribed "jeralog," which seems to have been his favored remedy for megrim, a shortened term for *hiera logadii*, a purgative treatment for melancholy and vertigo. He also prescribed bloodletting.[33] For Randall Young, Napier prescribed a mixture containing various ingredients, including cumin and fenugreek, to be boiled with milk. This seems to have been a variation on a much older recipe—for which there is fifteenth-century evidence—that called for cumin powder boiled in cow's milk until thick, and then laid hot on the head in a plaster.[34]

For others who consulted Napier, a megrim was one of a cluster of symptoms. In November 1598, Thomas Houghton described the extreme pain in his head and eyes as being "like a megrim." Houghton was obviously very uncomfortable: besides his head pain, he had "a great swelling" and no feeling in his right hand, arms, and side. Napier noted with interest that the man's foot was "most wonderfully swollen," along with "a great heat in his stomack & a hot water [tha]t commeth out of his mouthe." Though Napier wrote "megrim" in the center of the horary chart, the man's comment about the pain being like a megrim suggests that he used the term descriptively, assuming general knowledge of what it meant. Megrim itself would not normally have been associated with such extreme swelling, the brown color of which Napier blamed on choler and melancholy "broken out."[35] But Napier's identification of choler reflected the long held belief, discussed in chapter 2, that choleric fumes could cause megrim, and this was likely to produce pain on the right side. Having said that, on 31 May 1600, Forman saw Agnes Vale, a thirty-nine-year-old woman who also had megrim combined with a swollen arm, but this time on her left side.[36] In August 1598, Robert Vilveyne came to ask the astrologer what his disease was. Noting that the young man was "much payned w[it]h a megrim," Napier concluded that his problem was caused by "fleme and melancholy, mingled with red choler," a result of Venus being in Cancer.[37]

An anonymously authored booklet from the late seventeenth century, *The Great and Wonderful Prophecies of Mr. Patridge, Mr. Coly, Mr. Tanner, and Mr. Andrews*, gives us a taste of the kinds of highly specific—not to mention alarming—predictions that later pamphleteers produced in the name of astrology. It warned that in September, a "most hateful" opposition of Saturn and Mars would occur. This would provoke many "robberies, inhumane actions, and treacherous enterprises." Mankind would also be threatened "with strange *Distempers* of Body, as *Fevours*, occasioning *Megrim, Madness, Phranzies, Appoplexies, Lethargies*; with many other *Anonimous Diseases* and *Unnatural*, hard to be cured, and often terminate in *sudden Death*."[38] It would be easy to dismiss astrology, as manifested in sources such as this, but it was rarely so extreme an approach and sat well within the bounds of early modern medical culture. We have already seen how important astrological factors were in guiding the common practice of phlebotomy. Napier's ideas at the turn of the seventeenth century may have been astrological, but his framework for explaining megrim was largely a conventionally humoral one, and his treatments drew on a long tradition of herbal remedies. Apart from providing important evidence of migraine as a chronic disorder that waxed and waned, cases such as John Roughead's reaffirm the ongoing historical reality of this pain. It was extreme, it seemed deadly, it continued tormenting the person, and it came back, time and time again. We can also see how the onset of megrim, or a change in its character, could be interpreted within the context of significant events in the patients' lives, whether physical or emotional, a theme to which we will return in the nineteenth century.

Print, Pills, and Powders

Through print formats, medical knowledge became more widely accessible in the early modern period. In England alone, 2,700 editions of medical works intended for nonpractitioners were published between 1641 and 1790.[39] As we saw in the previous chapter, printed books blurred the boundaries between domestic and learned medicine and often included versions of recipes that appeared in household collections. These books were also used by professional practitioners, and they may have been particularly useful as stores of knowledge in rural areas. In 1690, Henry Williams, an apothecary in the remote village of Clynnog in northwestern Wales, owned both Philip Barrough's

Methode of Phisicke and Rembert Dodoens's *New Herball* on the shelves of his shop.[40] We might imagine Williams referring to these volumes when asked for a treatment for migraine. The customer might have left with Barrough's ointment made of oil of dill, ireos, white pepper, serpillum (thyme), castoreum (the secretion from a beaver's castor sac, used to mark its territory, and a common ingredient in early modern medicines), euphorbium, and wax, with instructions to apply it to the forehead and the muscles of the temples. More likely, perhaps, Williams simply might have supplied the raw ingredient euphorbium (a resin made from the euphorbia plant, commonly known as spurge), instructing the customer to mix it with vinegar and apply it to the opposite side of the head from their pain. If the patient complained of sudden pain, the apothecary could have dispensed myrrh and frankincense, again using Barrough as his authority.[41]

An apothecary's cashbook from the West Riding of Yorkshire in the first decade of the eighteenth century gives a sense of how much a migraine sufferer might have expected to pay for a simple treatment during this period. The cashbook details every patient the apothecary saw, visited, or provided a urine analysis for over an eight-year period. Though he didn't mention migraine by name, he often treated head disorders, using familiar descriptions for pain, such as "windy" or "beating" (recall Bartholomaeus's thirteenth-century description), and recorded a number of cases of headache accompanied by "rheumy eyes." Charging his patients either six- or ninepence, the apothecary offered two treatments. When John Lang's daughter came to him with a "pain in head," he took blood from the right foot, while for Christopher Lang's wife, who suffered "a windy pain in side & head," he bled from the left foot. In both instances, the patients paid sixpence. In April 1705, the apothecary saw another man with "sore rheumy eyes, pain in head" and prescribed a blistering plaster, again at a cost of sixpence. Yet he charged ninepence for the same treatment for Joshua Wright's girl, aged fifteen, who had a "violent pain in head with beating."[42]

Advertisements for preparatory medicines provide some of the clearest evidence of how the demand for migraine relief spilled out of homes and into the streets by the late seventeenth century. In 1695, the Licensing of the Press Act lapsed. First passed by the English Parliament in 1662 to reassert control over the press following the restoration of Charles II, this legislation aimed to prevent sedition and treason by requiring all books be licensed before their printing and distribution. The act had been difficult to enforce from the beginning, and it first lapsed between 1679 and 1685, but, after 1695, new period-

ical titles began to appear in greater numbers. The makers and sellers of medicines took full advantage of this new freedom to widely advertise their wares
in cheap newspapers. Two of the earliest and best known ones were the *Post
Boy* and the *Post Man*, established in 1695. These may have had a circulation
of three or four thousand each week, and both regularly carried an advertisement for Capital Salts.[43] Billed as "an admirable Remedy for the Diseases of
the Head, as Vertigo or Giddiness, Megrim, Head-ach, Lethargy, Apoplexy,
Epilepsy, Hysterick, Fits, Hypochondriack passions, all Vapours," potential customers were promised this "exquisite remedy" would prevent as well as cure
disease, help digestion, purify the blood, strengthen the heart and vitals, and
generally keep the body in good health.

One of the best-known medical empirics of the time was William Salmon:
astrologer; author of almanacs, domestic manuals, medical compendiums
and herbals; writer on anatomy, alchemy, religion, and surgery; and purveyor
of pills from various London premises. Salmon's *London Almanack* for 1701
carried advertisements for his Family Pills and Panchymagogue Pills, both of
which listed megrim as one of the diseases they could cure. "Panchymagogue"
meant a medicine that would purge all humors from the body, and Salmon
promised a "singular" cure against "Headach, Vertigo, Megrim, Lethargy,
Frenzy, [and] madness" (not to mention French pox, gonorrhea, sciatica, gout,
obstructions of the womb, alienation of the mind, dropsy, jaundice, leprosy,
and stubborn ulcers). Salmon's Family Pills offered relief for megrim "beyond
any Medicine ever yet known." He boasted:

> these *Family Pills* are the chief medicine now used, in the cure of all the afore-
> said diseases, not only in *England*, but in many foreign Countries and King-
> doms, being cried up and prized above all other Medicines whatsoever; in so
> much that in some thousands of Families, on most occasions they are the only
> Physick (and from thence they came to be called family pills) being known to
> be safe in operation, and certain in the end proposed; for no person curable,
> troubled with any of the aforesaid diseases, has failed of cure . . . and several
> hundreds, yea, thousands of People who have taken them, have given them this
> commendation.

Salmon seems to be playing directly to an audience tired of the constant
hunt for relief. He sent his pills by mail and promised that the person who
took them would no longer need to undergo "long, dangerous, and chargable
courses of Physick, suffer by bad medicines, and be driven time after time,
from one Physician to another." These Family Pills were gentle, friendly, and

operated according to the laws of nature. Moreover, they could be administered to children as young as age two, in which case he recommended disguising the medicine in an apple, honey, or a stewed prune. Adults could take the pills with a little beer, ale, wine, or broth, according to taste. While Salmon's Panchymagogue Pills cost eight shillings an ounce, the Family Pills could be purchased more cheaply: twelvepence a box, or five shillings an ounce.[44]

If Salmon failed to convince—or if his pills should, by some extremely unlikely circumstance, not live up to their billing—there were a number of other pharmaceutical choices for migraine that vied for attention in the explosion of cheap print. The *Post Boy* and the *English Post* regularly advertised "Medicinal Snuff or Cephalick Powder," which "seldom fails to cure the most inveterate and violent Aches or Pains in the Head, Vertigo or Dizziness, Megrim, lethargy, Sleepiness, Dullness, or Drowsiness." Not only this, but the miraculous powder could cure deafness, prevent apoplexy, or even remove mercury "lodged in the head by an ill course of Physick used for the Venereal Disease."[45] In 1704, a number of newspapers, including London's *Daily Courant*, the first daily in Britain, advertised a "True Head Snuff." This was "different from all other Snuffs" and warned potential purchasers of the dire consequences of taking other powders, which would only be "the Introducers of Ruin and Death." By 1705, this medicine had been renamed "the Grand Cephalick or Head Snuff."[46] Other options included head pills and tincture, Capital Liquid Snuff, Cephalick Errhine, Dr. Tyson's Snuff, Lower's Restorative Powder, and "the most Noble Volatile Smelling [Salts] Bottle in the World."[47]

Remedies could be purchased from a wide variety of tradespeople. In 1718, a customer could get Dr. Lower's purging Cordial Tincture, along with their cabbage, from Mr. Leening, the grocer, next to Little St. Helens Gate; from Mr. Hobson, the distiller; with their coffee from John, in Swithins Lane; or from Mr. Ford, the bookseller, in the short, but well-known, street called Poultry. In 1718, "the most famous Chymical Preparation in the World" could be bought at the Cocoa Tree Chocolate House in Pall Mall or the British Coffee House near Charing Cross, reflecting the well-known association of coffee culture with medical culture. Virtually all of the remedies advertised in pamphlets printed in London could be purchased along the central thoroughfares of the Strand and Fleet Street, with clusters of sellers around landmarks such as Charing Cross, St. Dunstan's Church on the Strand, and the Royal Exchange on Poultry and Cornhill. The area of central London directly east of St. Paul's Cathedral, in which many remedy sellers congregated, had been the traditional center for apothecaries since the medieval period. The streets around

St. Paul's Cathedral—Holborn, Fleet Street, and the Strand—were some of the capital's wealthiest, but this was also a hectic part of town, where marvelous animals, contortionists, giantesses, street vendors, and fire-eaters vied for the attention of passersby.[48]

The most famous, expensive, and long-established London apothecary shops were in the Royal Exchange, with many more around Cheapside and Poultry. The Royal Exchange itself was the capital's center of commerce and business, a "great place of noise and tumult." In 1711, Joseph Addison described "so rich an assembly of countrymen and foreigners consulting together upon the private business of mankind, and making this metropolis a kind of emporium for the whole earth."[49] The Exchange housed 160 shops, while, in the evening, a gaggle of "mumpers, the halt, the blind, and the lame; your vendors of trash, apples, plums; your ragamuffins, rake-shames, and wenches" replaced the crowds of merchants. Watchmakers, stockbrokers, newspaper vendors, and the sellers of patent medicines congregated outside the Exchange. In 1717, Mrs. Garway, with her supply of Lower's Restorative Powder, could be found there, dwarfed by the vast columns at the entrance of the Royal Exchange Gate. Printed advertisements always gave customers precise instructions about where their "exquisite" remedies could be found, using easily identifiable landmarks: "at the Golden Ball, next door but one to Tom's Coffee House, adjoining Ludgate"; "Adam's Toy shop in Spring-garden passage, going into St. James' Park"; "Mr. Ascough's toy shop at the sign of the Queen Arms, adjoining the Thatch'd House tavern in St. James's Street."

Navigating this area on a quest to purchase some medicinal snuff while in the throes of a throbbing, tormenting migraine would have been a nauseating prospect indeed. If we imagine the disorientation of such sufferers trying to get through these streets, the precise directions to particular locations take on a new significance. One of the advantages for customers in having these businesses clustered together, within a few streets, was that even if the particular remedy they wanted could not be found, or the details of an advertisement got lost, something else might be found nearby. St. Dunstan's Church on Fleet Street appears to have been a hotspot for medical salesmen and -women. Medicinal snuff, or cephalick powder, could be purchased "at Mr. Roper's bookseller, at the Black Boy over against St. Dunstan's Church" between 1700 and 1703. Some years later, Mr. Osborne sold "True Royal Snuff" from his toyshop at the Rose and Crown, by the same church. Between 1720 and 1724, customers were also directed here for "the Most Noble Volatile Smelling [Salts] Bottle in the World."

Some advertisements gave testimonials, along with addresses, implying that these users could be found and their endorsement checked. Potential customers for "True Royal Snuff for Purging the Head" were promised that directions on how to take the snuff, as well as "the dwelling places of several that have received benefit by it," would be inserted in the paper given out with the snuff.[50] Crucially, of course, this information would only be revealed after the vendor had pocketed the money. Sometimes the advertisement was for a service, rather than a pill or potion. One such puff piece (published a number of times between 1695 and 1713) contained the testimony of one William Fletcher, who had been cured of his "megrim, Giddiness or Swimming Pains in the Head" by Mr. John Moore at the Pestle and Mortar, Abchurch Lane, who had let his blood and given him a medicine. Fletcher's testimony described how he had been afflicted "so that oftentimes I was in danger of falling down as I Work'd or Walk'd which continued upon me for the space of 6 Years, and using divers medicines for my Cure without success." Fletcher had traveled from Enfield, twelve miles north of central London, to be bled in the nostril on one side of his head. A year later, he returned to be bled in the other side, leaving him "perfectly cured of that Vexatious and Troublesome Disease."[51] Whether or not William Fletcher was a real patient, the personal touch, and the detail of distance, promised that this was a treatment worth traveling for.

These purveyors of pills, powders, and phlebotomy were not marginal to a more orthodox and effective version of medicine happening elsewhere. For many people, this *was* medicine, particularly for urban residents, where the idea of a well-stocked herb garden, from which the ingredients for a recipe could be sourced, or for whom taking a journey to the warm, healing waters of somewhere like Buxton was an expensive and impossible fantasy. Pills and potions cost a few pence and were worth a try, because a consultation with a physician would set you back a guinea or two. Even those who could afford the advice of the best physicians regularly self-medicated. Yet the pufferies and the testimonies often proved to be empty promises. As Jane Cave's poem, "The Headache, Or Ode to Health," attested:

> In vain, the British and Cephalic Snuff,
> All patent medicines are empty stuff;
> The lancet, leech, and cupping swell the train
> Of useless efforts, which but give me pain;
> Each art and application vain has proved
> For ah! my sad complaint is not removed.[52]

It is easy to dismiss proprietary medicines as useless concoctions, shamelessly and cynically flaunted by quacks and charlatans, which were, at best, overpriced and ineffectual, and, at worst, downright dangerous. As Lisa Forman Cody has commented, the stereotype is that "eighteenth-century medical concoctions were made of nothing and good for nothing."[53] But, as Roy Porter has argued, the power of suggestion offered hope when other practitioners failed. Rather than dismissing those who purchased these treatments as gullible fools, we should acknowledge the worth of such sentiments. "So long as disease remained powerful," Porter explains, "so did all forms of healing."[54] Appreciating that there is a long history for migraine pills and potions is important, because it remains the case that many patients who are unable to access effective, regular medicines continue to turn to a range of self-help books, diets, homeopathy, natural remedies, and medical aids. In her recent memoir about migraine, Paula Kamen talks of the long and circuitous journey she took to find effective medication, and of the range of treatments outside the mainstream that followed constant failure. Alternative medicine, she writes, "appealed precisely because it was *not* Western medicine, which I had grown to revile and fear." Historians of medicine are used to talking about the medical marketplace, but Kamen uses a different, and revealing, phrase to describe this kind of world: the "marketplace of ideas."[55]As she states: "The absurdity wasn't that the 'cures' were alternative and increasingly offbeat. It was that, in my desperation and hope for a magic bullet, I would almost always try them."[56]

Tar-Water

Tar-water was one of the medical phenomena of the mid-eighteenth century. George Berkeley, a philosopher, Irish patriot, and bishop of Cloyne, revealed the secrets of his fashionable panacea in *Siris*. Tar-water could be made by pouring a gallon of cold water on a quart of tar (the kind that could be extracted from cedar and pine trees). This should be stirred thoroughly and left to stand for forty-eight hours to allow the salts and "active spirits" of the tar to infuse, before pouring off the clear water. Having initially heard of the drink being used against smallpox in the American colonies, Berkeley had tried it in his own neighborhood, first for smallpox, and then to counteract an increasing range of disorders as his confidence in it grew. Apart from being safe and cheap, Berkeley believed tar-water had multiple virtues. In comparison with many acids, it was "gentle, bland and temperate"; it quickened the circulation of the body's fluids without wounding the solids; its fine particles softened and enriched the sharp, vapid blood; it was not dangerous, like opium; it could warm and cool; and it "contains the virtues of the best chalybeat and sulphureous waters," without the need to observe a dietary regimen. Tar-water should be drunk daily: half a pint in the morning and at night, preferably warm. Berkeley saw tar-water as a panacea for the distress of the Irish nation—the answer to overcoming the poor health of his people.[57]

While the medical profession engaged in a pamphlet war against Berkeley, Thomas Prior's *Authentic Narrative of the Success of Tar-Water* collated over three hundred letters and testimonials regarding its ability to cure everything from ague and asthma to vapors and vomiting. Three of these narratives came from individuals who attested to tar-water's efficacy in treating megrim: Cornelius Townsend of Betsborough, County Cork; the Reverend Mr. Thomas Goodwin of Dublin; and an anonymous woman "cured of a megrim and inveterate headache."[58] Townsend's story described the state he had been in before discovering tar-water: "Such a costive constitution . . . my fundament was so inflamed with piles, that I was very apprehensive of a fistula, my flesh was bloated and very tender everywhere; I was subject to a palpitation of the heart, cramps, meagrims, &c. from all which (I thank God) I am quite free by the constant use of Tar-Water only." Commenting on the case of an anonymous lady, Prior added that several other persons had informed him that until they took tar-water, "they used to be seized with a dizziness in their heads on walking in the streets, so that they were obliged to catch hold of the rails as they went along to prevent falling."[59]

Some three decades later, another pamphlet of testimonials appeared. In 1771, an eccentric and imposing, but nevertheless cordial and cheerful figure had arrived in Dublin. Handsomely dressed in Turkish clothes, with a "pompous" gait and a huge black beard covering his chin and upper lip, Dr. Achmet Borumborad claimed to have fled to Ireland from Constantinople. Dr. Achmet, as he became known, gained the favor of prominent Irish physicians and members of Parliament, and he received a grant to establish hot and cold seawater baths for the use of Dublin's poor.[60] By the 1776 season, he boasted of admitting more than 1,900 people into his baths. Unfortunately for Borumborad, his career as a society favorite ended spectacularly: at a grand dinner for his patrons, after drinking copious amounts of wine, nineteen parliamentary men fell into his cold saltwater bath. After falling in love with an Irishwoman, Dr. Achmet revealed himself as Mr. Patrick Joyce from Kilkenny.[61] In 1777, before his undoing, Borumborad had published the details of 138 named cases from the Poor Baths Register. He insisted that he had been reluctant to publish the "many extraordinary cases" of those who had been relieved and cured at the Poor Baths, as such publications were justly considered "empirical gasconade, solely calculated to ensnare the ignorant and unwary." He felt accountable, however, for the expenditure of public money to provide free treatments for the poor in his baths.

As the testimonies to Berkeley's tar-water had done, Borumborad's anonymous *Report of the Cases Relieved and Cured in the Baths* gives a valuable insight into the health of Dublin's poor in the eighteenth century. In both his and Prior's pamphlets, a litany of chronic, debilitating pain emerges from the pages. In many cases, megrim was one of a number of diseases preventing patients from working. We find Charles McManus, of Mabbor Street, North Strand, who described "a weakness in my back, and Megrim in my Head, and violent Rheumatick Complaints in my Shoulders and Arms" following a fall. After being ordered into the baths by Dr. Achmet, "I have been fine ever since . . . and am, thanks to God, enabled to follow my business."[62] As James Bourke certified, "For three years I was most severely afflicted with a violent and inveterate scurvy, attended with ulcers in Legs and Arms, my Bones were also sore and racked with Pains, I also had a Megrim in my Head, and a great Dimness of Sight." Having become "loaded and almost overpowered with such a complication of disorders," and after trying a variety of other treatments without success, Bourke applied to Dr. Achmet. Like McManus, Bourke testified that he had been restored to perfect health and was now able to follow his trade once more.[63] Then we find Mary Bourne, who, for twenty years, had been "most severely afflicted with Pains in all my bones, a megrim in my Head, with Heats and Colds, and Swellings all through my body from a Contusion I received fifteen years ago." Having been reduced to a "mere shadow" of her former self, for five weeks Mary bathed and sweated at the hot baths, "as much as my weak state could bear," and found herself "perfectly freed . . . from all my long and dreadful complaints."[64] Bryan Green, having been for five years "most severely afflicted with worms, a foulness of stomach, and a megrim in my head," was enabled "to follow on my Business, and procure a comfortable subsistence for myself and Family" after being given medicine and using the baths. Borumborad also "freed" Catherine Desylva, who had been "severely afflicted with a great Giddiness and Megrim in my Head, and a near total loss of sight."[65]

When they are read together in this way, the testimonies in these two pamphlets appear formulaic and repetitive. Each of the *Report*'s accounts generally states the patient's name, residence, and the manner of their referral (usually by parish wardens or priests). The illnesses are outlined in great detail, to emphasize the failure of other treatments and the desperation of the applicant, before recounting the miraculous good effects of the baths, which enabled a return to work and resumption of family responsibility. To our eyes, this uniformity makes the narratives appear suspicious, but medical testimonials throughout the eighteenth century often aped the conventions of both legal courtroom terminology and the reporting of miraculous cures. Few of Borumborad's patients would have known exactly what had been written on their behalf regarding their cures, as most signed only with their mark, in the form of an X, but the impression of authenticity was nevertheless vital for readers. For instance, in witnessing her "extraordinary cure," Elizabeth Newton named "most of the inhabitants on the Coal Qay [*sic*], Mr. Redmonds, Publican, Mr. Quogh, publican &c. &c.," who all knew of her disease and its relief. As was the case with advertisements for proprietary medicines sold in London, the names and places included in testimonies pinned the stories down with an appearance of accountability and authenticity. Historian Hannah Barker has suggested that medical advertisements instilled a sense of trust through the use of testimonies, transforming a mode of writing originally applied to corroborate an exceptional religious experience into one that could be employed for a more commonplace and secular medical purpose.[66] While some historians have suggested that stories of miraculous recoveries mainly came from respectable members of society, the examples here support Barker's argument that testimonials were much more democratic than this.[67] In the case of Borumborad's Poor Baths, the witnesses were drawn from the illiterate poor, not only to convince the sick of his baths' value, but also to persuade wealthy patrons and politicians to continue funding and supporting his establishment, so it could still provide treatments free of charge. It is this necessary believability that gives an authentic glimpse not just into the experience of megrim, but of how life with chronic illness, and pain more generally, affected the lives of ordinary people in the eighteenth century. In some ways the comic, flamboyant figure of Dr. Achmet is a red herring, because what he was offering was a standard therapy that people from all walks of life had taken advantage of for centuries: using hot- and cold-water baths to treat a whole range of long-term ailments, including migraine.

Medicine by Letter

If you had the means to pay for a physician's advice, you did not need to leave your home to take advantage of the medical marketplace. To consult famous

Edinburgh physician William Cullen, you simply needed to enclose two guineas with your letter, and he would dispense his advice by mail. Physicians themselves also consulted the great doctor, hoping, by association with his name, to give their own prescriptions a greater air of authority. In April 1777, Dr. John Alves corresponded with Cullen regarding one of his patients, a Mrs. Baillie of Lamington, a village to the southeast of Glasgow. Alves had visited Mrs. Baillie, a member of a prominent Scottish Highland family, who had been unwell for some weeks. She had been feverish and initially thought that her complaints were "agueish." She improved gradually under Alves's regime of vomits, saline draughts, nitre, manna, and magnesia to settle her stomach, but she then "caught some fresh cold." The pain shifted to her temple and eyebrow and came and went periodically. At this point, Alves consulted Cullen about "the meagrim pain." Cullen thought it was simply a catarrhal infection following a badly managed cold. If the feverishness and megrim continued, he recommended that his colleague repeat the vomits or use a laxative. If the cough got worse, or was accompanied by chest pain, Alves should take some blood. If the megrim continued, Mrs. Baillie should immerse her feet and legs in warm water.[68] Three weeks later, Alves wrote to Cullen again, because, while Mrs. Baillie's fever and cough had abated, "what distressed her most was a daily return of the Meagrim which lasted for several hours." Although she initially had been taken out of bed and treated as Cullen had advised, Mrs. Baillie refused to allow the doctor to apply leeches to her temples. Nor would she take the "nauseating doses" of emetics. Dr. Alves had given her Peruvian bark (a treatment for fever) and valerian (an herb with sedative properties) to relieve her headache, which seemed to work for a while, but he had then received yet another letter from his patient. In despair, Alves begged Cullen, "You will please say what I am to do with this feverishness should it still hang about her, & with the hemicrania, should it continue or increase." As the spring weather had begun to improve, Alves wondered if Cullen would approve of Mrs. Baillie being allowed to go outdoors, in a chaise. He apologized for the questions, but it would give his reluctant patient (and her friends) "great satisfaction . . . [if] they know she is going on by your Directions."[69] On 7 May, Cullen replied, reassuring Alves that as long as Mrs. Baillie's feet and legs were well secured, and she took only the exercise that her strength would cope with, he saw no danger from either the cough or the megrim. Referring Dr. Alves to his earlier advice, Cullen hoped Mrs. Baillie "will not be so refractory as before."

Besides containing valuable evidence about the treatments that patients could expect to be prescribed for megrim in the eighteenth century, Alves's correspondence with Cullen illustrates how the meaning of megrim had changed by the seventeenth and eighteenth centuries. In the medieval and early modern periods, hemicrania was understood as a disorder in its own right, while, as we have seen in Napier's astrological casebooks, eighteenth-century advertisements, and the testimonials for Borumborad's baths and tar-water, megrim was often specified as being "in the head," as well as just one symptom that often appeared among a whole range of problems. Further-more, in the testimonials and advertisements, megrim often seems to be as-sociated more with dizziness than with pain. In 1627, the famous philosopher, author, and politician Francis Bacon had explained that "in every megrim or vertigo there is an obtenebration joined with a semblance of turning round," suggesting that some people, at least, considered the two terms to be inter-changeable.[70] "Obtenebration" meant a shadowing, or darkening, and Bacon believed this was caused by the weakness of the body's spirits. While humoral understandings of hemicrania, inherited from the classical period, denoted a pain on one side of the head, in vernacular English usage, the plural word "megrims" had come to be associated with depression or low spirits, or with an idea, a fancy, something done on impulse.[71] Philippe de Mornay's *Dis-course of Life and Death*, translated into English by the Countess of Pembroke, talked of "maigrims of the mind," while Puritan theologian Thomas Adams likened the ascending of vaporous humors through the veins or arteries to the "foggy mistes and cloudes" of ignorance, arrogance, and affectation that ob-scured and smothered "the true light of [men's] sober judgments," causing a "spirituall Migram or braine-sicknesse."[72] In French, the vernacular term *mi-graine* could also have the meaning of *pique*, or feeling irritated or resentful, which was more of an emotional or mental state, rather than a medical one. Indeed, famous French military surgeon Ambroise Paré (and his seventeenth-century English translator, Thomas Johnson) hinted at different meanings by emphasizing that migraine was strictly "a disease affecting one side of the head."[73] Poet and playwright Henry Brooke reflects this broader usage in his late-eighteenth-century tragedy, *The Imposter*:

> These are the very megrims of existence;
> The dizzy rounds of thought, that foundering drown
> In their own whirlpools.[74]

The common understanding that animals, particularly horses, could be subject to megrims complicates things further. When a horse was seized with "meagrims, sturdy or turnsick," it lost all balance or control. The animal "stops short, shakes his head, looks irresolute and wandering . . . in more violent cases he falls at once to the ground, or first runs round, and then sinks senseless."[75] This sense of megrim as occurring in the head, as well as the fuzziness of its association with a sense of dizziness, mood, or vertigo (seen as disorders of the head, rather than pains specifically) helps explain the emergence, at the end of the eighteenth century, of the new terms sick headache and bilious headache, which reasserted the link between headache and gastric symptoms that had traditionally been assumed by humoral models of hemicrania.

The language of migraine also became much more complicated and diverse on the European continent during the seventeenth and eighteenth centuries, a time of great interest in scientific classification, whether botanical or medical. For example, French physician and botanist Boissier de Sauvages identified ten different kinds of migraine (which he defined as violent, periodic head pain, often one sided or behind the eyes), including hysterical and ocular migraine, migraine caused by sinuses that were either obstructed or blocked by an insect, and a *migraine lunatique* that coincided with the phases of the moon. For Esther Lardreau, this "fastidious" enumeration reveals the sheer diversity of the language that was in use surrounding head pain.[76]

These ideas also had an important effect on the thinking of British physicians, as illustrated by one revealing exchange of letters. In late August 1781, Sir Charles Blagden—physician, Francophile, army surgeon, and Fellow (later to be Secretary) of the prestigious Royal Society of London—received a letter from his friend, Thomas Curtis, who was concerned about the health of his son. For more than a decade, the young man had suffered a "very peculiar kind of head ach," which had begun to return more frequently as he reached adulthood. Moreover, for the previous eight to ten weeks, the headache appeared to return "exactly periodically," every two weeks on a Wednesday "nearest the full or change of the moon." Curtis described his son's symptoms. A headache would come on with "a dizziness, or partial vision," and last for about half an hour, followed by a violent pain "sometimes quite through from the forehead to the Pole." The headache would continue for four or five hours, or until he fell asleep. When his son woke up, he would appear quite well, except for "a little languor." Curtis also noted that his son's breath could be "offensive," and he complained of wind in his stomach. Therefore, Curtis asked, might the cause arise from the stomach?[77] Blagden was not the first physician Curtis had consulted. In previous years, he had sought the opinion of well-known Bath physicians Abel Moysey and John Staker (a fellow member of the

Bath Philosophical Society, founded by Curtis), but their prescriptions had been ineffectual, aside from some temporary relief. So, as the family headed to the small and secluded (some said dreary) seaside village of Newton on the Bristol Channel in Glamorgan, South Wales, to see if sea bathing might benefit the young man, Curtis had written to his friend.[78]

Blagden responded swiftly to the letter. He apologized for an imperfect answer, produced from memory. As an army surgeon, he had only been able to take a few books directly related to military medical practice with him to Plymouth. Nonetheless, Blagden did remember that he had observed one of the young Curtis's headaches in London the previous year, and that his friend had mentioned the topic several times in conversation. Despite being away from his books, Blagden was confident that this was the kind of headache "better known in France by the name migraine, than among us by the corresponding word meagrim." Blagden's distinction between the French word *migraine* and the English term meagrim is telling. He explained that both migraine and meagrim were a corruption of the ancient word hemicrania, but they signified a different complaint, though "of a similar kind."[79] In proposing that the young man was suffering from the French type of migraine, Blagden did not elaborate on what he meant by the phrase, but it seems likely that he was aware of Boissier de Sauvages's classification of *migraine lunatique.*

Blagden was not convinced that the moon's phases were causing Curtis's son's illness, however, noting that while Wednesday, 6 June, had indeed coincided with the full moon, by mid-August, the young man's migraine would have occurred four days before the full moon. Blagden suspected the cause more likely lay in the young man's habits, or even in his expectation that the disease would return on a certain day. Blagden did not dismiss the lunar theory entirely, however, and thought the original impulse might have been from the moon. He noted that there were other states of the moon besides its phases that might produce an effect on the atmosphere, but nothing could be said with certainty until they had collected a sufficient series of observations. Blagden recommended recording the son's attacks until November. If the affliction continued to appear regularly on a Wednesday, it would, by that time, "be so near the quarter of the moon" that they could safely locate the problem in the young man's routine. If such were the case, Blagden would attribute the pain to "something of the nature of intermittent fever." If it turned out to be a lunar influence, he would suspect Curtis's son had "some tendency towards an epileptic affection," or at least a disorder of the nervous system.

If the young man's migraine returned on 12 September, the date of the next full moon, Blagden instructed that he should have twelve ounces of blood let a week later, on 19 September, and then try taking the herb valerian "in considerable doses," beginning with two scruples (forty grains), three times a day, and increasing the dose until his stomach could bear no more. We have already seen Dr. Alves prescribing valerian for Mrs. Baillie, as this was a fashionable choice in the late eighteenth century. Distinguished physician Richard Mead, author of the famous *Treatise Concerning the Influence of the Sun and Moon upon Human Bodies*, had recommended frequent use of the pulverized root of a young valerian plant for periodic diseases of the head.[80] This seems to have prompted Scottish physician John Fordyce to try it for his own hemicrania. Finding it of very great benefit, he recommended taking dram doses of valerian three or four times a day in his essay, *De Hemicrania*.[81] Valerian was not a new discovery, as it had long been known as an anticonvulsant. Moreover, the valerian family also contains spikenard, which, as we saw in chapter 2, had been a common ingredient in remedies for hemicrania since classical times. Both valerian root and spikenard have an earthy, musky odor, as well as sedative and relaxing properties.

Given Curtis's and Blagden's discussion about the moon, it is significant that valerian had appeared in Mead's work. Although overt zodiacal astrology had fallen out of fashion by the eighteenth century, an ongoing belief in the influence of the sun and moon on human bodies was most clearly, and influentially, represented in the work of royal physician Richard Mead, who used Newtonian physics to explain how "lunar action" caused distention of the vessels in the body, particularly resulting in diseases of the head. Mead proposed that illnesses manifesting once or twice a month should be treated by "evacuating" measures, such as bloodletting, plasters, or vomiting, if not to cure, then at least to ease the patient.[82] As Meadian medical astrology remained an important part of military medicine throughout the century, Blagden's professional background as an army surgeon helps explain his ready acceptance of lunar influence as a possible cause for migraine, interwoven with some of the most up-to-date of medical theories coming from the continent.[83]

The exchange of letters occasioned by the illness of Thomas Curtis's son provides important evidence for when and how the French word *migraine* came to be adopted in the English language. This was not simply an alternative name for meagrim, but a more advanced understanding of the disorder altogether. The letters between Blagden and Curtis hint at the vibrant cross-Channel exchange of ideas and knowledge that characterized elite science and medicine in this period and would continue to be influential during the nineteenth century, as English-speaking physicians began to adopt nervous theories to explain migraine's pathology.

In 1780, famous Swiss physician Samuel Tissot discussed migraine in an eighty-three-page chapter in his *Traité des nerfs*. Tissot distinguished migraine from the three other types of headache (he added a fourth variety to the usual triad, which he called *le clou*, or *l'ouef*) by the severity of the pain, its periodicity, its recurrence independent of accidental causes, and its distinctive symptoms—as a pain that occupied the temple, ear, eyebrow, and eye, and either the right or left side of the head.[84] Tissot argued that migraine was the result of a sympathetic communication between the nerves of the stomach and the head.[85]

Nervous diseases seemed to be the price of modernity, wealth, and social progress. In his famous polemic on the nation's fitness, *The English Malady*, physician George Cheyne blamed intemperance, sedentary lifestyles, sensual pleasures, and the pollution of urban living for a whole range of nervous disorders. Those who engaged in works of imagination, memory, study, and thinking were most prone to maladies such as vapors and low spirits, because their nerves were "finer, quicker, more agile and sensible, and perhaps more numerous" than in other people. As society progressed, Cheyne worried that the bodies and constitutions of each generation would become "more corrupt, infirm, and diseas'd."[86] Later in the century, William Cullen was the first English-language writer to elaborate a clear medical position regarding neuroses—diseases that affected the functions of the nervous system—though his classification certainly drew on the work of many before him. Cullen's classification quickly became out of date, but his emphasis on the centrality of the nervous system, rather than the blood vessels, as the chief determinant of health was significant. He acknowledged that neuroses were a potentially pointless category, since almost every disease might be called nervous.[87]

In 1778, English physician John Fothergill urged his colleagues to take sick headache more seriously, noting that although "it occurs very frequently, [it] has not yet obtained a place in the systematic catalogues." Fothergill observed that sick headache chiefly affected those who were "sedentary, inactive, relaxed, and incautious respecting diet." This type of headache, he argued, proceeded from the stomach. Melted butter, fatty meats, and black pepper were common culprits in causing sick headache. This meant meat pies, containing all of these ingredients, were particularly dangerous, "as fertile a cause of this complaint as anything I know." The wrong quantity of food could also produce the same effect, and acid bile would "excite this sick-headach in a violent degree."

Sick headache was the result of repeated errors in diet or dietary conduct, which weakened the digestive powers and disordered the animal functions. Over time, a regimen of drinking mineral waters would help, but there was no point in turning to the materia medica without correcting the faulty diet.[88] Fothergill's writing, particularly when viewed in the context of concern about the nation's health, illustrates how nervous theories about migraine, which updated old humoral ideas about a sympathetic relationship between different parts of the body, could be allied with the concept of disease as attributable to failings of individual character, as well as to one's constitution. Such ideas also reveal that the association of migraine attacks with particular types of food has a very long history.

Conclusion

In May 1782, a year after Curtis and Blagden had corresponded about migraine, a flamboyant character graced the King's Theatre Masquerade in London. Gliding his way past the Venetian sailor, the gentleman in a coat of two different colors, and the usual "unremarkable" costumes of some eight hundred attendees, the dashing figure of the High German Doctor introduced himself to the gathering as "Le Sieur François de Migraine, Docteur en Médicine."[89] Throughout the eighteenth century, the cultivation of French language and conversational skills had been an essential element of an English gentleman's identity and of civility in polite society. By the end of the century, however, commentators concerned with national character were increasingly seeing the adoption of French elegance and delicacy as a threat to the strength and sincerity of English masculinity. In his *Comparative View of the French and English Nations*, John Andrews commented that if the English were to indulge in the company and attention of women "to excess," as the French did, "what we might gain in delicacy and refinement, we might lose in manliness of behaviour and liberty of discourse; the two pillars on which the edifice of our national character is principally supported."[90]

Masquerades were first held at Somerset House by the French ambassador, the Duc d'Aumont, in 1713 (while, outside on the Strand, peddlers offered up their miraculous remedies). Such events, like the one attended by Le Sieur François de Migraine, had been all the rage since the 1760s. These were notorious social gatherings, lavish expressions of parody, debauchery, excess, and "perverse foreign fashion."[91] So whom did our attendee represent? To call someone a High German Doctor in the eighteenth century was definitely to accuse him of quackery. A caricature (attributed to Sir William Bunbury) of

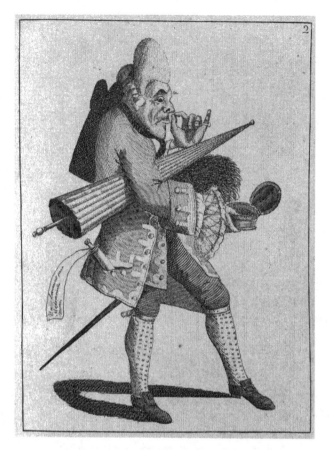

Fig. 4.2. Monsieur le Médecin, attributed to Sir Henry William Bunbury, 1771, accession number 2011.88(3). Metropolitan Museum of Art, the Elisha Whittelsey Collection, Elisha Whittelsey Fund, 2011

Monsieur le Médecin, with his carefully powdered wig, his snuff, and his parasol, gives a sense of what our masquerading character may have looked like (fig. 4.2).

Le Sieur François de Migraine is worth taking seriously, because he illustrates an important change in the understanding of migraine. Something was happening to migraine in the late eighteenth century. It had begun to gain a personality of its own, an identity that went beyond mere symptoms and theories about its causes. Esther Lardreau has described France as the homeland of migraine: "[It was] a grimacing image of the various fractures in the country, be they social or sexual. It was the disease of intellectuals, the disease of ill-married women, the disease of the bourgeoisie."[92] For English observers, its new association with flamboyance, with wilting Parisian nervousness and effeminacy, made this fresh kind of nervous migraine suspect. In the summer heat of August 1787, for instance, the writer of the *General Evening Post's* "Parisian Intelligence" column claimed that "half Paris had the *migraine*, and no lady of fashion could be prevailed upon to quit her boudoir."[93] It is telling that in 1819, out of more than twenty letters that Frederica, Duchess of York, wrote about her health to famous society physician Sir Henry Halford (best known for ministering to mad King George III), all were in English, apart from two. The latter were the letters recounting the migraine she had suffered on a recent visit to Windsor. The episode apparently required her to pen these missives in French.[94]

Throughout the early modern period, there is much evidence for migraine being a chronic disorder that affected the lives of people across the social spectrum, as well as many examples of the varied medical markets that promised relief in the form of baths, tonics, pills, powders, and tinctures. Le Sieur François de Migraine illustrates the culmination of a gradual but important shift in the way people saw migraine. Shifting from a humoral disorder denoting pain in one side of the head, we now see megrim emerging as a much more fluid concept. A megrim could certainly be an extreme, debilitating pain, but it could also be a fuzziness, or a sensorial disturbance. By the late eighteenth century, migraine was coming to be understood as a nervous complaint that could be caused by an emotional event, such as grief, or one that affected a particular kind of person. What is fascinating is how the first real evidence for not taking migraine—and those who had it—too seriously emerges not from discussions about gender per se, but from gendered anxieties about national character. In the wider culture, migraine seemed to provide an apt metaphor for certain assumptions about French national character in the unsettling political climate of the late eighteenth century.

CHAPTER FIVE

"The Pain Was Very Much Relieved and She Slept"

Gender and Patienthood in the Nineteenth Century

✳ ✳ ✳

Elizabeth, the Girl Who Dropped Trays, 1895

In April 1895, Elizabeth, a sixteen-year-old servant from the small village of Burbage in rural Wiltshire, southern England, traveled eighty miles to central London. She sought the help of physicians at the National Hospital for the Paralysed and Epileptic in Queen Square. Her casenotes, which can be found in the thick bound volume of casenotes and treatment cards for prominent neurologist John Hughlings Jackson's female patients during 1895, reveal something of her first meeting with the doctors and the story she recounted about her illness. Elizabeth described how she had been experiencing St. Vitus Dance (rapid involuntary movements) on her left side, headaches and pains in her eyes, sickness, and nervousness. The headaches occurred two or three times every day and lasted for five minutes at a time. They particularly affected her left side, at the back part of the top of her head. Noise, or sometimes reading in the morning, was most liable to bring on an attack. Elizabeth had experienced spells of giddiness and twice felt weakness in her hands in the mornings. She described episodes in which she could only see the left side of her visual field, or the left half of objects. This hemiopia (or half vision, to which we will return in the following chapter) could come on suddenly or gradually, from the periphery, though she had never seen zigzags or vomited. While she said that she had never experienced any illness other than "nettle rash" (hives), she had known sickness and pains in her head ever since she could remember. These worsened when she went to school, and particularly as she learned to read. By all visible measures, Elizabeth appeared healthy. Her admission report describes "a bright intelligent healthy looking girl of 16." She was not anemic, and she showed no outward appearance of disease. Both her facial expression and her behavior appeared "natural," and her muscles were strong and normal in size. The only thing a careful observer might note was the "constant flexion and extension of the left fingers with a rough rhythm & having an amplitude of almost half an inch."[1] For the past month, she explained, she had been unable to keep her left hand still.

Elizabeth also recounted a particular event, which the physician recorded in the margin of her hospital casenotes. One day, while carrying a tray full of things at her employer's house, the spoons on the right-hand side of the tray had suddenly disappeared from her vision. Making a dash to catch them, she "dropped the lot." We might imagine her employer's reaction to such an apparent episode of clumsiness. It is likely, for a start, that the cost of replacing the breakages would have come directly out of Elizabeth's pay.[2] Any repeat of such an incident would certainly endanger her employment, not to mention her chance of receiving a good reference to take onward. Her predicament helps explain the young woman's decision to travel to London for help. Elizabeth described her home life to the physician, underscoring further the significance of her trip in hope of a cure. She was one of eleven children. At first, she said they were all healthy, but when pressed further, she admitted that one sister had neuralgia in her face. It turned out that another sister did, too. A brother, age fifteen, had water on the brain. Her mother was alive and healthy, and Elizabeth had always been well fed and clothed, but the family was poor. "The house was unhealthy," the notes record, "very draughty and damp— moss grew up the walls. Drains are carried straight into a stream." From such a description, there is little doubt that the family would have relied heavily on Elizabeth's ability to work to bring money into the household.[3]

This chapter explores how, in the nineteenth century, physicians developed new theories about head disorders, including sick headache, bilious headache, megrim, and hemicrania. Rather than focusing on the character and location of pain (as had been common in humoral explanations), they based their ideas on the presumed cause and physiology of pain within the body, and, in so doing, increasingly made assertions about the gender and class of people subject to such conditions.[4] Women, especially exhausted mothers and working women, came to be seen as migraine's "martyrs." By the 1860s, researchers—keen to develop theories about migraine and its causes and test potential treatments—could take advantage of the availability of inpatients in specialist settings, such as the National Hospital for the Paralysed and Epileptic.

Like Elizabeth, people often traveled great distances to access care at the

National Hospital in the hope they might be treated and return to the working lives that chronic illness was making impossible. The casenotes and reports produced in institutional settings as varied as lunatic asylums and court trials reveal how ordinary people explained the onset of illness within the context of their lives, the profound effect of migraine on work and relationships, and the sometimes disturbing experiences of institutional patienthood. There is no doubt that neurological laboratories and hospital wards in places like London's National Hospital were the crucible for some of the most advanced neurological breakthroughs in modern medicine, but it is also true that these developments came at a human cost, as people in pain willingly submitted to exploratory ideas, therapeutic fashions, and experimental pharmacological mixtures.

Weak Nerves and Bad Habits

Around the turn of the nineteenth century, the terms sick headache and bilious headache began to appear more regularly in medical texts. This was a commonsense way to denote a headache accompanied by nausea, giddiness, and an aversion to food. During the first decades of the nineteenth century, physicians made clear links between sick and bilious headaches and emerging theories about the function of nerves and the brain. In 1807, influential Scottish naval physician Thomas Trotter rejected the shackles of nosological systems such as Cullen's and bundled together all the diseases commonly known as "nervous, bilious, stomach, and liver complaints, indigestion, low spirits, gout etc." into his *View of the Nervous Temperament*, in which he aimed to prevent physicians from making serious mistakes, such as diagnosing physical and mental debility as typhus (as a naval surgeon, preventing fever was one of Trotter's passions). The need for this work was urgent, he explained, as the demographics of nervous complaints had changed. "No longer confined to the better ranks in life," they were "rapidly extending to the poorer classes" in commercial, civilized society. The fashion for drinking tea, Trotter suggested, was in large measure responsible for the increasing prevalence of "nervous, bilious, spasmodic, and stomach complaints" among the "lower ranks of life." Hemicrania, he argued, was one of a number of nervous signs that revealed a predisposition to, or the existence of, nervous disorders, particularly in young women with "gouty parents."[5]

As we began to discover in the previous chapter, and as Trotter's polemic against tea further suggests, nervous symptoms such as hemicrania were increasingly being seen as the result of errors in modern lifestyles. Although I have found no evidence that any specific link was discussed at the time, it is worth noting that in the eighteenth century, commodities such as coffee and chocolate—now so often recognized as migraine triggers—became fashionable, not just among wealthy consumers, but throughout society. Nevertheless, as we saw with John Fothergill's railing against meat pies, physicians were increasingly focused on diet's relationship to migraine more generally. Writing for an American audience in 1819, James Mease declared the stomach to be the "seat and throne" of sick headache, a disease of "high living, over-eating, late hours . . . late suppers, indolence, and relaxing habits."[6] In the 1840s, well-known London physician Theophilus Thompson described sick headache as one of many symptoms (including heartburn, sleepiness after meals, dietary intolerances, timidity, hypochondriasis, intellectual "cloudiness," or even a tendency to suicide) that could be attributed to dyspepsia, or indigestion.[7] For Thompson and his contemporaries, these symptoms were the result of modern habits, such as a sedentary life, full meals on an empty stomach, confined air and high temperatures, disturbed sleep, anxious and prolonged study, "unsatisfied ambition, and perturbed passions." The language here is important. Sick headache, and those experiencing it, were by now being consistently dismissed, ridiculed, and belittled. If only sufferers would remedy their bad habits, such pronouncements implied, they would have little need for medicines.

In 1825, fashionable English physician Caleb Hillier Parry made an important intervention when he rejected the popularly accepted view that impaired function in the liver or alimentary canal was the cause of sick headache. Instead, Parry blamed "excessive determination of blood" to the branches of the internal carotid artery supplying blood to the brain. Parry's very modern claim nevertheless employed a treatment that was centuries old. He recommended "spontaneous bleeding from the nose, or other similar remedies applied to the head."[8] A few years later, French physician Henri Labarraque argued that migraine was a disorder of the nervous system in the head, which came in several varieties, provoked by a sympathetic transmission of irritation from the eyes, stomach, or sinuses. Labarraque's treatments took careful account of the patient's constitution and the variety of their migraine. He recommended removing sources of irritation from the stomach, such as coffee and tight clothing. Persons with an irritable stomach should have a diet of white meats and fish, green vegetables, and water. Paying close attention to ancient authors, Labarraque also recommended age-old therapeutic measures, including bleeding, vomiting, and the application of a theriac plaster to the stomach.[9] By 1848, Marshall Hall proposed that compression of the veins in the neck could obstruct the flow of venous blood away from the head and cause a whole range of "apoplectic, paralytic, epileptic, syncopal, or maniacal seizures," of which milder forms might include sick headache and "sick giddiness."[10] We can see in these examples how classical theories about animal spirits, vapors, and humors were being replaced with modern physiological explanations for a whole range of disorders, including sick headache, that were now being located primarily in the nervous system. At the same time, old ideas about treatment persisted. By the middle of the nineteenth century, biliousness, too, was being seen as an outdated concept in relation to migraine.

Martyrs

Between February and May 1854, the leading British medical journal, *The Lancet*, published a five-part essay by Patrick J. Murphy on the subject of "Headache and Its Varieties." Headache, Murphy explained, was a complaint for which medical men were "almost daily consulted." Murphy believed general confusion on the subject had led to unsatisfactory—and, in many cases, harmful—treatments. He singled out the idea of bilious headache as a particularly defective and stereotyped one. "I have never yet met a physician who could define what bilious meant," he commented, "least of all a bilious headache." He had been prompted to address the subject in response to the declaration by Dr. Graves, an American, that it would require "a good monograph" to satisfactorily classify disorders of the head.[11] Murphy proposed that classifying headaches was a relatively simple matter. There were five ordinary types of headache, of which two (anemic and congestive) were intracranial, while three (neuralgic, rheumatic, and periosteal) were extracranial. The extracranial category could be diagnosed easily by its "peculiar characters." Thus the important thing was to be able to identify the two types of intracranial headache. To do this, a physician needed to determine whether a patient's headache was caused by a *deficiency* of blood within the cranium, which would produce the most common anemic type, or by a *surplus* of blood, leading to a congestive headache.[12]

In classifying headaches this way, Murphy did not entirely reject classical conceptions of headache, but he did repackage them. He explained that anemic headache was the type commonly known by names such as cephelea, vertigo, megrim, or giddiness. Echoing William Buchan's ideas about malnourished wet nurses who suckled babies for too long, Murphy explained that anemic headache often affected "mothers in the lower classes of life," whose minds and bodies had been weakened by daily toil, disturbed sleep, and insufficient nourishment, while their bodies were "hourly drained by lactation."[13] In such cases, Murphy recommended a nutritious diet, including plenty of meat to restore the nervous system. Because megrim was caused by a deficiency of blood, it was thus fundamentally different from a sick headache, caused by "congestion." Nevertheless, young women were martyrs to sick headache, too, which occurred when menstruation was either scant or stopped altogether. In this case, blood should be taken. A third kind of headache in Murphy's classification was what he called neuralgic headache, which he deemed synonymous with the hemicrania of "old authors." This, again, was "*peculiar* to females," occurring from puberty until the end of their menstrual periods, and was "undoubtedly hysterical" in origin.[14]

Murphy's classification of headaches reveals two important changes in the way physicians were thinking about migraine in the middle of the nineteenth century. First, he divided sick headache, megrim, and hemicrania into separate disorders, based on what he believed to be their different causes. Second, Murphy insisted these were all illnesses that primarily affected young women, and he clearly linked them to hysteria. During the eighteenth century, physicians had dismissed the overt gynecological assumptions that had characterized older ideas of "hysteric passions," "suffocation of the womb," or "fits of the mother" and instead explained women's apparently greater tendency to suffer from hysteria as the result of weaker and more delicate nerves. As Mark Micale argues, however, the nineteenth century witnessed the reverse, so that women's dysfunctional bodies again became the source of nervous failure.[15] Murphy's ideas illustrate how this trend fed directly into changing ideas about headaches as a problem affecting women.

Sick Headaches at the Old Bailey

At this point, the report of a criminal trial might seem a strange place to look for evidence of the history of migraine. Yet, as social historians such as David Turner have argued, legal records like these, with their forensic intrusion into the minute details of people's daily lives at home, at work, and on the streets, allow us to vividly see "the calamitous effects of disability" on personal relationships, working lives, and general well-being, not just for those who stood trial.[16] For example, on 21 December 1864, George Kempt, the subwarden at the House of Correction, Coldbathfields, went to the cell of prisoner George Phillips. The previous day, Kempt had warned Phillips that the prisoner had wrongly stacked his books on the shelf, with the "Lord's Book" on the top, rather than on the bottom of the pile, as required. When Kempt entered the cell, he took Phillips's stool away, "as I wanted to sit down, having a sick headache —the stool was not required by the prisoner." As Kempt stooped, however, Phillips struck him a "violent blow" on the chin and inflicted two wounds on the subwarden's face with a knife.[17] George Kempt's unfortunate need to sit down at the precise moment he was supposed to be inspecting a prisoner's cell demonstrates the deeply inconvenient intrusion of the subwarden's bodily weakness into the scene, as well as the opportunity it provided for a dissatisfied prisoner to avenge a slight.

Yet we digress. The *Proceedings of the Old Bailey*—texts of trials at London's central criminal court—also provide important evidence of how changes in the language of sick headache, biliousness, female headaches, and hysteria could play out in real life. In 1844, Jane Milburn, a charwoman, appeared at the Old Bailey, having been indicted for stealing a spoon, valued at five shillings, from her master, Augustus Ironmonger. Milburn had taken the spoon to a pawnbroker, but the crest on the item had raised his suspicions, and he had handed her into custody. William Webb testified on her behalf. "I have known the prisoner twenty-three or twenty-four years," he explained. "She is not insane, but is so affected with sick headache, that at times she is not capable of knowing right from wrong."[18] She was found not guilty, because the strength of Mr. Webb's testimony seems to have convinced the court of the effect of her sick headaches on her mental capacity. Milburn's case reflects an observation made by historians of crime and punishment: courts often gave sympathetic treatment to defendants who provided strong evidence of suffering and incapacity.[19]

The vocabulary used by different parties in the case of laundress Ann Noakes in 1880 illuminates the gap that had emerged between lay and professional understandings of headache disorders. While ordinary people continued to use the older terms sick headache or bilious headache in the narratives they told of their own lives, or of the people they were called on to defend or accuse, doctors who gave professional evidence were looking at these symptoms, particularly in women, in a very different way. Noakes, a widow with four children, stood trial for the willful murder of her youngest son, William. Amy Risbridger, who had worked with Noakes for four months, described how Ann's health was in "a dreadful state," but she would not contemplate giving up work, for fear that her children would end up in the workhouse. "When she could forget her trouble," Risbridger said, "she was as nice and cheerful a woman as I ever worked with," but "she used to complain of her head very much at times—she had got a sick headache—at those times she used to say that her trouble was too much for her to bear." Another witness, fourteen-year-old Emma Dibstall, gave a similar testimony: "[Noakes] said her head was so bad she could not bear her trouble . . . she was a very hardworking woman, standing at the tub till late at night." Risbridger remembered that Noakes had been attended by a Dr. Walters for "loss of blood, some complaint of the womb." John Walters, MD, was called to give his testimony. He explained that he had seen Noakes constantly, finding her weak, in poor health, pale, bloodless, and complaining "of great headache and restlessness at night." He told her that she needed to rest, and that the treatment would not work unless she could "lay up." The friends, families, and fellow workers who testified in defense of Noakes portrayed a hardworking woman, dealing on a daily basis with sick headache as a chronic problem that threatened not only her own mental state, but her ability to keep her family together. Noakes's long working hours seemed to contribute to the failure of her health. For Risbridger, the knowledge that Noakes was receiving treatment for "some complaint of the womb" was incidental to the way she saw her friend suffering from pain in her head and fearing for the welfare of her family. Dr. Walters saw her sick headaches as the symptom of a deeper disorder of her reproductive system, but Noakes simply could not afford to follow his order that she must rest if his treatment was to have a chance to work. Walters concluded that Noakes had been suffering from homicidal mania, and that "she would not know she was doing a guilty act" in killing her child. The court found the laundress not guilty on the grounds of insanity.[20]

The cases of Jane Milburn and Ann Noakes illustrate how, as biliousness fell out of favor during the middle of the nineteenth century, physicians became more confident in linking migraine to hysteria, epilepsy, problems in women's reproductive systems, and insanity. Although these Old Bailey records are extreme cases, they are evidence of how changing medical ideas and the language medical practitioners used to override more common understandings of illness had real effects on people's lives, particularly for women.

In 1878, F. Arnold Lees talked of the "megrim of hysterical ill-nourished women." In the 1885 Cavendish Lecture, J. S. Bristowe designated megrim as just one of "many functional diseases of the nervous system," including various forms of "insanity and epilepsy, chorea, neuralgia, and hysteria." There was no clear demarcation between these disorders, but "emotional persons, and persons of marked hysterical tendencies" were more liable than others to suffer from such affections.[21] In 1888, James Ross argued for a close relationship between hysterical headache and true migraine, describing the former as "frequently limited to one spot, and feels as if a nail were being driven through the skull; hence it is often called *clavus*." According to Ross, menstrual periods and mental worry increased the severity of the headache, while "amusement and anything which engages the attention" would end an attack.[22] Ross nevertheless warned of mistaking hysterical clavus for migraine. True migraine, Ross explained, was not only hereditary, but generally followed the female line, from mothers to daughters. This inheritance would not necessarily show up directly, as hemicrania. Rather, headache was just one possible manifestation of a "neurotic tendency," along with epilepsy and insanity.[23] As Joanna Kempner has observed, nineteenth-century authors like Ross had become adept at making arbitrary distinctions between medical categories.[24]

Migraine, Neurology, Psychiatry

Nervous diseases were a large and unwieldy category. Although a symptomology of seizures and periodicity seemed somehow to connect disorders such as paralysis agitans, epilepsy, tetanus, migraine, and hysteria, the links remained stubbornly resistant to explanation. In attempting to unravel the web of connections and theories relating migraine to a host of other problems in the late nineteenth century, it is important to realize how often investigations into malfunctioning minds and bodies overlapped. Nerves were dealt with in a variety of institutional contexts, and, significantly, there was no real division between neurology and psychiatry throughout the nineteenth century.[25] William F. Bynum has described lunatic asylums as "museums of neuropathology" for patients with a whole range of diseases of the nervous system, including neurosyphilis and epilepsy, in addition to those we would now classify as mental illnesses.[26] Alienists, as asylum doctors came to be known in the 1860s, were interested in boosting the status of asylum medicine by dedicating themselves to a broad range of problems: mental pathology, psychology, physiology, and neurology.[27] One of the most important settings for early research on the brain was the West Riding Lunatic Asylum, a site of "fruitful interchange" for neurologists, psychiatrists, physicians, and pathologists. The *Reports of the West Riding Asylum* (the predecessor to the journal *Brain*) reveal a whole range of experiments on physiology, specialist diagnostic equipment, and pharmacological preparations, such as chloral hydrate and amyl nitrite. John Hughlings Jackson and Thomas Clifford Allbutt, both prominent commentators on migraine, were part of this circle.[28]

An experiment in treating migraine with cannabis at the Sussex County Lunatic Asylum illustrates the exploratory culture at the intersection of neurology and psychiatry. In the asylum's 1871 *Annual Report*, Richard Greene, the assistant medical officer, reported on *Cannabis indica* (Indian hemp) as a potential treatment for migraine. Unlike many other contemporaneous remedies—for example, digitalis—it appeared that cannabis could be taken in large doses "without producing any unpleasant effects" and did not require "the exercise of any fortitude by the patient." Although there is some evidence for employing cannabis as a treatment for headaches and migraine in the Middle Ages, the more modern use of cannabis for migraine seems to derive from John Clendinning's 1843 proposal, mentioning "cannabis sativa of India" as a favorable alternative to opium, which had a wide range of unpleasant side effects.[29] In 1870, Scottish psychiatrist Thomas Clouston was awarded the Fothergillian Gold Medal for his experiments with opium, potassium bromide, and cannabis to treat acute mania in patients at the Cumberland and Westmorland Asylum.[30] In 1871, the same year when Richard Greene was experimenting in Sussex, Francis Anstie suggested using between a quarter and a half grain of "*good* extract of cannabis," rather than strong narcotics such as belladonna (deadly nightshade) and opium, as an "excellent" remedy for migraine in children.[31]

At the Sussex asylum, Greene had only been in his job for a few months, following the retirement of Charles Lockhart Robertson, who was also the editor of the *Journal of Mental Science* (later the *British Journal of Psychiatry*). Under Robertson, the Haywards Heath Asylum had been well known for its experimental approach. Robertson and his assistant medical officer, S. W. D. Williams, had regularly contributed to *The Lancet* and the *British Medical Journal* on subjects such as the use of Turkish baths, the sedative action of cold wet sheets in treating mania, the nonrestraint of patients, fractured ribs, and the therapeutic use of digitalis. Despite these contributions, the Haywards Heath staff believed county asylums were under "constant reproach" from both the medical and general press for doing little to advance knowledge of mental diseases.[32] So, in the year Greene arrived, a new feature had been added to the Sussex Asylum's *Annual Report* to record novel and successful treatments. In 1871, experiments included the use of potassium bromide and amyl nitrite in the treatment of epilepsy, and ergot of rye for insanity.[33]

Greene commented that migraine was an illness "over which medicine has no control." Substances such as arsenic, quinine, injected morphia, or alcoholic stimulants were "perfectly valueless" as a permanent cure, or even, in most cases, as temporary relief. Greene had often used cannabis previously in his work with patients in lunatic asylums and claimed that it nearly always produced some benefit. Greene discussed his treatment of six cases of migraine (four women and two men). In each instance, cannabis given as an alcoholic extract seemed to reduce the severity and frequency of the migraine attacks. In the only doubtful case, the patient admitted to not having taken the medicine regularly but added that "a double dose when the headache was coming on often relieved it." One woman had experienced migraine for upward of twenty years. After taking half-grain doses of cannabis in the morning and night for five weeks, "great improvement followed." Increasing the dose to one grain reduced the severity and frequency of the headaches still further. Greene lamented that if only he had been able to persuade the patient to give up the "wretched stimulants" of tea and coffee, even greater relief might have been obtained. He concluded that although cannabis was not a cure for migraine, it rarely failed to improve even the most apparently hopeless cases.[34]

Greene's experiment in treating migraine with cannabis brought together changing ideas about the brain, concerns about the professional status of medicine in provincial asylums, attempts to find pharmacological treatments for a range of mental and neurological illnesses, and a growing recognition that migraine was being particularly poorly treated. During 1872, the major medical journals carried several reports on the use of Indian hemp and guarana (which contained large quantities of caffeine) for the treatment of sick headache. At St. Thomas's Hospital, Dr. Charles Murchison's experience with guarana was "not very favourable," while Dr. John Murray at Middlesex declared it "sometimes of great value . . . at other times equally valueless." By the end of the year, the editors of the *British Medical Journal* concluded that guarana—which, in France, had been used for migraine for some time—should "be brought prominently before the notice of the profession," and that more extended trials were needed.[35] Both the Sussex experiment and the reports from other hospitals bring migraine squarely into the bounds of an uncomfortable historical reality: therapeutic experimentation, however well-meaning or ultimately beneficial, relies very heavily on the bodies of poor and vulnerable patients.

The National Hospital

Queen Square in central London is almost hidden in the narrow space between the world-famous Great Ormond Street Hospital for Children and the tourist hotels of Bloomsbury. At its center is a quiet, leafy garden—a space of calm in the midst of central London—overlooked by buildings housing neurological research and imaging laboratories, the National Hospital for Neurology and Neurosurgery, and the University College London Institute for Cognitive Neuroscience. A plaque on the wall of the Queen's Larder tavern explains that this place has been associated with healing since King George III stayed privately on the square while under the care of Dr. Thomas Willis. Author Robert Louis Stevenson described the square, set apart from the bustle of Bloomsbury, as "a little enclosure of tall trees and comely old brick houses . . . it seems to have been set apart for the humanities of life and the alleviation of all hard destinies."[36] An act of Parliament had placed the center of the square in the care of the residents.

In 1860, the square witnessed the opening of the National Hospital for the Paralysed and Epileptic. The early hospital had eight beds for women, and its aim was to provide an alternative, less stigmatizing care facility than an asylum for patients with chronic neurological conditions, such as paralysis and epilepsy. It was to cater to patients from a poor or humble background who would be unable to pay for other kinds of medical treatment in private establishments. One of the criteria for admission was that the patient must be considered curable. If this changed, then the patient would be discharged, to be seen at the outpatient department instead. From the beginning, epilepsy and paralysis were the most common admissions to the National Hospital. The hospital provided specialized care and a dedicated space for neurological research in the center of London, and it soon outgrew its original building. The Hospital's board purchased the lease of the building next door from artist William Morris, allowing its capacity to be increased to sixty-four inpatient beds. Patients had use of a library, gymnasium, bathrooms, and day rooms attached to the wards. Physicians saw patients in consulting rooms, and the hospital had a small laboratory at the rear. In 1862, John Hughlings Jackson joined the consulting staff, visiting outpatients at their homes and inpatients twice a day. By 1870, when William Gowers was appointed as medical registrar, the hospital had ten physicians. The doctors at Queen Square, including John Hughlings Jackson, William Gowers, and David Ferrier, would become known as some of the fathers of English neurology.[37]

Elizabeth, the servant whose case opened this chapter, was admitted to the National Hospital on 10 April 1895. Her hospital casenotes follow a set format, giving details of the physicians involved in the case, her name, sex, age, and address. Most patients also received a diagnosis.[38] Fuller sections followed, outlining family history, the patient's previous health, the symptoms of their current illness, the comments of any family members present, and their physical and mental state during the consultation. The physicians paid a great deal of attention to the patients' own descriptions of their symptoms, particularly when related to problems with speech, hearing, eyesight, weakness, dizziness, paralysis, and headaches. Elizabeth seems to have been the only female in-patient with migraine in 1895, and it is likely she attracted Jackson's interest because of the accompanying twitch in her left hand. For the physicians, symptoms of migraine and sick headache seem to have most often been worthy of attention when they promised to reveal a possible relationship to epilepsy, as well as the potential presence of lesions in the brain that might account for its pathology, a theme to which we will return in the next chapter.[39]

When the patients were women, the physicians asked questions about their reproductive history, the health of their children, and their menstrual cycles. Casenotes often included photos, cards tallying the fits or attacks day by day, and printed diagrams on which the location of pain and sensory symptoms in the head and body could be marked. The volume for 1895, in which we find the casenotes for Elizabeth, contains details of seventy-three patients. While Jackson oversaw the patients' treatment, their day-to-day care was in the hands of the hospital's house physicians. Two-thirds of the women and girls in 1895 were under the care of A. J. Whiting, and each patient also had a named clinical clerk—often one of the other house physicians. The volume gives a useful snapshot of the variety of disorders the physicians considered. There were ten cases of disseminated sclerosis, thirteen of epilepsy, seven of neurasthenia, and six of peripheral neuritis, as well as a variety of tumors, cases of paralysis (including two infants), neuralgia, myelitis, fits, and chorea. In 1895, the hospital admitted girls as young as ten months old, and women into their sixties. They were the daughters of bootmakers, hat blockers, warehouse porters, bakers, bricklayers, an innkeeper, and a laundress. Elizabeth was the youngest of seven female servants admitted in 1895, but other patients' jobs included housekeeper, governess, nurse, and cook, as well as the wives of a baker, clerk, coachman, licensed victualler, carpenter, spinner, traveler, printer, and one "theatrical." The majority of the women were from London or its surrounds—including one coming directly from the Newington workhouse. Others journeyed much farther across England. An eleven-year-old girl traveled more than two hundred miles from St. Columb in West Cornwall, while other women came from rural Lincolnshire, Norfolk, and Shropshire.

It is likely that Elizabeth got to know some of the other women who were admitted around the same time. There was Isabel, whose sister explained that her sibling had been quite well up until five months previously, when she fell down suddenly. Sometimes Isabel foamed at the mouth and bit her arms, refusing to answer questions or speak. Isabel complained of a lump in her throat that "nearly chokes her sometimes." On 1 May, her notes record that when Isabel had a fit, the physicians took "no notice, and deliberately avoided an examination." The fit apparently "ceased spontaneously in less than a minute," leading the physicians to conclude that these attacks were "favoured by the presence of one or more doctors." The doctors complained that Isabel could not be trusted to give reliable statements when having her vision tested, and she appeared to lie about whether she could hear a tuning fork placed on her teeth. Although her casenotes record multiple fits, Isabel was discharged. Elizabeth was also joined by Lily, who had a history of epileptic fits that had initially been brought on by fright after her brother was brought home dead from drowning, an incident that itself was caused by a fit. Lily was discharged and sent to the hospital's convalescent home in East Finchley, north of London, on 28 April, apparently against her will. A comment on her notes asks, "Why was she sent here?" Then there was Eliza, diagnosed with alcoholic neuritis, who had given up working eight weeks earlier because of the pains in her feet and legs. Eliza denied she was an alcoholic, "but her friends give a different account," telling the doctors that she would drink half a pint of brandy a day. Elizabeth was discharged on 5 June, having remained "quite free from migraine or twitchings for several weeks." She, too, was recommended for referral to East Finchley.[40] These casenotes, as partial records of conversations physicians had with their patients and observations made about their lives give a moving glimpse of the patients' own voices as they tried to explain their illness, often through the contexts of family history, work, and daily life.

Although there are relatively few inpatient cases where migraine was the primary diagnosis, the physicians often recorded headaches, particularly sick headaches, as relevant to a patient's personal and family history for a variety of disorders. One sixteen-year-old boy, diagnosed with epilepsy in 1877, noted that his mother was subject to headache, and his thirteen-year-old brother had sick headaches all his life. The boy himself explained that ever since he could remember, he had "suffered from headaches which were brought on by over-exertion or over excitement, noise, or indigestion."[41] A young woman from Stevenage, whose illness did not receive a diagnosis, recalled that she had been liable to severe sick headaches her whole life, but she had never felt giddy until about ten weeks previously. The doctor's notes recorded that one Saturday, she had a bad "sick headache," and, on the following day, felt "ill generally." On Monday, "she noticed a sort of 'swimming in the head' as soon as she got up & on stooping over the wash hand basin she pitched forwards." She had to be very careful going down stairs, and during the one-mile journey to a doctor, she found she could not walk straight: "Objects before her appeared dancing about, not moving in any particular direction. After her walk the sense of giddiness was much greater, so that she could not look upwards." The next day, she continued to feel ill, giddy, and "shook much."[42] These symptoms continued for almost two weeks, her head was hot, and she could not eat.

In a case study published in *The Lancet* in 1874, we meet Thomas R. This account is filled with the everyday realities of coping with the type of symptoms common to migraine. We first meet Thomas being sick in his own backyard and then collapsing on his stairs. Later, Thomas described how he frequently dropped things: "If he places his stick [in his left hand] in order to open the garden-gate with his right, the stick often falls out." His illness affected his work as a tailor—one day he severely burned his insensible left hand with a hot iron—and his impaired vision affected his perception of the world around him. He saw the word "land" rather than "Midland" painted on the side of a cart, remarking to his son that "Liver" was a strange name. His son pointed out that the word was Oliver.[43]

In a now classic article from 1982, sociologist Michael Bury discusses the concept of chronic illness as "biographical disruption." Grounding his observations on work with patients with rheumatoid arthritis, Bury notes that when professional medical knowledge about a disorder is incomplete or based on practical trial and error, individuals have to rely on "their own stock of knowledge and biographical experience" as a way to cope with illness and answer questions such as "why me?" and "why now?"[44] We can see this process occurring in these historical case records, where the incomplete knowledge of the professional met the lived experience and worldview of the sufferer. Patients at the National Hospital frequently explained their migraine attacks as having a distinct cause, often a significant event in their lives. One thirty-six-year-old woman described how she had given birth to a full term but still-born child three months earlier. After a few days, as the fever that accompanied her breast milk coming in subsided, she began to experience pains on the left side of her head. At first the headaches lasted for a week. Now they lasted half an hour or so, but with no more than an interval of an hour between the headaches, and she was sick every few days. After being given quinine, calomel, and a full diet, she was discharged, seemingly improved.[45] Janet, a forty-five-year-old cook from Hampstead in London, reported that despite never being very strong and remaining in delicate health since the age of twenty-three, she had worked all her life until being admitted to the National Hospital in February 1899. Thirteen years earlier, in 1886, she "had some teeth out under gas," and a week later was seized with a headache that came on over two days. She fainted, and then was sick repeatedly for twenty-four hours. The pain, always in the right side of the head, "was of an agonising shooting nature" and lasted a week each time. After five weeks in the Women's Hospital and a month at a convalescent home in Brighton, she had felt well, but six weeks later she experienced a similar attack. Since then, this had happened every two weeks. She had a "striking feeling of *bien être*" just before the attacks began, and felt "remarkable well" afterward. While it was commonly understood that migraine tended to improve around the time of the menopause, for Janet the attacks had become much worse since "the change." Now she never recovered between attacks and had "a constant feeling of pressure on the top of her head." As the attack came on, she saw "zigzag flashes of light on a normal visual field of the left eye" and "similar flashes and black spots in the right eye." Recognizing that the "exciting causes"—what we now would term triggers—for her attacks included heat, excitement, and tiredness, Janet benefited from the diet and rest during her sixty-nine days as an inpatient at the National Hospital. She even put on a few ounces of weight before being discharged as "improved."[46]

The language available for people to describe experiences of pain and disorientation was both shaped by and a reflection of the social and cultural environment in which they lived and worked. Emma Jane, a forty-two-year-old woman seen by Jackson in 1892, described noises in her head and ears that sounded "like an engine letting off steam."[47] William Gowers's casebook records the admittance, in September 1898, of Augustus, a fifty-four-year-old cabdriver from Hammersmith, who had long been affected by headache, staggering, and general weakness. As many others did, Augustus considered himself healthy. He was married, with nine children (of whom five survived, well and strong), had always been strong, and never had any serious illness. Yet, for twenty years, Augustus had experienced attacks of severe pain in the left side of his head, followed by severe vomiting, dimness of vision, and an inability to fix his sight on anything. These attacks, occurring from every few weeks to months, usually lasted for twelve to twenty-four hours. Eleven years earlier, in 1887, he had been forced to give up work and took to his bed "on account of the almost daily occurrence of the headache, giddiness, and vomiting." During attacks, "he used to stagger & had a feeling like that of seasickness of the stomach." On that occasion, he spent six months at the National Hospital. He got better, and for the next nine years had only occasional attacks until, sixteen months ago, he again began to experience them daily and had been "laid up" ever since. The cabdriver's casenotes described his symptoms:

> He rises from bed feeling quite well. So soon as he begins to walk about he experiences a tight feeling beginning behind the right ear but soon becoming localised over the left side of the head. The tight feeling begins to throb and an intense headache comes on generally confined to the left side but sometimes spreading over to the right. He has a feeling at the pit of the stomach as if he is going to be sick. He has to lie down to relieve the pain & if he is unable to rest directly the pain comes on he staggers about & is giddy & the attack will last much longer than if he rested. His eyes are so painful that he keeps them closed. Occasionally he has seen flashes of light. After 4–12 hours pain he begins to vomit and brings up bile. The vomiting lasts several hours and when it ceases the headache goes and he feels quite well.[48]

Accounts like Augustus's and Janet's reveal the effect of migraine on working lives and the unpredictable nature of chronic illness. Janet considered her overall health to be "delicate," while Augustus seems to have separated his experiences of migraine from what he considered to be his general good health and strength, a pragmatism in the face of unavoidable, expected problems that sociologist Jocelyn Cornwell has termed the notion of "normal illness."[49] Both Janet and Augustus had experienced periods of remission, seeking help only when the symptoms had become so bad that they had once again been forced to stop working.

Some patients journeyed long distances to see the neurologists at Queen Square. In 1891, a twenty-three-year-old carpenter traveled more than 250 miles from Penzance, in far southwestern England. For nine years, George had been subject to attacks that initially affected his vision, followed by a pricking sensation that began in his fingers. The feeling traveled up his arm to the shoulder, across the chest, to his mouth, and ended, around a quarter of an hour after his vision first dimmed, with a severe pain in the temples that continued until he went to sleep. Sometimes, when the sensation reached his mouth, George found he was unable to speak clearly enough to make people understand what was happening. These attacks occurred about three times a month, leaving him weak and ill for two or three days afterward. The casenotes describe a "healthy looking man." After seventeen days in the hospital without an attack, he was discharged, with a month's medicine, as his case was deemed to have "improved."[50]

The casenotes of Jane—a thirty-year-old woman who traveled 140 miles from Gorleston, on England's east coast, and was admitted under Dr. Thomas Buzzard in May 1881—provides important evidence of the options for self-medicating migraine in the late nineteenth century. Jane had experienced headaches since she was ten years old, though she could not think of any particular cause. The attacks came on suddenly, with pain in the right eye, spreading to the forehead, and then over the right side of the head. Attacks would last a whole day, with vomiting several times an hour providing no relief. She had been prompted to seek specialist treatment after noticing some months earlier that her right eye did not look straight forward after some of the attacks, but turned slightly outward. In January, this had worsened. After one attack, her right eye "looked very much outwards and the eyelid completely closed," so she could not open it. Although her eye had improved, it had never been "quite well" since. Jane had tried "all kinds of diets, starving herself & lived once on toast and water for a month." This did no good. She had taken patent medicines and chlorodyne, and tried "Pulvermacher's and other appliances."[51]

Chlorodyne was one of the most famous nineteenth-century patent medicines, initially created by Dr. J. Collis Browne, an army surgeon, around 1850 to treat cholera among the troops, but it was soon marketed by rival brands, such as Freeman's chlorodyne. Sold in tablet form, the medicine was a compound of morphine hydrochloride, cannabis extract, nitroglycerin, hyoscyamus (henbane), chili oil (now more commonly known as pepper spray), and peppermint oil.[52] Pulvermacher's sold a variety of flexible chain belts, which were attached to a galvanic battery. Marketed as a cure-all for nervous and chronic diseases, the belts promised that "Electricity, Nature's Chief Restorer," dispensed with the need for medicine.

Under Dr. Buzzard, Jane was prescribed a range of substances, including hydrocyanic acid diluted in soda water to stop her vomiting, and then, an hour later, chloral and potassium bromide. Her casenotes recorded that the "pain was very much relieved and she slept." Although the pain continued throughout the next day, it was much less severe and "bearable." The following morning she felt well, apart from a sinking feeling in her chest and throat. Three days later, Jane was given gelsemium, commonly used as a treatment for neuralgia. On 22 May, after only two weeks in the hospital, Jane received the news that one of her children was ill. The following morning, one of the attacks began, giving the physicians an opportunity to see the effects on her eyes. Their observations, and Jane's treatment, had to be cut short, however, as she returned home to her family.

Hydrocyanic acid had long been used in preparations such as cherry-laurel water and could be made by distilling the leaves of *Prunus laurocerasus*. In 1789, William Cullen had noted the powerful sedative effects of this highly poisonous substance. Although widely rejected in the eighteenth century because of its toxicity (the acid's vapor could quickly kill rabbits, cats, and dogs), it had returned to the materia medica in the nineteenth century as an antispasmodic and a more efficient sedative than opium. Potassium bromide and chloral were also sedatives commonly used for treating epilepsy.[53] In 1872, Dr. Samuel Wilks was effusive about potassium bromide's value for treating sick headache (apparently his own), as "it can scarcely be superseded by a better remedy."[54]

Pharmaceutical Cocktails

Annie, a thirty-two-year-old butcher's daughter (she indicated no occupation of her own) from Wimborne, in Dorset, could tell when a headache was coming on, as black dots danced about in front of her eyes for a day or more. She also experienced shivers. The pain nearly always attacked the right side of the head, and it usually began in the morning. At first the headaches had struck once a month, but now they came every week, lasting over two days. When the headache was at its worst, around twelve hours after it began, she vomited. For two years, Annie had experienced persistent pain on the vertex (the top surface of her head), which felt tender under pressure and was worse on some days. There was little in her family history to explain her illness. Although her father had heart disease, and a sister was anemic, her mother and five brothers were healthy, and the family was "not nervous." From the age of twelve, she had suffered with disease in her right hip. The abscess had been opened, the joint had been excised, and it had "discharged constantly until two years ago." Four months earlier, the hip had been very painful, but now it was better. Annie felt that the healing of her hip two years previously was significant, because the head pain commenced "just at the time when the hip ceased discharging and she associates these two facts." Before coming to Queen Square, Annie had tried many different treatments, including tonics, quinine, antipyrin, phenacetin, and bromides. Until three or four months ago, two fifteen-grain powders of antipyrin would stop the headache: this had been better than anything else she had tried. Annie was admitted to the hospital on 17 March 1899, under the care of William Gowers. On 28 March, she was able to give the physicians a clear description of her attack, as she had experienced a vertical "thumping pain" up the right side of her face and had been sick in the night.

She was put on a diet of milk, eggs, and bread. Although she felt better the following day, Annie then came down with influenza. Two weeks later, she reported that she had had a constant headache every day since, never being free from pain for more than five minutes. Every morning she would have "nettle rash" on her arms, legs, and neck. On 21 April, the casenotes record that she had been sleeping better since 12 April, when digitalis had been added to her nighttime medicine.[55]

During her stay as an inpatient, Annie received an astonishing array of pharmacological substances and experimental treatments. On 17 March, the physicians began with chloralose, an anesthetic and sedative. The following day she was given a mixture of diluted phosphoric acid, liquid strychnine, liquid trinitrine, and tincture of gelsemium. This combination is significant, because it is an early version of what would become one of William Gowers's most famous legacies, a migraine treatment known as Gowers' Mixture, which contained nitroglycerine, sodium bromide, gelsemium, strychnine, nitric or hypobromic acid, and chloroform and was in use until the 1970s. For Gowers, the most important element was the trinitrine, in the form of nitroglycerine, which acted as a potent vasodilator.[56] Two days later, on 19 March, Annie was prescribed fifteen grains of antifebrine, a treatment for fever and pain. Over the next few weeks she was also dosed, in various mixtures, with calomel (mercury chloride), potassium bromide (an anticonvulsive and sedative often used for epilepsy), brandy, migranin (a preparatory medicine), more trinitrine, morphine, chloral (a sedative with hypnotic effects), senega (a stomach irritant), antipyrin (an analgesic known to cause rashes and cyanosis), cannabis tincture, phenacetin (an analgesic), and two potent plant extracts—digitalis (from foxglove) and belladonna (from deadly nightshade). Annie was also given exalgine, a substance often prescribed for neuralgia and migraine, although its safety and dosage had been much debated during the 1890s, after several cases of poisoning. On 29 May, Anne received cannabis for the last time. A day later she was discharged, after becoming "mentally affected" for the previous three or four days. She had "imagined that the other patients were always talking about her and discussing her private affairs." She had also taken a "strong dislike" to the night nurse and night sister and seen "funny wriggly animals round the bed." Regretfully noting that she had previously been of "a particularly nice disposition," the physicians discharged her. It is hard not to conclude that this change in her personality must have had something to do with the cocktail of drugs that she had been given over the previous six weeks.

Conclusion

In 1897, Samuel Potter's *Handbook of Materia Medica* recommended antipyrin as "the most single valuable remedy for headache, especially in migraine." Depending on the type of symptoms or the constitution of the patient, the book also suggested the use of phenacetin, belladonna, cannabis, camphor, croton-chloral, caffeine, valerian, ammonium chloride, potassium bromide, ergot, menthol, arsenic, aconitine, amyl nitrite, sanguinaria, nux vomica, cimicifuga, or a rubber bandage.[57] In contrast, a volume of standard pharmaceutical formulas published by *Chemist and Druggist* in 1904 simply listed antifebrin, phenacetin, and caffeine as the three recommended substances for treating migraine.[58] Behind this authoritative, simple statement lay a history of theorizing, guessing, and experimentation on patients like Annie. Desperation sent them to famous neurologists such as William Gowers, John Hughlings Jackson, and their colleagues, but the role that the patients' pained bodies played in the development of these new drugs was swiftly forgotten as the casebook pages turned to record new life stories. It was, of course, the "objective" work of Gowers's brain that was immortalized in his eponymous migraine mixture, not the subjective pain of bodies like Annie's.

During the nineteenth century, there had been radical changes in how migraine was thought of and treated. For centuries, physicians and patients had shared a common language and perception of megrim, bilious headaches, and sick headaches that reflected the long legacy of humoral theory. As physicians embraced nervous physiological theories from the eighteenth century onward, however, they increasingly presented their patients as holding "deep-rooted," "loose," and "conventional" notions that made the latter's statements untrustworthy. By the middle of the nineteenth century—at least in professional medical discourse—migraine had become an affliction firmly associated with a whole range of functional nervous disorders, in particular, the problems of exhausted young women. Institutions such as the Sussex County Lunatic Asylum and the National Hospital provided physicians with a wide range of opportunities for neurological, psychiatric, and pharmaceutical innovation, and migraine was just one of many ailments that attracted researchers' interest. As professional and lay medical knowledge diverged by the end of the century, new explanations and treatments for migraine that emerged from such settings laid the foundations for twentieth-century approaches to migraine's relationship with class and gender.

In the early twenty-first century, the lawn in the center of Queen Square is shaded by trees and encircled by wooden benches dedicated to patients, doctors, and staff of the hospitals that surround it. Plaques commemorate inspiring clinicians, night sisters, nurses, beloved babies, teenagers, grandfathers, and residents, as well as staff from the Homeopathic Hospital who were among 118 people killed in the Trident air disaster in 1972. At the southern end of the garden, a life-sized statue of Sam the cat jumps over a wall, and an ice cream van parks just past the children's intensive care ambulance. Patricia Finch's sculpture of a mother holding a baby, and the hum of the Mobile MRI Scanner Unit outside the National Hospital, remind visitors of the discoveries, grief, fear, and joy that this remarkable corner of London must have witnessed. It is here that patients, relatives, and staff have waited, contemplated, wept, rested, and endured. It is not possible to follow Elizabeth, Janet, Augustus, and Annie after their discharge from the National Hospital. We cannot know whether their relief from migraine was short lived, or how their future lives played out as they continued to try and manage work, families, and illness. As they descended the hospital's steps onto Queen Square, perhaps they, too, sat for a while in the garden, gathering their strength before returning into the throng of the metropolis.

CHAPTER SIX

"As Sharp as If Drawn with Compasses"

*Victorian Vision, Men of Science, and the Making
of Modern Migraine*

Mr. Beck's Aura, 1895

In June 1895, Dr. William Gowers presented a portrait of a bearded older man, sitting underneath a strange zigzag arc that looked almost like a halo, to the audience of the British Ophthalmological Society's prestigious annual Bowman Lecture (fig. 6.1). At the bottom of the picture, the artist, Mr. Beck, had explained that this was his migraine aura: "The phenomenon shows itself in the butiful colours of the rainbow circuling round the head in the zig-zag form as appeared before me siting in my room." The self-portrait was one of many he had produced during his five years as an outpatient at the National Hospital for the Paralysed and Epileptic in London. Beck had first been treated in the hospital at the age of sixty, and he had presented the collection of drawings to Gowers in the form of a book. Gowers recounted Beck's explanation of another aura that occurred when he sat down to dinner with two friends: "The zig-zag spectrum, coloured red and blue, suddenly appeared, surrounding the edge of the plate before him." Beck had hesitated, and then continued, "As I looked curious and nervous, Mrs. B—— said, 'Why do you not carve?' On taking my eyes off the plate I said to them, 'The zigzag rainbow colours are gone out of the window.' This was the first time my wife and friends believed I saw something very extraordinary."[1]

Gowers confessed that he did not quite know what to do with Mr. Beck's drawings. Beck, Gowers explained, was possessed "with the idea that these spectra were objective things, and he delighted in depicting them in the fashion of an engineering draughtsman." Yet the visions were not real, and Mr. Beck posed a conundrum. By trade, he was a mechanical engineer and an inventor. Thus Gowers considered him "a member of our own profession."

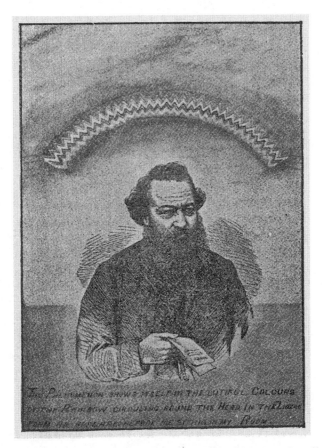

Fig. 6.1. Mr. Beck's "Arched Spectrum," figure 8 from W. R. Gowers, "Subjective Visual Sensations," 1895. Courtesy of the Wellcome Library, London, licensed under CC-BY

Their precise execution rendered Beck's illustrations "in some points trustworthy," but the "rather quaint descriptions" of his perception of the aura as a real thing—not to mention his desire for the drawings to be brought to the notice of Queen Victoria (we can well imagine the laughs that would have rippled through the gentlemanly audience of the Ophthalmological Society at this statement)—meant that his drawings could only be seen as a "curious" record, rather than an authoritative one.

As he continued his lecture, Gowers turned to another set of sketches, also of migraine aura, that were the work of a physician named Hubert Airy. He emphasized the reliability of these elaborate and precise illustrations, their accuracy supported by notes that Airy had made at the time. Airy's observations, Gowers believed, had "very great weight" as scientific records that could help show how vision worked, because they gave rare evidence of visual activity, rather than loss. As he concluded his lecture, Gowers reminded his audience once again of Hubert Airy's entirely "trustworthy" diagrams. Gowers donated both Beck's book and Airy's images to the Ophthalmological Society as a "unique collection of facts," which he hoped might attract others to add similar items.[2] A few months later, the secretaries of the society used the letters pages of the *British Medical Journal* in an appeal to members of the profession to contribute written accounts, drawings, and diagrams of the visual symptoms of migraine to the nascent collection, so "valuable information might be obtained."[3]

The first half of this chapter traces the discussions about transiently defective vision that elite men of science and medicine, such as Sir John Herschel, David Brewster, Hubert Airy, and Edward Liveing, engaged in during the second half of the nineteenth century. In doing so, it examines how one image of a single symptom—Hubert Airy's diagram of his aura—came to define an accurate, authentic, authoritative migraine experience. The dominance of Airy's image is significant, because it eclipsed other drawings (such as Beck's) and, hence, other ways of representing migraine, which were largely forgotten. This chapter argues that Airy's depiction of aura needs to be understood as a scientific "working object."[4] A working object, as historians Lorraine Daston and Peter Galison have argued in their important study of the history of the idea of scientific objectivity, is an "image of record" (often published in large format, on expensive paper, in color) that makes collective empiricism possible. Working objects teach scientists "what is worth looking at, how it looks, and perhaps most important of all, how it should be looked at." Airy's knowledge was objective in the sense that he insisted human frailties and foibles (in his case, the distraction of pain and nausea) had not contaminated the production of the aura.[5] Airy's image, and those drawn by other men of science, helped create the idea that a particular type of migraine was a characteristic of a scientific person. Understanding how this came about, at the same time as physicians talked in general of migraine being a problem of young women, helps reveal how certain notions of gender, class, and intellect became central to understandings of migraine into the twentieth century.

Scientific Vision

As we have already seen, there is occasional evidence, though little that is definitive, of disordered vision being associated with migraine for centuries.

The banns of a fifteenth-century itinerant leech described "mygreyn" as taking "half a man's head and causing him to lose the sight of his eye." In 1627, Francis Bacon's use of the word "obtenebration" to imply a darkening or shadowing is also suggestive, if ambiguous. Eighteenth-century physicians from continental Europe were the first to discuss visual symptoms as part of the migraine experience in any great detail. In 1780, famous Swiss physician Samuel Auguste David Tissot devoted a long chapter to the study of migraine in *Traité des nerfs et leurs maladies*. He identified migraine as occupying only one side of the head, principally the front, in the eye and the temple, and also as being distinguished by the violence of the pain and its frequent recurrence. Tissot described the case of a thirty-two-year-old Austrian military officer, who had experienced migraine since the age of nine:

> It starts in the eyes; when I least expect it, I see all of a sudden, more on one side than the other, like a person who has looked at the sun. This lasts about ten minutes; followed by an arm and a leg of the same side, one day on one side and one day on the other, they fall asleep. I feel shivers as if there were ants; I have the same feeling in the mouth and tongue, and during this time, I have a lot of trouble speaking. This lasts about half an hour; then the pains in my head begin, but only in the temples, where they persist with great strength for seven or eight hours. When I can vomit, this relieves me.[6]

London physician John Fothergill's account of sick headache, dating from December 1778, is commonly seen as the first clear English-language account of migraine being associated with visual disturbance. In his treatise on sick headache, Fothergill recounted "a singular kind of glimmering in the sight; objects change their apparent position, surrounded with luminous angles, like those of a fortification. Giddiness comes on, headache, and sickness."[7] In 1802, William Heberden portrayed hemicrania as "what follows that mist before the eyes which makes a part of every object invisible."[8] More than two decades later, Caleb Hillier Parry described how he often experienced a "sudden failure of sight," particularly when he was tired, with a semiopaque cloud "on one side of the direct line of vision," lasting from twenty to thirty minutes. Its upper part "appeared bounded by an edging of light of a zig-zag shape, and coruscating nearly at right angles to its length." This was still perceptible with both eyes shut. Although Parry never experienced headache, these clouds seemed to be connected to the state of his stomach.[9] In the 1830s, French physician Gabriel Andral noted that patients often experienced a troubled sense of vision: "Dazzling lights are very commonly seen, and sometimes the sight is even lost for a time before the migraine commences."[10] Andral's theo- ries were reprinted in England's medical press, but, apart from these few oft- quoted examples, British physicians seem to have taken little notice of visual symptoms and did not assert a clear relationship between migraine and dis- tortions of vision until much later in the century. They seemed much more interested in making assumptions about migraine in relation to women's re- productive problems. To understand how, when, and why visual disturbances became an integral part of the common language of migraine in English—not until the 1870s—we must look beyond the medical sphere, to the science of light.

On 30 September 1858, the day after the close of that year's annual meeting of the British Association for the Advancement of Science, Sir John Herschel, renowned British mathematician, astronomer, chemist, and inventor of the term photograph, gave a lecture on "Sensorial Vision" to the Philosophical and Literary Society of Leeds. It was a very personal talk, following a difficult decade for him. Herschel's health had declined, and he increasingly turned to opium and laudanum to try and reduce his pains.[11] In his lecture, Herschel spoke of "ocular spectra," which he explained as temporary disturbances to sight, including the impressions produced by strong light on the retina of the eye. Herschel also talked about the images of faces that he saw, "sometimes ten or a dozen appear in succession," as well as the landscapes he visualized more rarely, but much more distinctly, when his eyes were closed.[12]

There was another class of ocular spectra for which Herschel did not have an explanation, but for which the meaning of "spectra"—as something ghostly, unsubstantial, or unreal—seems fitting. One morning, while he sat at his breakfast table, he had been startled by a "singular shadowy appearance" that appeared at the outside corner of his left field of vision. As it advanced into his full field of view, it "appeared to be a pattern in straight-lined angular forms, very much in general aspect like the drawing of a fortification, with salient and re-entering angles, bastions and ravelins, with some suspicion of faint lines of colour between the dark lines." These visual impressions ap- peared to be geometric and regular; sometimes the forms were perfectly sym- metrical, in a lattice pattern. Very occasionally, Herschel saw "complex and coloured patterns like those of a carpet." He spoke of the "Turkscap pattern" he had witnessed in 1855, when under the influence of chloroform, as two surgeons operated on an abscess in his leg. Herschel told his audience that although he had mentioned these visions to several people, he had only ever met one other person to whom the phenomenon had occurred, although she always found that a violent headache followed, which Herschel did not experience.[13] He speculated on what these effects might be. They were evidently neither dreams nor memories, nor could they be fleeting impressions on the retina. Perhaps, he mused, the sensorium—the part of the brain that responded to and interpreted stimuli—possessed a kaleidoscopic power to form regular patterns. Herschel apologized for saying so much about himself and his personal experiences, but he believed that the nature of these things would only be discovered if individuals put their personal experiences on record.[14]

Herschel's private diary, now held at the Royal Society of London, contains more evidence of the visual disturbances that he discussed in Leeds. In June 1846, he had woken in the morning, and as he lay trying to remember his dream, a large, well-defined, ivory-colored circular spectrum "began to appear and grew every instant more vivid till at length it grew so bright I became alarmed & opened my eyes." Since the sun was not shining into the room, and there was no other object that would explain the impression, Herschel closed his eyes to watch it: "It faded rapidly after one or two alternations of colour to bluish & purple as a natural spectrum would have done."[15] In the margin of his diary, he drew the shape he had seen. Herschel seems to have experienced a range of different effects, including a double halo, one that was entirely black, and the "perfect Turkshead pattern" he mentioned in the lecture, "as sharp as if drawn with compasses."[16] In 1865, during a "feverish night." Herschel described "visual impression of a most beautiful landscape," complete with trees and boats on the water. In the decade after his lecture in Leeds, as he continued his work on sunspots, Herschel's visual disturbances became more frequent and were an uncomfortable reminder of his aging senses. In July 1866, the fortification pattern appeared two days in a row. "I suppose I shall go blind," he concluded.[17]

Other men of science besides Herschel had written of their visual defects, but his discussions were more than personal musings on visual fragility. Instead, they provided opportunities to theorize about the physics of light and optics and the physiology of vision. In 1824, William Hyde Wollaston described how, after taking some "violent" exercise, he "suddenly found that I could see but half the face of a man whom I met; and it was the same with respect to every object I looked at. In attempting to read the name JOHNSON over a door, I saw only SON.... This blindness was a shaded darkness ... without definite outline." Wollaston thought these temporary episodes of half blindness were far more common than generally recognized and commented that he had recently heard of two more cases of the disease: a friend who had regularly experienced it for sixteen or seventeen years, whenever his stomach was "deranged" through indigestion, and another man who suffered half blindness and a headache, always lasting about twenty minutes.[18] For Wollaston, his incidences of "diseased vision" over a period of twenty years afforded him a chance to contribute to a long-running debate about the structure of the optic nerves within the human body.[19]

A few years after Herschel's lecture in Leeds, the natural philosopher and inventor of the kaleidoscope, David Brewster, also thought that hemiopsy, or half blindness, might shed light on the workings of human vision by establishing the optical condition of the eye during such episodes. Because "there is neither darkness nor obscurity" during an ordinary case of hemiopsy, Brewster deduced that the retina must still be sensitive to light, but not to the lines and shades of the pictures it was receiving. Thus Brewster rejected any idea that hemiopsy was connected to cerebral disturbance and instead argued that it was a result of distended blood vessels in the retina: in his case, a result of straining to read the small print of the [London] *Times* newspaper.[20] Brewster's comments on hemiopsy prompted the Astronomer Royal, George Biddell Airy, to write to the editors of the *Philosophical Magazine and Journal*. He, too, had been frequently attacked by hemiopsy—at least twenty times, and "probably much oftener." As Wollaston and François Arago had done, Airy commented that he knew of other cases: an acquaintance had suffered from it over a hundred times, while another friend blamed mental anxiety or the pressure of business for his attacks. Airy drew a sketch to explain what his hemiopsy looked like: a series of zigzag arcs, radiating from a central point of origin, to show its expansion across the visual field for over twenty to thirty minutes. Airy likened the zigzags to "the ornaments of a Norman arch," only somewhat sharper and becoming deeper over time. He couldn't decide whether the disease affected both eyes, or whether the "tremor and boiling" on one side was simply so oppressive that it cancelled out the vision in the other.[21]

One way to see these discussions about ocular spectra is as part of a long association of physical frailty with genius, overwork, and the stimulation of reading and writing. In the eighteenth century, William Buchan had declared intense thinking to be "so destructive to health, that few instances can be produced of studious persons who are strong and healthy." Even a few months of intense study might "ruin an excellent constitution" by inducing a train of permanent nervous complaints, including gout, stone, jaundice, indigestion, hypochondria, and consumption. Long bouts of thinking often induced "grievous head-achs, which bring on vertigoes, apoplexies, palsies, and other fatal disorders." Buchan advised that those who found their eyes sore, particularly after working by candlelight, should bathe them in cold water with a little added brandy.[22] There was better news for astronomers, however. In *The Infirmities of Genius*, physician Richard Robert Madden declared that natural philosophers, particularly astronomers, were the least likely to fall victim to an early death because of their passion. Looking at the stars, it seemed, quite literally elevated the mind of a great man above the trivial concerns of humanity when he contemplated the magnificence of space, invigorating both thoughts and body.[23]

If the association of genius with physical infirmity was commonplace into the nineteenth century, these personal accounts of hemiopsy are striking in how carefully they denied any other kind of suffering apart from visual disturbances. David Brewster pointed out that his attacks "were never accompanied either with headache or gastric disturbance."[24] George Airy, too, observed that "in general, I feel no further inconvenience from it," although his friends often experienced "oppressive head-ache" after a visual disturbance.[25] Wilfred Airy's preface to his father's autobiography reaffirmed the Astronomer Royal's strong constitution and good health.[26] So what was hemiopsy to these men? It certainly wasn't a symptom of migraine or sick headache, as far as they were concerned. Rather, visual disturbance provided this generation of analytically minded men, often seen as the first modern scientists, with opportunities to gain insight into pressing questions about light, optics, vision, and the very workings of that most mysterious organ, the human brain. The strength of their attentive powers, the sensitivity of their vision, and the accuracy of their observations, unencumbered by the distracting effects of pain, was part of what made them authoritative as scientists.

Hubert Airy's Aura

In September 1866, two months after John Herschel confided to his diary his fear that he would lose his eyesight altogether, Hubert Airy, the Astronomer Royal's son, paid a four-day visit to Herschel at his home. Twenty-eight-year-old Hubert was a physician and, like both his father and John Herschel, often experienced visual disturbances. Airy and Herschel began to correspond on the subject. In February 1868, Airy visited the older man again. We can imagine them spending hours discussing and comparing their visual experiences, interspersed with excitement about the recent outbreak of spots on the surface of the sun. After Airy's departure, as Herschel returned to poring over his figures of the Orion nebulae, another fortification pattern "suddenly came on": an arc of red, blue and black. In May 1868, Hubert Airy sent his descriptions and pictures of the fortification spectrum he saw to Herschel. Herschel was impressed by the white pictures on a black background. Later in the day, as he read a book on the terrace, Herschel again realized he was witnessing a spectrum of his own. As usual, it obliterated his vision below and to the left of the visual field. "How strange!" Herschel commented in his diary entry, as he contemplated the apparently direct relation between the delivery of Airy's drawings and his own attack later in the day.[27]

Herschel's discussions with Hubert Airy, and perhaps seeing the younger man's own visual disturbances drawn in such detail, seem to have reassured the elderly astronomer that his symptoms did not mean inevitable blindness. Herschel continued to observe and study his own sensory experiences, recording the details in his diary, particularly the colors and shapes he saw (fig. 6.2). On 22 June 1869, the fortification pattern appeared twice:

> Colours red & black or red & yellow & black with little blue & at moments only black and white. Also a sort of chequer worked filling in in rectangular? patches & a carpet-work pattern over the rest of the visual area. The second & far the brightest largest & most beautiful in colouring was turned to the right. . . . Colours very vivid—red, blue, yellow, black, not sure of any green.

"Since I wrote to you," Herschel explained to Airy in a letter later that year, "I have been very frequently visited with the phenomenon in a greater or less degree." Although his visions no longer seemed to contain the vivid colors and distinct forms that he had earlier described, they now included some new features, such as "patches of a kind of coloured chequer work in some of the corners of the fortification forms." The vision always began "with a small glimmer *near* the middle of the field of view, and spreads out." Having carefully observed many of these events, Herschel was now confident that "it sometimes opens out from left to right, and sometimes from right to left."[28] Hubert Airy was convinced that these visual experiences promised to reveal something new and exciting about the workings of the mind, as well as being ones that natural philosophers such as Brewster, Herschel, and his own father were uniquely well qualified to comment on. These were men trained "by their habits of accurate observation to contemplate attentively any strange apparition, without or within." As men used to intense eye work, they were especially suited to the study of visual derangements, and they were an important

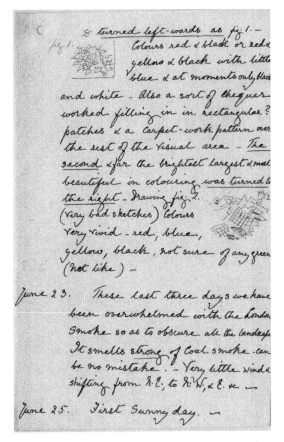

Fig. 6.2. John Herschel's diary, 22 June 1869, MS 583/4. © The Royal Society of London

source of evidence for the physician who, "unless personally subject to the malady, must depend, for his acquaintance with its phenomena, on the imperfect or exaggerated accounts of patients untrained to observe closely or record faithfully."[29] If natural philosophers were best placed to document such happenings, then, as a medical doctor, it was incumbent on Airy to assess their significance.

No doubt gaining confidence from Herschel's endorsement of and interest in the topic, on 17 February 1870, Hubert Airy presented his work on vision to a meeting of the Royal Society in Cambridge.[30] Rather than using the term ocular spectra, Airy preferred "transient hemiopsia" and, more specifically, "teichopsia"—literally "town-wall vision"—to describe the visual effect of angular bastions and fortifications. Airy devoted most of his paper to his personal experience of this visual phenomenon. He had first encountered it as a student in 1854, at the age of eighteen:

> In its height it seemed like a fortified town with bastions all around it, these bastions being coloured most gorgeously. If I put my pen into the space where there was this dimness, I could not see it at all, I could not even distinguish the colour of the ink at the end. All the interior of the fortification, so to speak, was boiling and rolling about in a most wonderful manner as if it was some thick liquid all alive.

Airy blamed "toilsome reading" for his attacks, particularly if he had not taken enough exercise. He had experienced hemiopsy a hundred times, and possibly many more, at intervals from a month or two right down to twice in an hour. In great detail, Airy recounted the expansion of the shape, initially from a blind spot in the center of his vision, enlarging at first with a "slow rolling heaving swaying motion to and fro," then with a rapid flickering tremor, until finally the edge of the cloud reached the edge of his vision and his sight was gradually restored from the center, twenty to twenty-five minutes after it began. Unusually, Hubert did admit to more than just visual weakness. As the boiling reached its height, he would feel the gradual onset of a headache, accompanied by nausea that would last for five or six hours. Nevertheless, Airy was careful to emphasize that in the early stages of the attacks, he felt no discomfort at all, and his mental faculties were free to observe the visual phenomenon "closely and carefully."[31]

So why did Airy think that indulging in a recital of his personal experiences was worthy of presentation to the Royal Society? Because, he concluded, this teichopsia was more than "merely" a disease. It could be regarded as "a veritable 'Photograph' of a morbid process going on in the brain."[32] Airy's use of the term photograph was sure to gain the attention of his audience, and it acknowledged the importance of his discussions with Sir John Herschel. These were people who understood scientifically objective photographs to be more than just pictures. They were a way to make invisible phenomena visible, such as ultraviolet light or the movement of birds in flight. Because photography was automatic and mechanical, it promised to break free from human interpretation, temptation, and will.[33] If the teichopsia itself was the photograph, then Airy saw himself as the camera. Our duty, he concluded in his paper, was to collect and record such facts, "in confidence that they will

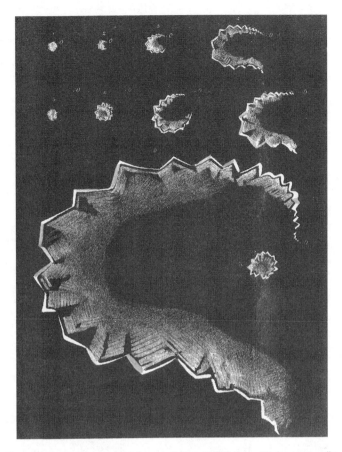

Fig. 6.3. "Diagram of Transient Teichopsia," plate XXV, from Hubert Airy, "On a Distinct Form of Transient Hemiopsia," 1870. © The Royal Society of London

arrange themselves into a theory sooner or later." That theory was to arrive sooner than even Airy might have imagined.

Airy's diagrams of his transient teichopsia were at the heart of his presentation in Cambridge (fig. 6.3), and they would also be dramatically reproduced when his lecture was published in the society's *Philosophical Transactions*. The plates were printed by London lithographer G. West & Company, who often produced images for the Royal Society's publications and specialized in large pullout plates.[34] That Airy's striking black background in these drawings echoed the astronomical interests of his audience, particularly Herschel, is unlikely to have been a coincidence. At the cutting edge of mechanically reproduced illustration, Airy's diagram took its place alongside some of the most famous scientific imagery of the time. From the moment of its publication, Airy's undeniably beautiful and instantly recognizable image embarked on a life as the standard bearer for judging authentic, accurate migraine experiences.

A Modern Megrim

Another young physician, Edward Liveing, was in the audience for Hubert Airy's presentation at the Cambridge meeting, and he was distinctly impressed by the young physician's careful observations, minute descriptions, and "excellent" drawings of the spectral appearances.[35] For several years, Liveing had been collecting material on a group of disorders he thought to be closely related, and he believed that the use of the word megrim in English had "cramped [rather] than extended our knowledge of a class of disorders" understood much more comprehensively in Europe. Liveing felt that in order to catch up with their continental colleagues, English physicians needed to better understand the natural and intimate alliance of a family of functional disorders that included sick, blind, and bilious headaches, epilepsy, asthma, and angina pectoris, all of which were characterized by paroxysms, or fits.[36] In this respect he disagreed with English physician John Addington Symonds, who, in his influential Gulstonian Lecture in 1858, had argued that sick headache was distinct from the hemicrania, or migraine, that had been "described so graphically and minutely by French authors." Migraine was characterized by the location of the pain and its intensity, recurrent nature, sense of anguish, "dimness of sight, or partial blindness," and noises in the ears (or even deafness).[37] Liveing did not believe it necessary to adopt a foreign term, however, so he proposed a revival of the vernacular English word megrim. In 1873, Liveing published *On Megrim*, a treatise that has come to be seen as a foundational moment in modern understandings of migraine.

Liveing was particularly struck by seventeenth-century English doctor Thomas Willis's description of a disease that could "pitch its tent very near the confines of the brain, and long besiege its Regal Tower yet not take it, leaving the faculties of the soul sound enough."[38] Rejecting the gastric and bilious theories of writers such as Fothergill and Tissot that had been so dominant in the late eighteenth and early nineteenth centuries, Liveing understood megrim as a nervous affliction, one of a group of disorders caused by the tendency of an unstable nervous system to gradually and irregularly accumulate tension, and then explosively discharge this "nerve-force" in a "nerve-storm." For a time, equilibrium would be restored, but then the cycle would begin again.[39] Based on clinical observation, Liveing saw the paroxysms of migraine, epilepsy, or asthma as analogous to sneezing, coughing, or vomiting.[40] Liveing also drew on continental ideas about the importance of emotion as a causative factor in the timing of attacks. He quoted Tissot: "It does not seem in fact to matter much what the character of the emotion is, provided it be strongly felt."[41] Liveing often provided examples from his patients' accounts, where they explained how fright, anxiety, mental distress, and anger preceded their attacks. Liveing also noticed that strong emotions—such as anxiety, dread, depression, ill humor, or "reckless despondency"—could either accompany or act as premonitory symptoms of an attack.[42]

When working men suffered from megrim, Liveing blamed the exhaustion of "excessive hours of labour" or close confinement in "the unwholesome and ill-ventilated workshops and dwellings of our crowded towns." In these cases, the treatment was obvious, if difficult to administer: a nutritious diet, a check on the causes of exhaustion, and the prescription of tonic and restorative remedies. For men of "a somewhat higher social grade," excessive brain work was generally to blame. This included studying, literary composition, and work in legal chambers or the countinghouse, as well as the strain from prolonged anxiety and disappointments that accompanied ambition, competition, and the excitement of university, business, and professional life. For women, the emotional causes of megrim lay in "the narrower sphere of domestic life, in the anxious forecasting and much serving, which slowly undermine the nervous energies of many wives and mothers." Under the accumulating weight of family cares, the female nervous system was in danger of breaking down. In short, Liveing emphasized that nervous strain affected men and women differently, acting on the intellectual faculties in men and the affective faculties in women. Any medical treatment would be useless unless underlying errors in the "moral and material conditions of life" were corrected through rest, diet, exercise, and, ideally, a change of locality or climate. When women were affected, Liveing felt that medical men were duty bound to insist on a temporary absence from home. The implication was not just that these women did not have anyone around them who was competent to help, but, since they were so used to relying on their own resources and experience, even when there were people with "latent capabilities" who could assist, the women would rarely delegate tasks. Enforced separation left others

with no choice but to take on this responsibility.[43] By identifying women themselves as being at fault, Liveing's work opened the door for twentieth-century
ideas about the migraine personality.

Yet it is the focus on the experiences of intellectual men that stands out
from Liveing's account. Andrew Levy has suggested that Edward Liveing created a "cultural portfolio" for migraine.[44] In particular, his ideas about the
kinds of people who were particularly at risk from megrim had both class and
gender implications that would persist into the twentieth century. Throughout *On Megrim*, Liveing referred to Hubert Airy's paper, and he found plenty
of opportunities to diagnose the men of science who had talked of their visual
disturbances in previous decades. Liveing believed that John Herschel, who
had recently died, suffered from the "purely visual" form of megrim. George
Biddell Airy, he suggested, had "simple visual megrim without headache,"
while Hubert was "liable to the same affection together with nausea, headache,
and perhaps other symptoms." The father-son relationship of George and
Hubert Airy was particularly important, as the influence of heredity added
weight to Liveing's argument about the close affinity of different forms of
nerve-storm seizure.[45]

In *The Lancet*, a review of Liveing's *On Megrim* noted the "excellent chromo-
lithograph" of Airy's spectral images, which had been taken from the original
publication of Airy's paper in *Philosophical Transactions*. Liveing reproduced
one of Airy's images from the 1870 paper as a double-page pullout, in full
color, placed at the end of the volume, between the index and the analytical
table of cases. Airy's image was more than illustrative, since Liveing used it as
a standard against which to judge other patients' accounts.

In the same year as Liveing's *On Megrim* appeared, another Cambridge
physician, Peter W. Latham, published two lectures he had given at Adden-
brooke's Hospital on the topic of "nervous or sick headache," and he later
defended his ideas in the *British Medical Journal*.[46] Latham advanced a different theory from Liveing. He believed that migraine's visual aura could be
explained by a contraction of the blood vessels of the brain, and the headache
that followed was brought on by dilatation of the same vessels. Influenced by
recent work on the sympathetic nervous system, Latham suggested that the
cause of sick headache could be attributed to a range of problems resulting
from "exhausted powers" and functional disharmony that could irritate the
nerves. This could include violent emotions or gastric derangement; hence
the apparent relationship of sick headache or bilious headache with the stomach or intestines.[47] "Perhaps in an University town," Latham commented, the

disorder "may be more prevalent among males than in other places." As Liveing had done, Latham devoted substantial space to reprinting scientific discussions about visual disturbances. He, too, prominently reproduced one of Hubert Airy's diagrams, including it as the frontispiece to his book. Liveing's theory of nerve-storms and Latham's vascular theory came to define two separate schools of thought about the causes of migraine during the late nineteenth century.[48] But in other respects, there were striking similarities in the way they foregrounded the visual disturbances affecting intellectual men. Whichever side of the theoretical fence you fell on—vascular or nervous— Airy's personal experience was presented as a visual shorthand for the accurate representation of migraine, a disorder that had suddenly gained cultural and medical prestige through its association with genius, science, and the intellectual elite.

The Social Profile of Megrim

In the decades after 1873, supporters of Liveing's and Latham's theories would fall into two camps. Proponents of Latham's vasomotor theory, believing that migraine was caused by a contraction of the vessels of the head and anemia of the brain, tended to deny the resemblance between migraine and epilepsy, and they rejected the idea that the two disorders could pass into one another. On the other hand, Liveing's epileptic hypothesis of migraine—that its cause lay in an as yet undiscovered lesion in the pons and medulla—was widely supported.[49] Notably, Liveing's ideas about neurosis would influence Thomas Clouston and John Hughlings Jackson's attempts to relate migraine to epilepsy. Jackson's study of Thomas R. from London's National Hospital for the Paralysed and Epileptic is a good example.[50] Jackson presented the case as an instructive example of hemiplegia, or one-sided paralysis, due to a lesion in the brain. He suspected that somewhere in Thomas's head, there was a "grave" lesion, probably a clot. In particular, Jackson was looking for a lesion that might explain migraine.[51] The case, he proposed, might help explain those "remarkable" cases of migraine which involved symptoms of temporary hemiopia and one-sided sensation disorders.

In an influential article considering the relationship between migraine, gout, and epilepsy, Clifford Allbutt hypothesized that all three of these disorders were characterized by a gradual increase in tension and a sudden release of energy. Allbutt praised physicians such as Edward Liveing, Francis Anstie, and German physiologist Emil du Bois-Reymond for reasserting migraine's place among the neuroses and rescuing it from the humoral doctrine of biliousness. Allbutt believed that the presence of migraine was a useful test for an inherited neurotic diathesis, or susceptibility, within families. "Migraines in such cases are like springs here and there in the land, which indicate the main direction of the subsoil water," he explained. Hemiopia, vertigo, vague dreads, yawning, sensations of bitterness or thirst, and constipation were all "shadows" of migraine, whether or not they were accompanied by hemicrania.[52]

One of Liveing's theories was that the excessive generation or retention of uric acid in the body might be a possible culprit in migraine.[53] In the following decades, this idea that a toxic condition of the blood might poison nervous centers and cause megrim gained traction, and it helped account for migraine's apparent relation to gout. The main proponent of the uric acid theory was London physician Alexander Haig, a keen supporter of Liveing, who believed that a huge array of functional and organic diseases, including migraine headaches, were the result of excess uric acid in the body.[54] For Haig, a "uric acid headache" was the same thing as Liveing's megrim. The high blood pressure produced by uric acid obstructed the peripheral vessels and acted on the "unyielding membranes of the brain," which accounted for the pain. Haig suffered from migraine himself and described his own flickering fortification pattern: a "flashing of light on quickly rippling water." He believed he could produce migraine "at pleasure" by using drugs such as acids, opium, antipyrin, or mercury to produce a fluctuation in the body's excretion of uric acid, and, more importantly, quickly cure it (in around an hour) by raising the acidity of the urine to prevent excessive excretion of uric acid. Both Haig's children suffered from headache with aura until, he claimed, they had been cured by diet. Haig proposed that "poisoning" by eating meat and drinking tea produced headache, particularly in persons with large arteries supplying blood to the brain, which also explained the intellectual superiority of migraine sufferers.[55] Haig recommended taking calomel or morphine at the time of an attack to clear uric acid out of the blood and to prevent an accumulation of uric acid between attacks, particularly by avoiding animal foods, soups, and extracts.[56]

During the late nineteenth century, migraine was discussed in relation to a whole range of nervous disorders. Perhaps the most significant of these was neurasthenia. The term had been coined by New York neurologist George Beard to describe an "American disease" of nerve weakness, or nerve exhaustion, that affected the "in-door classes" and "brain-working households," particularly in professional men, who were burned out by the pace and pressure of life in modern civilized countries.[57] Neurasthenia could manifest as an array of symptoms, including dizziness, tiredness, insomnia, headaches, digestive disorders, tooth decay, and general illness. Beard was careful to distinguish the new, modern disease of neurasthenia from illnesses that had been around for centuries, such as epilepsy and hysteria. Importantly, Beard saw neurasthenia as a physiological, rather than a psychological disorder, an accompaniment to modernity that helped make it culturally acceptable, even respectable.[58]

Sick headache played an important role in Beard's neurasthenic concept as both "a symptom and a safety valve." It allowed nervousness to manifest itself and, if not too severe, prevent the development of worse affections. Sick headache was often the most visible symptom of nervous exhaustion and, for Beard, was something of a red flag. Patients would come to him convinced they suffered no other symptom, before further examination revealed "an army of troubles which had annoyed and followed them for years." These symptoms would come and go, brought on by emotional disturbance, confinement in hot or airless rooms, or mental labor.[59] Because of the subjectivity of the symptoms, Beard observed that neurasthenic patients often had difficulty persuading others of the seriousness of their ailments. While the patient who experienced an attack of sick headache could be "without hope," friends "laugh at his fears and ridicule him for talking or thinking of his symptoms."[60] Noting that *Cannabis indica* had "revolutionized" treatment of sick headache, he even went so far as to suggest it offered a permanent cure. Beard predicted that cannabis would soon become one of neurology's "major divinities," and he used it for a variety of neurasthenic and allied afflictions. While Beard recommended caffeine for temporary relief at the beginning of a sick headache attack, he warned that excessive drinking of tea or coffee could provoke a sick headache, to which he gave the name caffeinism.[61] Beard argued that although neurasthenia was more frequent in women, it was to be found "in great abundance" in both sexes, "and in both men and women of intellect, education, and well-balanced mental organizations."[62]

Liveing had emphasized that for men, ignoring the warning signs of sick headache risked more formidable attacks of apoplexy, epilepsy, and mania.[63] By the 1890s, physicians in Britain were falling over themselves to diagnose all manner of frightening social and hereditary ills arising from modern life. Thomas Clifford Allbutt, an influential supporter of the neurasthenia label, believed nervous disorders extended to wage earners throughout society, even to inmates of the workhouse.[64] James Crichton-Browne, who for ten years had been director of the West Riding Lunatic Asylum, believed that although men were more prone to organic diseases of the nervous system, women suffered more from functional disorders, including "epilepsy, neuralgia, hysteria in all its protean shapes, chorea, migraine, [and] neurasthenia."[65] W. Bolton Tomson articulated an evolutionary argument for the apparent correlation between the rise of neuroses—including megrim—and modernity. "Neurotic patients abound in all highly cultured communities," he observed. "From the standpoint of the evolutionist, instability of the highest nerve centres is due to their being the most recently evolved, and is therefore a necessary evil accompanying an intellectual advancement."[66]

In 1888, in an article for *The Lancet*, Samuel Wilks wrote:

> The migrainous patient frequently belongs to the most cultivated and intellectual class of society, and is of the temperament called neurasthenic, whilst the epileptic, in my experience, belongs to a lower grade, and is generally the stupid one of the family; if indeed, his fits are not associated with other grave defects of his nervous system. There is no lunatic or idiot asylum without its numerous epileptics, whereas some of the best descriptions of migraine are to be found in the *Philosophical Transactions*, given by the authors themselves.... I will not go as far as to absolutely endorse an opinion expressed by more than one observant medical man, that migraine is never met with amongst the lower orders, although it is difficult to conceive how such services as those of policemen or engine-drivers could go on were it at all common amongst the working community.[67]

Samuel Wilks has been described as the grand old man of British medicine. He was a prolific author, originator of the term Hodgkin's disease, president of the Royal College of Physicians of London, and physician extraordinary to Queen Victoria. He was also a great believer in the value of potassium bromide to treat his own migraine.[68] Here, however, he exploited the cultural cache that migraine had accumulated to denigrate the sufferers of epilepsy. In his comments, gender was invisible, but his assumptions about working people suggest a profound ignorance of and lack of care for the lives of the people on whose experiences advances in neurological understanding and pharmaceutical innovation relied in institutions such as London's National Hospital. Wilks's prejudice toward epilepsy, masquerading as medical insight, also ignored the observations and the critique of dangerous working conditions that had been an important part of Edward Liveing's account of migraine.

If there was one point that physicians did agree on, it was that migraine was hereditary and usually appeared at a young age. Estimates of the prevalence of migraine within families had gradually increased over the preceding half century. In 1858, Symonds reported that 44 percent of the people with migraine stated that one or both parents had the disorder. In 1873, Liveing estimated 50 percent, and by 1912, one researcher suggested nearly 100 percent.[69] In childhood, the symptoms were often abdominal, with pain, vomiting, and constipation. Once the condition was established, it continued throughout adulthood before diminishing around the age of fifty, or with the ending of menstruation for women. It was not clear why this should be, but one theory held that as the arteries hardened with age, the patient would become protected from the vasomotor disturbances that seemed to provoke the symptoms.[70] This nervous inheritance was not necessarily direct; it might appear in one generation as migraine, and in another as asthma. The question of morbid heredity was made more complicated, prominent British psychiatrist Henry Maudsley explained, because of the tendency for nervous diseases to "blend, combine, or replace one another." Epilepsy in the parent might manifest as insanity in the child, or vice versa. A whole range of incarnations, including neuralgia, suicide, mania, melancholy, or remarkable artistic talent, might reveal a familial predisposition to insanity. So, too, "neuralgic headaches or megrims, various spasmodic movements or *tics*, asthma and allied spasmodic troubles of breathing will oftentimes be discovered to own a neurotic inheritance or to found one." Maudsley saw the neurotic diathesis as fundamental, but it had various outcomes. This was particularly the case with "functional" diseases that displayed no evidence of an organic pathological state.[71] For children of a nervous disposition, school was a particularly dangerous place to be in such a formative period. While British children seemed to be less at risk from "over-exertion of the mind" than their counterparts in France and Germany, James Crichton-Browne railed against the "evil consequences" of educational pressure and brain fatigue, which could cause headaches, sleeplessness, night terrors, epilepsy, and hallucinations among the young. Indeed, he saw schools as veritable factories of stupidity.[72] As we will see in chapter 8, these discussions about the relationship between health, intelligence, and nervous inheritance would take on new significance in the twentieth century, as concerns about national degeneracy became a powerful influence in medicine, policy, and public opinion under the guise of the eugenic movement.

The late nineteenth century witnessed a number of contributions on the importance of gender in determining a person's tendency to migraine, and this discussion inherited a distinct stereotype. We find it first in the late eighteenth century, when William Buchan talked of wet nurses who suckled babies for too long as being particularly prone to hemicrania. In the 1850s, Patrick Murphy evoked the lower-class female martyr, her body "hourly drained by lactation." In 1873, Edward Liveing identified seamstresses and "poor women exhausted from over-suckling" as the particular victims of megrim.[73] It is significant, therefore, to find precisely the same categories in George Beard's discussion of neurasthenia. For Beard, it was overworked housewives who were most prone to neurasthenic melancholia, as well as "mothers, worn by repeated child-bearing and prolonged lactation."[74]

Edward Liveing criticized writers who assumed, with insufficient evidence, that women constitutionally had a greater predisposition to nervous affections than men, but he admitted that it did seem as if women were "slightly" more likely to have megrim than men. Helpfully, Liveing quantified "slightly" as a ratio of five to four, and he recognized that for many women, migraine recurred each month, with menstruation. While admitting a "distinct catamenial influence," Liveing nevertheless considered this to only be a minor factor, compared with a nerve-storm.[75] For her Paris MD thesis, "Sur la migraine," Elizabeth Garrett Anderson had observed the women who attended her medical practice in 20 Upper Berkeley Street, London, and St. Mary's Dispensary for Women and Children, which she had opened in 1866. Although she found that migraine attacks often recurred during menstrual periods, Garrett Anderson did not venture an opinion on whether that made women inherently more susceptible. The main message was still that the disease often attacked "the most intelligent members of a neurotic family." In 1872, Dr. Lawson, of St. Mary's Hospital, curtly dismissed the need for any discussion, as "he does not think [sick headache] is more frequent in one sex than the other, and he is not aware that menstruation affects it in the slightest." The main duty of the physician, Lawson seemed to suggest, was simply to not make any promises to the patient that their complaint would not occur again.[76] For Samuel Wilks, gender was important, primarily because he believed that men and women should be prescribed different treatments: potassium of bromide for men, and the milder guarana for women (quite possibly reflecting Latham's recommendation that guarana was most useful for sick headache in persons "of a hysterical temperament").[77] In *Neurotic Disorders of Childhood*, Benjamin Rachford went further than most writers in commenting on the intersections of gender and class. Among the "poor and uneducated," he believed that migraine was four or five times as common among women as men. It was particularly prevalent among factory girls and tenement dwellers, because of their "indoor life, [and] lack of fresh air and sunlight." Unwholesome food and general ill health also contributed to a tendency toward migraine. Among the "rich and refined," however, women only slightly predominated, perhaps due to the influence of menstruation as a precipitating factor. For Rachford, the explanation for this gender and class disparity was thus not primarily biological, but social. Since laboring men tended to lead physically demanding outdoor lives, they were unlikely to experience migraine.[78]

William Gowers's two-volume *Manual of Diseases of the Nervous System*, published in 1888, has been called "the greatest large textbook on the subject ever written, and ever likely to be written."[79] Under the category of "General and Functional Diseases," Gowers devoted a chapter to migraine (he preferred the French term to the English word megrim), distilling state-of-the-art migraine knowledge at the end of the nineteenth century.[80] For Gowers, the "essential" and most distressing component of migraine was the headache. He described how the pain begins in a small spot and "often has a boring character, as if some instrument were being forced into the skull," before spreading across one side of the head and, often, both sides. Or it begins at the back of the head and extends forward to the temple, or in the middle of the head and then down one side, sometimes even to the neck and arm. To deal with migraine, increased rest, regular meals, and good diet were paramount. If drugs were required, Gowers recommended nitroglycerine, taken regularly during the intervals between attacks (similar to the way bromide was prescribed for epilepsy), rather than during the attack itself, when it was unlikely to be effective and might make the attack worse. During the migraine, "a good dose" of bromide could relieve pain, along with a tincture of Indian hemp. Other treatments included valerian and asafetida (as recommended by Latham). Strong tea and coffee, or a few drops of caffeine, might also provide relief. Gowers was dismissive of ergotin, since "all that a full dose ... does is to lessen the throbbing intensification of the pain." Guarana had been generally disappointing, electricity "is not often of service," faradism was harmful, and the value of galvanization "doubtful."[81]

Gowers was pessimistic that migraine's pathology could be revealed. Reminding his readers of the two chief theories, he considered Liveing's nerve-storm proposal to be a "somewhat inapt metaphor," but he was even less convinced by Latham, as "the difficulties in accepting the vasomotor explanation of the sensory symptoms are so great that it could only be admitted as a tenable hypothesis if there were no other explanation of the coincidence of the two phenomena." As far as Gowers was concerned, the physiological cause of the headache remained obscure, but seeing migraine as a derangement of nerve cells of the brain better explained its relation to other neuroses. Gowers placed great importance on the connection of migraine to other "neurosal" diseases, because of the possibility of a transition from one disorder to another, including neuralgia, laryngeal spasm, angina seizures, and "paroxysmal insanity." Epilepsy was of special interest, due to the common features it shared with migraine.[82] At the end of his life, Gowers revised his ideas about the relationship between migraine and epilepsy in *The Border-Land of Epilepsy*, now considering it extremely rare for one to develop into the other. Any conjunction between them must be indirect. Although both diseases were characterized by premonitory symptoms, these varied so greatly in duration and character that Gowers now believed the two conditions could not be related.[83]

Conclusion

For many modern neurologists, it is the 1870s—the combination of Liveing's magisterial treatise and Airy's beautiful depictions of aura—that marks the arrival of modern, neurological migraine. Mervyn Eadie argues that "Hubert Airy's one original neurological publication resulted in migraine with a visual aura becoming transformed from an occasional and relatively unimportant curiosity into a significant clinical entity in the medicine of English-speaking countries."[84] John R. Levene similarly describes Hubert Airy's paper as "the first truly systematic and comprehensive account [of migraine] to appear in the literature."[85] As we will see, Airy's image did not just ensure that migraine aura would be included in modern ideas about this disorder. It came to define a very narrow model for what a reliable first-hand representation of migraine should look like, even though there are a wide variety of manifestations of visual aura, including dots, clouds, a corona, or a simple loss of vision.[86] The value accorded to Airy's image came at the expense of other kinds of migraine experiences, including Mr. Beck's, and continues to have a profound effect today on the way neurologists *see* migraine.

Liveing's synthesis gave migraine a coherence and prominence in English-language medicine that it had not had before the 1870s. Yet, as neurologist and historian Mark Weatherall argues, Edward Liveing's theories are much more than "an ancestor to neural concepts." Claiming Liveing's account as the birth of modern neurological migraine requires us to "divest it of all its contemporary richness and depth."[87] One of the most overlooked aspects of Liveing's analysis has been his nuanced account of migraine's relationship to gender and class, which acknowledged the effects of poverty, overwork, and emotional strain in poorer communities. For Liveing, men of intellect were only one of several social groups that could be affected, but his prominent emphasis on Airy's aura, and other physicians' personal investment in the idea that migraine was a disorder of male intellectual superiority, minimized important insights that also had to compete with the social implications of a possible relationship between migraine and epilepsy, and the considerable influence of the concept of neurasthenia. While the diagnosis of neurasthenia largely disappeared by the 1920s, the idea persisted that a nervous disease might affect well-educated men under pressure at work, as well as women worn down by the anxieties of domestic responsibility. Twentieth-century ideas about migraineurs grew directly out of the cultural and social profile of migraine and the intellectual space that the demise of the concept of neurasthenia left vacant.

Throughout the late nineteenth century, observations about migraine's relationship to gender and class relied on stereotypes, anecdotal evidence, and assumptions gleaned from clinical experience. Victorian physicians, such as Hubert Airy and Alexander Haig, intermingled their personal experiences with their physiological and therapeutic observations. Migraine had to be a disease of intellect, drive, and ambition. Otherwise, how would they explain their own disposition (not to mention that of their children)? William Gowers's reluctance to admit Mr. Beck's images to the realm of trustworthy diagrams of aura showed how fervently some physicians believed that only a particular kind of person—a scientist or a physician—could be relied on to produce accurate accounts of lived experiences.

More than anything, the history of migraine in the second half of the nineteenth century, explored in this and the previous chapter, reveals how physicians shaped and then came to police the emergence of migraine's modern boundaries. Through their theories, discussions, and practices, these doctors defined which symptoms were in and which were out, as well as whose voices and subjective experiences were taken seriously, and whose were ignored. Ideas about migraine, and its relationship to other disorders, were shaped in large part by assumptions about class, gender, and education, as well as by the valorization of particular kinds of physiological experience. In his hugely influential treatise, William Gowers repeated Liveing's diagnosis of migraine's causes, including excessive brain work, fatigue, labor carried out in hot and crowded rooms, anemia, and excess lactation. Thus, while Gowers's publications present an undeniably *modern* account of migraine, containing most of the features that we recognize today, his work nevertheless cemented a key set of ideas about gender and class that had been developing over the nineteenth century.[88]

CHAPTER SEVEN

"A Shower of Phosphenes"

Twentieth-Century Stories and the Medical Uses of History

Discovering Hildegard of Bingen, 1913

In 1913, a young scientist and historian, Charles Singer, was in Germany researching precursors to modern theories of contagion.[1] In the library at Wiesbaden, a small city on the east bank of the river Rhine, he consulted the illuminated twelfth-century manuscript *Scivias*, which described twenty-six religious visions seen by Hildegard of Bingen, the celebrated abbess of the St. Rupertsberg convent.[2] When he saw the images in this extraordinary manuscript, he abandoned his work on contagion and devoted his attention to the stars, crenellated shapes, shining lights, fortification figures, and concentric circles that characterized the miniature illustrations of Hildegard of Bingen's religious visions (fig. 7.1). Writing about the moment later on, he recalled that he "recognised at once that the figures . . . resembled descriptions by patients of what they had seen during attacks of migraine."[3] Convinced that he was looking at scintillating scotoma and noting that Hildegard had admitted to long periods of illness, Singer retrospectively diagnosed a functional nervous disorder—specifically, migraine.[4]

In this chapter, I argue that Hildegard's migraine is a twentieth-century story that could only be possible after medical men began to regularly link visual aura with migraine in the late nineteenth century. Even though our ideas about migraine have changed considerably in the century since Singer made his observations about Hildegard, the idea of her migraine has endured, attaining the status of medical fact. Some medieval scholars have used Hildegard's migraine as evidence in attempts to settle questions about her remarkable life, including whether she was the designer of the *Scivias* illumi-

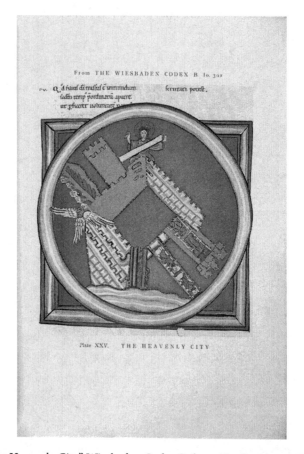

Fig. 7.1. "The Heavenly City," Wiesbaden Codex B, from Charles Singer, *Studies in the History and Method of Science*, 1917. The Wellcome Library, London, reproduced with thanks to Andrew Singer and Nancy Underwood, copyright holders

nations. Contributors to blogs and websites have proposed that Hildegard should be adopted as a patron saint of migraine and migraineurs.

Yet Hildegard's was not the only story about migraine's history to emerge in the first half of the century. I begin by examining Sir Lauder Brunton's proposal, dating from 1902, that trepanning had been an ancient treatment for migraine. The chapter concludes with the case of Anne Conway, another retrospectively diagnosed sufferer, whose migraine label dates from the 1930s. Physicians have often been tempted by the possibility of diagnosing historical figures with named modern conditions, using clues gleaned through the interpretation of texts, artifacts, images, and commentary. Was King George III's madness actually porphyria? Did Nietzsche have syphilis? Were Vincent Van Gogh's illnesses and suicide caused by epilepsy, neurosyphilis, bipolar disorder, schizophrenia, or the effects of absinthe? Since the eighteenth century, a variety of disorders—including madness, tertiary syphilis, vertigo, Ménière's disease, meningitis, dementia, aphasia, or stroke—have all been proposed as the cause of author Jonathan Swift's cognitive decline.[5] Historians, by contrast, have tended to dismiss a technique that seems to reduce the lives and minds of individuals to the expression of disease. Roger Cooter, for example, has disparaged retrospective diagnosis as "inherently condescending."[6] A good example of what's at stake is the discussion of whether women in the Middle Ages can be said to have had anorexia. Medieval historian Caroline Walker Bynum has criticized any assumption that we can apply secular or medical explanations to behavior previously regarded as religious. She explains that a number of medieval paradigms existed for not eating.[7] Other historians have pointed out that the validity of any diagnosis depends on which modern definition of an illness is chosen. I am not particularly concerned with whether or not Hildegard or Conway had migraine by any modern definition. Rather, I am interested in the role these stories have played in the creation of a particular way of thinking about migraine in the twentieth century.

It is no coincidence that all three of the stories considered in this chapter (trepanning, Hildegard, and Anne Conway) emerged in the first decades of the twentieth century. Historian Sally Shuttleworth has argued that medical writers have often used clinical legends for their own ends. When endowed with the authority of a professional diagnosis, these historical stories become transformed into cases.[8] Hildegard of Bingen's and Anne Conway's migraines are good examples of this phenomenon in practice. By examining how these three very common narratives in migraine's history first emerged, and showing the links between the three cases, this chapter illuminates the power of historical accounts to provide a grounding for uncertain medical knowledge. Moreover, they illustrate how influential such stories can be, particularly once they become detached from the sometimes tenuous evidence and contexts in which they were created.

Trepanning

If there is one stock stereotype in the history of migraine, it is that trepanning is one of the most ancient and enduring treatments for migraine. The word "trepanation" comes from the Greek *trypanon*, meaning "a borer." The word "trephine" dates from the seventeenth century and comes from the Latin *tres* (three) and *finis* (ends). Both denote the technique of removing bone by scraping, sawing, drilling, or chiseling.[9] The earliest known trepanned skulls date from around 10,000 BCE, in North Africa. There are accounts of the technique of drilling holes into skulls as a therapeutic measure in the Hippocratic corpus, when it was used mostly in cases of fracture, as well as for epilepsy or paralysis. In the second century, Galen also wrote of his experiments with trepanation on animals in his clinical studies.[10] But in general, the reasons for trepanning remain unknown, and there is a distinct lack of definite examples, particularly in relation to migraine. A fifteenth-century Ottoman source suggests that physicians may have treated chronic migraine surgically, by sectioning the superficial temporal artery, but this certainly does not imply trepanation.[11] While some neurologists have suggested that there is evidence "trephination was performed . . . as late as the seventeenth century," in his *London Practice of Physick*, published in 1685, Thomas Willis stated quite clearly that although William Harvey had suggested it, actually opening the skull with a "trepand iron" had been "tried as yet by none."[12] There is, however, one known example from the seventeenth century. A barber surgeon, Wilhelm Fabry von Hilden, used trepanation for chronic headache and as a treatment for depressed fractures, but recent authors have acknowledged that there is little evidence to suggest that trepanning has been carried out for migraine.[13] So where did this persistent idea come from?

In 1902, the *Journal of Mental Science* published a lecture by Sir Thomas Lauder Brunton, physician to St. Bartholomew's Hospital in London. He was well known for his work on pharmacology.[14] Brunton's lecture on visual and sensory perception was an eclectic mix of ocular and neurological theory, armchair anthropology, excitement about the potential of wireless telegraphy, and interest in the organic and pharmacological causes of defective vision. In it, he discussed premonitions, telepathy, hypnotism, and hallucinations before moving on to epileptic and migrainous aura. Brunton believed migraine was the result of both arterial contraction and dilatation, a theory that could account for the varied phenomena of migraine if the arterial spasms extended far enough down the artery to affect the centers for hearing, taste, smell, and vision.[15] One of Brunton's proposals was that superstitious visions of fairies "were nothing more than the coloured zigzags of migraine modified by imagination," and, in some cases, by an abnormal condition of the eye. That these fairy sightings were so often accompanied by the jingling of bells, he elaborated, was further evidence of nerve center stimulation causing auditory hallucinations. Adding some amateur ethnography into the discussion, Brunton went on to suggest that sick headaches were perhaps more frequent "amongst highly sensitive members of civilised communities, but it is probable that they have existed at all times and amongst all peoples, and wherever they have been present they may have led to visions."[16]

This observation led Brunton to his next suggestion: the openings bored into Stone Age skulls when the person was alive had been made during episodes of migraine. Paul Broca, a French physician, surgeon, and anthropologist, caused considerable excitement during the 1870s when he confirmed that ancient skulls recently discovered in Peru and France had been opened surgically during life, and that those individuals had survived long enough for the bone to begin to heal. According to Broca, the procedure might have been performed during childhood for some religious or social reason. He theorized, on the basis that Neolithic peoples could not have had any real understanding of the brain, that these skulls had been opened in order to release evil spirits.[17] Thus it was only a small leap of imagination for Brunton to suggest that these surgeries had been undertaken to cure migraine. "To any sufferer from sick headache the first idea that suggests itself is that the holes were made at the request of the sufferers in order to 'let the headache out,'" Brunton observed, "for when the pain of headache becomes almost unbearably severe, an instinctive desire sometimes arises either to strike the place violently in the hope of relieving the pain, or to wish that some operation could be done to remove the pain." In some ways, trepanning *does* seem an entirely logical response to the intense pain of migraine headache. As Andrew Levy notes: "It is the right external drama, proportionate to the drama inside. . . . The migraining head wants to be cut open; it longs to be cut open."[18] But apart from referring to French surgeon Just Lucas-Champonnière's 1878 study of trepanation, which claimed that some South Sea islanders still performed this procedure, Brunton's conjecture about trepanning for migraine was as entirely speculative as his thoughts on fairies: the product of a heady mix of amateur anthropology, medical antiquarianism, post-Darwinian racial theorizing, emergent knowledge about the brain, and fascination with the prospect of modern cranial surgery. Nevertheless, his theory soon gained a life of its own.

By 1913, William Osler was stating as fact that trepanation operations had been used "for epilepsy, infantile convulsions, headache, and various cerebral diseases believed to be caused by confined demons."[19] By the 1930s, the specific association of trepanning with migraine had become well established. In an article in *The Lancet*, T. Wilson Parry reasoned that the large numbers of trephined skulls found throughout France could not all be accounted for by epilepsy. He therefore proposed that the procedure had become "instituted as a rite for the casting out of other devils." According to Parry, the next class of demons to be tackled would be disorders with "exasperating" head-symptoms, including "persistent chronic headache, migraine, chronic neuralgia with acute exacerbations, alarming attacks of giddiness, with or without singing in the ears, and distracting noises of the head."[20] From these almost entirely unsubstantiated hypotheses, the notion of trepanning for migraine has become so commonly accepted that it now is one of the few things many people think they know about migraine's history. It is somewhat ironic, as we will see in the next chapter, that the only substantial evidence we *do* actually have of surgeons cutting holes in skulls for migraine comes from the twentieth century.

Still, we need to return to Brunton, because his historical musings did not end with trepanation. He went on to compare the "striking similarity in form" of the long zigzag lines of people in some of Gustav Doré's famous illustrations for Dante's *Inferno* to Hubert Airy's illustration of scintillating scotoma. Brunton's article included Airy's diagrams of his transient teichopsia, recycling this imagery for a new generation, three decades after their initial publication. Significantly, however, Brunton was not only reaffirming the value of Airy's image as an accurate depiction of migraine aura, but also using it as a standard with which to retrospectively diagnose migraine as the inspiration behind a work of art. Airy's image now had a new authority. Rather than being a representation of one person's subjective experience, it had become a tool for diagnosis. This proved to be a significant shift.

Diagnosing Hildegard

Hildegard of Bingen, born to a wealthy Rhineland family as the youngest of ten children, had been dedicated to a religious life by her parents, a common practice during the medieval period. In 1112, at age fourteen, she joined the community at Disibodenberg, along with Jutta, the daughter of another wealthy family, who was six years her senior. From a very early age, Hildegard had experienced waking visions and what she referred to as "so great a light that her soul trembled," but she did not know how to fully describe her experiences. When she was in her early forties, after her tutor Jutta's death, "the great pressure" of these pains propelled Hildegard to explain her visions in writing. Through long periods of illness and self-doubt, Hildegard worked for a decade on the text that would become *Scivias*, a staunchly theological work combining ethics, biblical commentary, history, and cosmology with the record of her prophetic waking visions. In 1148, she received papal approval to continue writing—the only woman of her time to be granted this authority. *Scivias* was completed in 1151, having been further delayed by Hildegard's purchase of land at Rupertsberg to found her own convent. In the following years, she attracted widespread fame as a celebrated visionary, preacher, and reformer.[21]

Let us now jump forward to the Wiesbaden library in 1913, where Charles Singer was utterly captivated by the images in *Scivias*. He enthusiastically shared his discovery with his friend, Swiss physician and historian Arnold Klebs, who wrote back to him in the summer of 1913: "I was very glad to have the chance to see those beautiful reproductions of the Hildegard manuscripts . . . and the more I think about it the more I become convinced that you have discovered an eminently interesting subject." Three weeks later, Klebs wrote again, reminding Singer that he was anxious to receive a set of Singer's photographs of the *Scivias* images.[22] Singer returned to England and presented his argument that Hildegard had been a sufferer of migraine to the Historical Section of the Royal Society of Medicine in November 1913. In his talk, he showed colored reproductions of the *Scivias* manuscript's illuminations. One member of the audience, Dr. Richard Hingston Fox, spoke as a sufferer of migraine himself and felt Singer had proven his case. Fox also suggested to Singer that "the blue colours in the pictures were as important as the red, both these hues, as well as others, being characteristic of migrainous spectra."[23]

Singer's ideas about Hildegard brought him professional recognition. William Osler, a supporter of trepanation theories and, by now, Regius Professor of Medicine at Oxford University, urged Singer to publish his research. In 1914, he invited Singer to take up the Philip Walker Studentship in Pathology at Oxford. From then on, Singer was able to devote virtually all of his time to the history of medicine and science.[24] In June 1914, Charles and his wife Dorothea returned to Germany to consult the *Scivias* manuscript once again. By late July, as political tensions with France grew, travelers checks could no longer be paid in German currency. The Singers quickly left for Holland, and Charles described "a most trying journey across the line of German mobilisation" with a small party of English citizens and Americans. With little money, the couple had been forced to abandon their luggage. Singer's bags had contained the only copy of his essay about the Hildegard manuscript. So, after he arrived back in England, Singer rewrote the article from memory. "I rather think I improved it," he later commented.[25]

Singer's rewritten article, "The Scientific Views and Visions of Saint Hildegard (1098–1880)," was finally published in 1917 as the first chapter of his edited collection, *Studies in the History and Method of Science*. His theory about the migrainous, pathological basis for Hildegard's religious visions constituted only a four-page coda to a fifty-five-page chapter devoted, in the main, to explaining Hildegard's ideas on scientific subjects, including the structure of the universe, the microcosm and macrocosm, anatomy, physiology, birth, death, and the soul. Singer argued that Hildegard's writings about her religious visions, which she experienced "neither in sleep, nor in dream, nor in madness. . . . But wakeful, alert," provided further evidence for his diagnosis. It seemed clear to Singer that Hildegard's repeated complete recoveries, her prolific activity between attacks, and her long life indicated migraine. "In the 'more typical' of her visions," he wrote, "the medical reader or the sufferer from migraine will, we think, easily recognise the symptoms of scintillating scotoma."[26]

A decade after Brunton had used Airy to point out the migrainous features of Doré's illustrations for Dante's *Inferno* in 1861, it was not just the aesthetic similarity between the *Scivias* illuminations and Airy's diagrams that would have attracted Singer. Wrapped up in the authority of Airy's diagrams, as we have already seen, was the strong association of migrainous visions with genius, scientific vision, and the intensity of (men's) intellectual work. Like many of his peers, Singer believed history played a meaningful role in explicating the very nature of medicine and science, and, by taking ideas out of their contemporaneous religious milieu, they could be secularized as science. Singer had developed a firm belief in the early chronology of scientific development and insisted that the past should be interpreted in the light of present knowledge.[27] This was exactly what he did in diagnosing Hildegard's migraine. Compared to the "dark degradation" of her twelfth-century contemporaries, Singer believed Hildegard was important because she was beginning to approach a rational explanation of the world. He promised his readers that if they could look past the "bizarre and visionary form" in which she presented her theory of the essential similarity of macrocosm and microcosm, they would find a systematic and skillful elaboration of a scientific philosophy. Minus its religious underpinnings, Singer believed Hildegard's was a commonsense approach that gave meaning to the facts of nature.[28] His migraine diagnosis was crucial to this transformation, by retrospectively endowing the abbess with a disorder that had become accepted in late-Victorian expectations of the physical and mental constitution of a scientist. Using his medical knowledge to interpret the unusual patterns in Hildegard's religious imagery as the manifestations of a neurological disorder enabled Singer to sideline Hildegard's theology and replace it with science as the basis for her philosophy of the world. In effect, Singer was using migraine aura to induct Hildegard into a select, and very eminent, group of men who had (accurately) observed and drawn their visions. Hildegard had earned a place in Singer's broader project of identifying a story of progress from the superstitious darkness of the Middle Ages to the light and reason of modern science. For Singer, such a presentation was an urgent exercise in scientific humanism, a means of addressing the problems of his own age, which seemed to be experimenting dangerously with rampant scientific and technological progress, as well as with democracy.[29]

Singer published a second version of his Hildegard commentary in 1928, in a collection of essays that laid out his by now fully formed theory of the history of scientific progress. *From Magic to Science* traced the collapse of ancient science into the "swamp of magic," as well as the first attempts to recover "from that hideous slough." Hildegard represented the moment when science left the Dark Ages and the dawn of modernity had begun. The 1928 version of his earlier article included new captions for the colored plates, which confidently highlighted the migrainous features of the imagery to readers.[30]

In the years that followed, readers of Singer's work identified with his depiction of Hildegard as a neurologically troubled genius. In 1932, Lieutenant Colonel R. H. Elliott delivered a lecture to the Medical Society of London with the title "Migraine and Mysticism." Dismissing Hildegard's science as "crude," he nevertheless took Singer's diagnosis as medical fact, referring to Hildegard as "a woman of an extraordinarily active and original mind . . . and with a marvellous ability for depicting the numerous sensations to which her migraine gave rise." What particularly interested Elliott about Hildegard, however, was the effect the *Scivias* imagery had on his own patients, who recognized "without hesitation features of their own migraine attacks," even though her drawings and paintings were nearly eight centuries old. The golden light and the bluish-white fortification patterns were "immediately recognised by any patient who sees these phenomena today." His patients' responses left Elliott in no doubt that Hildegard herself had painted the miniatures. In image after image, Elliott picked out the stars, zigzags, rotating circles, wavy lines, and areas of darkness as confirmation of the abbess's migrainous life. The connection, moreover, confirmed the social and cultural status of his patients. Those who experienced the richest of symptoms, he suggested, were the "clever intellectual people endowed with the creative type of mind." In Hildegard, Elliott saw "an extraordinary example" of this. Warming enthusiastically to his theme, and interspersing it with observations from encounters with his own migraine patients, Elliott went on to suggest that Moses, Jeremiah, Ezekiel, Daniel, Paul of Tarsus, St. John the Divine, and Zoroaster could all have been diagnosed as migraine sufferers, on the basis of their religious visions.[31] Reading Elliott's published lecture now, it is difficult not to dismiss his enthusiastic diagnosis of a swathe of biblical and religious figures as condescending, if not entirely ridiculous, but his claims illustrate two important points. First, Elliott showed how the idea of migraine as a disorder characterized by aura, and associated with creativity, intellect, and visual disturbance, had become commonly accepted since the 1870s. For Elliott, the effects of aura were *the* defining characteristic of the disease. Second, Elliott demonstrated how a sense of history had become part of his clinical encounters. Hildegard's images seemed to speak across the centuries and made what was, in the 1930s, a very recent understanding of migraine appear timeless.

Despite Elliott's enthusiasm, and the reprinting of Singer's article in 1928 and again in 1958, the idea of Hildegard's migraine faded as physicians interested in functional nervous disorders turned to examining the physical and emotional effects of wars. Medical theories about migraine fragmented as researchers suggested a whole host of roles for pituitary swelling, brain swelling, allergies, endocrine organs, psychology, and, in the 1940s, the vascular system. Then, in the late 1960s, a young neurologist, Oliver Sacks, was inspired to write a new book about migraine (taking just nine days to do so) after reading Edward Liveing's *On Megrim*. Sacks was entirely convinced by Singer's argument, agreeing that the *Scivias* images were "indisputably migrainous." Yet he went further than Singer, reducing the abbess's allegorical interpretation of her ecstatic inspiration to an entirely physiological process. Hildegard had simply experienced "a shower of phosphenes in transit across the visual field, their passage being succeeded by a negative scotoma."[32]

Sacks's discussion of Hildegard concluded the chapter in which he argued that although aura lay at the very heart of migraine, it had not received sufficient attention since Liveing's work in the 1870s.[33] Sacks did not dismiss vascular changes as an explanation for the cause of migraine headaches, but he argued that this theory did "nothing to explain the origin of migraine *attacks*."[34] Sacks's championing of Singer's ideas about Hildegard's migraine used history to stake a claim for the authority of neurology to account for migraine at a moment of real flux in the medical consensus, when vascular theories gave way to neurological ones (to which we will return in the next chapter). Sacks also used a black-and-white line drawing, based on the *Scivias* miniature of "The Heavenly City," as the book's frontispiece for every edition, with a caption explaining that the figure is "a reconstruction from several versions of migrainous origin." Although revised over time, the book's opening paragraphs also consistently emphasized this long history, boldly stating that none of the chief features, phenomena, experiences, and triggers of migraine had changed in two thousand years.[35] Hildegard's apparently timeless migraine experience, and the recognition of aura in her visions, anchored a new neurological model of migraine in a very long history.

Hildegard's Migraine and Medieval History

In her own words about her illness, Hildegard described her eyes as "so afflicted with a clouding over that I was unable to see any light," and of herself as being "so pressed down by the weight of my body that I could not raise myself. . . . So I lay there, all day and all night overwhelmed by these intense pains." She also described how God allowed "excruciating airs" to course through her whole body, and how the "marrow in my bones dried up so much it was as if my soul must be released from the body."[36] We can be sure that Hildegard would not have recognized the neurological formulation of migraine with which she has been retrospectively endowed. Instead, Hildegard saw her illness as a divine punishment from God. This is not to say, however, that Hildegard did not have an understanding of *emigranea*. As we have already seen in chapter 2, some of the most vivid expressions of medieval humoral ideas about it can be found in her *Causae et Curae*.[37]

Singer's theory concerning Hildegard, as revived by Sacks, has posed a challenge for medieval historians. For some, the authority of a medical diagnosis simply established Hildegard's migraine as a clinical fact. For example, in her 2010 study of pain in medieval culture, Esther Cohen talks of Hildegard taking to her bed "with violent migraines" when her will was crossed, though in the letter to which Cohen refers, Hildegard described "a grievous illness."[38] Other medieval historians have been more critical of the diagnosis. In a 1985 article, historian Barbara Newman dismisses the idea that a physiological cause might account for Hildegard's spiritual inspiration, referring to it as a "reductionist error" to be avoided.[39] By contrast, Sabina Flanagan, in her 1998 book on Hildegard, believes Oliver Sacks has not gone far enough, since it was possible to identify every illness that Hildegard described as a manifestation of migraine. Furthermore, Flanagan argues, these experiences of illness correlated with Hildegard's production of visionary writings, allowing a better understanding of how the abbess assumed her prophetic role.

Migraine had provided her with "a wonderfully adaptable instrument."[40] If, for Flanagan, the diagnosis is a methodological resource in understanding the relationship between Hildegard's illness and her creativity, for Newman it is a red herring Flanagan uses to protect Hildegard against accusations of charlatanism. On the other hand, Newman asserts that Hildegard's declarations about her chronic debilitating illnesses needs to be understood in the light of medieval ideas about intense religious experience and feminine incapacity, as well as the hagiographic conventions of the time.[41]

Perhaps the strongest supporter of Hildegard's migraine diagnosis has been art historian Madeline Caviness, the first recent scholar to make a serious case for Hildegard's role as the designer of the *Scivias* miniatures. Caviness drew on Singer's migraine thesis, as well as her own experiences of migraine aura, in support of her assertion that Hildegard is "surely as much the author of these pictorial ideas as she is of the words that she also did not physically write." Caviness's empathy as a fellow sufferer who recognizes the distinctive jagged-edged and crenelated forms, black clouds, and "tiny light points that make the contours shimmer" is an important element of her rationale. She contends that the visual cues in the *Scivias* illuminations are "the most persuasive arguments for Hildegard's close personal attention to the execution of the illuminations, since she was the one with migraine and knew these effects at first hand."[42] Medieval manuscripts were often produced by trained artists and scribes under instruction from authors. Even if Hildegard did not actually mix the paints or apply the brush for this "deluxe illuminated copy," Caviness suggests that "the authentic rendition of these visual auras is thus best attributed to Hildegard herself . . . unless we suppose that an illuminator was found to work on the Rupertsberg *Scivias* who also had migraine." Essentially, Caviness implies that *only* someone who had personally experienced migraine aura could have designed these images. For Caviness, establishing Hildegard's role as the designer of the illustrations in *Scivias* is crucial, because it constitutes "the last area of Hildegard's multimedia outpourings that has been denied to her by recent scholars."[43]

Neither Caviness's empathy, nor her art historical expertise in arguing for the inseparability of image and text in *Scivias*, is in question, but understanding the circumstances behind Hildegard's diagnosis reveals her argument to be a circular one. In order to claim that Hildegard suffered from migraine, Charles Singer had to assume she had an integral role in the production of the illuminations in *Scivias*.[44] When Caviness applied a migraine argument to support her assertion that Hildegard was directly involved in creating the

Scivias miniatures, the medical evidence already included this integral assumption. Independently, both the physiological element (Hildegard's manuscript illustrations are evidence of migraine) and the historical element (Hildegard was responsible for the images) in this argument are plausible, but if we have to assume that Hildegard had direct responsibility for the illuminations in order for the migraine diagnosis to make sense, we can't then say that *because* Hildegard had migraine, she must have been the illustrator.

Nevertheless, as Caviness's work reminds us, we also cannot (and should not) deny that since Singer's first presentations of his ideas about Hildegard in 1913, patients have recognized their own experiences of migraine aura in the *Scivias* miniatures. In May 2012, Pope Benedict XVI formally canonized Hildegard. In October of the same year, he proclaimed her a Doctor of the Church, in recognition of her teachings. Hildegard is only the fourth woman to receive this honor. Her life has also been the subject of a feature film, and, in Germany, a system of alternative holistic healing bears her name. Given her reputation, it is perhaps no surprise that contributors to an online forum recently discussed whether Hildegard would make a good patron saint of migraine. As one member has commented: "I'm sure we can use all the saints we can get. I don't think we found an 'official' migraine saint. I didn't check the archives but I think some of us just decided that Hildegard would be a good choice."[45] If we wholly consign her diagnosis to history, we also deny the real meaning people continue to derive from the association of Hildegard with migraine.

Anne Conway

For over twenty years, a seventeenth-century noblewoman experienced pain on one side, then the other, and, often, over the whole of her head for two, three, or four days at a time. In his famous discourse on diseases of the brain and nerves, published in 1664, celebrated physician Thomas Willis described how this anonymous woman could not bear "light, speaking, noise, or of any motion, sitting upright in her Bed, the Chamber made dark, she would talk to no body, nor take any sleep, or sustenance."[46] As the attack began to wane, she would lie down in a "heavy and disturbed sleep," from which she awoke feeling better. The humors flowing in the meninges of the woman's brain, it seemed to Willis, had gripped her head with an "habitual and indelible vice."

Anne Conway's migraine diagnosis first appeared in a paper by Sir Gilbert Roy Owen, following the publication of Marjory Hope Nicolson's edited collection of Conway's letters in 1930, which also revealed her identity as Willis's patient. Owen was keen to determine what had ailed Conway so strongly that she had needed to consult such an "imposing array" of physicians as William Harvey, Thomas Willis, Robert Boyle, Kenelm Digby, Jan Baptist van Helmont, and Valentine Greatrakes. Although he accepted that any modern medical suggestions would come "too late to aid" Conway, Owen had asked the opinion of famous American neurosurgeon Harvey Cushing, who initially favored a "pituitary origin" for her disease. The suggestion that Conway had migraine came later and seems to have been Cushing's way of sitting on the fence. He changed his original pronouncement after seeing further evidence and explained that a diagnosis of migraine "covered a multitude of sins." Indeed, Cushing's was not the only suggestion for what might have been Conway's problem. Ernest Sachs ruled out brain tumor, and Nicolson herself thought of hyperthyroidism. Others had suggested syphilis, though this was contradicted by Willis's account. Neurologist Carl Rand was tempted to say Conway exhibited the effects of childhood meningitis, though he admitted this might have been based on an old wives' tale. For his part, Owen seems not to have made a firm decision about the cause of the "paines, violent and continuall" that dogged her to the end of her life.[47]

Despite the equivocation and uncertainty in Owen's article, modern neurologists and literary scholars seized on Conway's possible migraine as medical fact. Her rise to prominence as a celebrated migraineur is interwoven with the status Willis, her physician, has gained as a founding father in neurological history for his work on cerebral blood flow. He was also the first person to use the word "neurologie" in print.[48] In Edward Liveing's eyes, Willis's comment that head pain was sometimes an "innate and hereditary" debility, often "delivered from the parents to the children," cemented his position as an early authority on megrim.[49] Yet neither Willis, nor Conway, made any connection between her illness and migraine. For Willis, the only real significance of the term hemicrania, which he only used once in his text (poet Samuel Pordage, who translated Willis's *De Anima Brutorum* from Latin into English in 1683, rendered Willis's "hemicraniam" as "meagrim"), was to identify the location of pain if it was in the side, front, or back of the head.[50] In her own writing, Conway described how her "old distemper" had greatly increased after surviving smallpox. Nevertheless, Willis's vivid account of this "invincible and permanent" illness has come to be seen as a classic early description of chronic migraine, and the noblewoman has become one of the most well-known of history's migraine sufferers.[51] Modern confidence that Willis's account is accurate enough to enable Conway's symptoms to be diagnosed is both reinforced by, and a confirmation of, his anachronistically endowed status as a neurological pioneer and authority.

For Willis, headaches were a very blood-filled affair. He did deal directly with head pain in the treatise containing Conway's case, where he explained how humors within the body pushed, pulled, and watered the nervous fibers, "irritating them into painful corrugations." He believed that increased blood flow across the skull was responsible for headache pain, which could be light or vehement, sharp or dull, and either short, continual, or intermittent, Its approaches might be "periodical and exact" or, at other times, "wandering and uncertain." Blood poured onto the sensitive membranes of the brain by "many and greater Arteries," bringing "hurt to the Meninges" when the blood, or serum, passed through all the arteries at once. His observations about the flow of cranial blood were a significant precursor to the vascular theories of migraine that became so important from the nineteenth century on.

In common with her contemporaries, Conway tried every possible treatment, although in vain. She had consulted English doctors, traveled to Ireland and France, taken the air in several countries, and purchased medicines from the "Learned and the unlearned, from Quacks, and old Women." She had ingested dangerous mercurial powders, visited baths, and drunk spa waters. She frequently had her blood let, including once from an artery. Yet "the contumacious and rebellious Disease, refused to be tamed, being deaf to the charms of every Medicine."[52] If we are to give Conway a role in the history of migraine, we should do so by witnessing the vast range of treatments she tried and her commitment to a quest for relief.

Hildegard of Bingen and Anne Conway have been seen as women whose intellectual powers seem to transcend the constraints of their own times. Hildegard would have been "extraordinary in any age," Barbara Newman has argued, but for a woman of the twelfth century, her "achievements baffle thought, marking her as a figure so exceptional that posterity has found it hard to take her measure."[53] Both Conway and Hildegard sometimes acted as if they were men, and their modern migraine diagnoses serve to enhance this sense that there was something exceptional going on in their lives and their minds. The men in Conway's life, Andrew Levy suggests, were aware that "the mix of Conway's acumen with her distress was what made her extraordinary." He goes further still, identifying a "migrainy metaphysics" to her posthumously published writings.[54]

Conway and Hildegard are some of the best known in a long list of famous historical figures who have been retrospectively diagnosed with migraine in the twentieth century. Once released into the wild, these diagnoses, at first tentative, speculative, or based on a particular narrow reading of evidence, soon become accepted as truth. Another famous case, concerning artist Pablo Picasso, is a salutary lesson in the perils of treating retrospective diagnosis as a parlor game. In 2001, two Dutch physicians proposed that Picasso could have had migraine aura without headache, based on the visual appearance of some of his artwork, notably in the vertically fragmented depictions of faces.[55] A decade later they admitted, with some embarrassment, that their suggestion had not been based on research in biographies, letters, or memoirs of either Picasso or his contemporaries.[56] Nevertheless, the theory had spread, and their retraction was too late.

For Lewis Carroll, the question has not been so much whether he was afflicted with migraine himself—diary entries show that he did—but whether his experience directly inspired his novel about Alice's adventures in Wonderland. Dr. John Todd, a British psychiatrist, was the first to make this suggestion in 1955. Although neurologist Joseph N. Blau has since implored that this piece of neuromythology be laid to rest, the popularity of the link between migraine and Alice grew.[57] In their 1999 article, Klaus Podoll and Derek Robinson reveal a previously unseen sketch from Carroll's family magazine, *Mischmasch*, showing the figure of a standing man with parts of the right-hand side of his body missing, and a diary entry from 1856, which recorded Carroll consulting eminent ophthalmologist William Bowman about his eye problems. If Carroll had experienced aura as early as the 1850s, as this evidence seems to suggest, then Podoll and Robinson believe the thesis that migraine was the inspiration for *Alice in Wonderland* is strengthened once again.[58]

Literary scholar Andrew Levy has reflected on the personal significance of knowledge that famous sufferers such as Anne Conway, Charles Darwin, Ulysses S Grant, Virginia Woolf, Pablo Picasso, and Rudyard Kipling all succeeded in spite—perhaps, even, *because*—of their struggles with migraine. They have given him a sense of validation, a community to help guide him through his own pain, and a sense of "metaphysical stability." Whether some of these "old practitioners," as Levy calls them, actually had migraine, either in their terms or ours, was less important than the recognition, pattern, or clarity he finds in their examples. Levy states that "playing detective" with Lewis Carroll's biographical materials is an entirely unnecessary pursuit, "rendered irrelevant" by simply reading *Alice in Wonderland*, a book he considers possibly the best literary representation of migraine in history. For Levy, what matters is that men and women like Hildegard, Picasso, and Carroll "all went down the same deep well that the migraine sufferer reaches." It can be tempting to think that there might be some profound link between migraine and creativity, but, as Levy acknowledges, the numbers of famous migraineurs simply do not add up. We cannot see the "gifted men and women who never got a chance to nurse those gifts because they were too occupied to do anything but nurse their pain."[59] As novelist Mary Sharratt points out quite bluntly, "the migraine sufferers I know in my own life regrettably report that they've never beheld wondrous visions."[60]

Conclusion

"Of all the common and much-dreaded nervous diseases we recognise," J. M. Aikin lamented in the *Journal of the American Medical Association* in 1902, "none are less perfectly understood than migraine; nor is there any other nervous disorder which is so disastrous to the physician's ability for treatment . . . it is easy to say what [migraine] is not, but difficult to define what it is."[61] The casual way in which Singer could choose a diagnosis for Hildegard, or Owen and his colleagues could speculate about Conway, is in stark contrast to the much more difficult—and consequential—decisions physicians faced in their everyday practice. Away from the pursuit of historical cases, the first decades of the twentieth century were characterized by physicians' pessimism about the possibilities for curing migraine, their frustrating interactions with the real patients who sat in their offices, and their inability to explain the disease's causes or mechanisms, not to mention the ongoing disagreement as to what migraine even was when faced with a multiplicity of idiosyncratic symptoms.

Had Hildegard von Bingen traveled across the centuries and been able to visit a physician in the 1930s, R. H. Elliott confidently declared that "she would have consulted her doctor and have been sent to an ophthalmic surgeon."[62] Reflecting on his own long career from the vantage point of the 1980s, Macdonald Critchley (who died in 1997) remembered the "inordinate" emphasis that had been placed on the visual factors of migraine during the 1920s and early 1930s.[63] In his 1924 Savill lecture, Arthur Frederick Hurst identified an ocular origin for the majority of migraine cases, and he summarily dismissed other theories. If a toxic idiopathy was present, he had never seen any evidence that it provoked attacks; anaphylactic theories were attractive but "extravagant"; glandular theories, "purely speculative." Hurst believed even very small errors of refraction were able to produce migraine, especially in highly strung, clever people with "a very irritable migraine storm centre." Drugs such as luminal and bromide might have some effect on migraine, but they would simply not be required if one's eyesight was corrected.[64]

A discussion held at the Royal Society of Medicine in 1927 demonstrates that basic questions—what migraine was, what symptoms should be included in the category, how it related to other disorders, and how to treat it—all remained unanswered. Leading the debate, Dr. C. P. Symonds proposed that migraine needed a clearer definition, in order to facilitate methodical investigation. It might be convenient, in a clinical context, to include headaches that resulted from disordered nasal sinuses or headaches that followed injuries to the head under the category of migraine, but for the purposes of scientific investigation, Symonds proposed that *only* recurrent headaches accompanied by visual or sensory disturbance should be considered. Moreover, these disturbances must be short lived, as well as followed by a complete recovery. How migraine headache *felt* was also important: it should be "throbbing, bursting, or splitting" in character. These clinical characteristics were so well defined, Symonds explained, that using them would ensure a correct diagnosis. By this logic, Symonds excluded sick headache, it being what he considered an incomplete migraine. No doubt drawing murmurs of surprise from some of his audience, Symonds proposed that headaches caused by eyestrain also did not count as migraine.[65]

Symonds's audience had plenty to say about his definition. Dr. A. F. Hurst insisted that eyestrain was the most important and common factor in migraine, by virtue of its increasing the constitutional and, often, inherited irritability of the central nervous system. He also accepted that fatigue and toxemias, as well as endocrine activity during menstruation, increased a person's likelihood of experiencing migraine attacks, but he urged anyone who thought eyestrain was unimportant "to find another oculist, or, if necessary, a series of oculists, to examine their migrainous patients."[66] Dr. J. Kingston Barton rejected this insistence on the importance of eyestrain and thought that the old authors had been correct when they grouped migraine, asthma, and skin affections together with inherited gout. Mr. Herbert Nott and Dr. Agnes Savill supported Symonds's proposal of "a floating toxin in the blood" as migraine's probable cause. Dr. J. A. Ryle changed the subject again, asking why migraine and other "explosive" disorders such as asthma, epilepsy, and gout were incurable. Dr. W. R. Reynell suggested that only when the problem of epilepsy was solved would they know more about migraine. Somewhat wryly, Dr. F. W. Collingwood observed that as he had been subject to migraine his entire life, his worst attacks had followed "debates in which controversial questions have arisen." He might well have regretted attending that particular meeting of the Royal Society.[67]

Apart from the profound disagreement about migraine's causes, Symonds's comment about clinical convenience is a revealing hint that physicians were using migraine as a diagnosis to placate patients.[68] One of the unfortunate results of seeing migraine as a label of convenience, rather than of accuracy—or, in the words of Harvey Cushing, as a diagnosis covering "a multitude of sins"—was to compound what already were disputed understandings of migraine's identity and destabilize any conviction that it was a legitimate—or even a real—illness. Writing in the *British Medical Journal* in 1927, E. Miles Atkinson presented a vivid picture of how a lack of clarity and a proliferation of theories about migraine affected patients and their relations with medical professionals:

> Every medical man frequently has to deal with the type of case to which I refer. Some of the patients suffer almost constantly, and look ill, run down, and tox-aemic; others have violent attacks of headache with periods of freedom ... some suffer in silence as far as any reference to a medical man is concerned; others seek remedies everywhere. If they have sought medical advice they will probably have been investigated for bowel trouble, menstrual disorders, errors of refraction; and possible sources of toxaemia such as septic teeth.

For his part, Atkinson believed frontal sinus disease was the cause of head-ache, and he again emphasized how crucial the presence of aura was for an accurate diagnosis. A pain might be a true hemicrania (i.e., a one-sided head-ache), but if the "typical battlemented spectra of migraine are absent," it only mimicked what he considered to be migraine.[69] Visual experiences defined migraine, because they were the only symptom that gave any certainty to a diagnosis.

Neither Hildegard of Bingen nor Anne Conway could visit an early twen-tieth-century physician's office, or cause the kinds of diagnostic difficulties that occurred when patients had inconvenient symptoms, such as nausea or pain. Singer and Owen were free to highlight whichever elements of the avail-able evidence supported their theories and ignore those that did not. In 1913, Hildegard's diagnosis was contingent on the understanding that aura was an essential feature of migraine. By 1937, Conway's diagnosis was even less certain. As Marjorie Lorch has noted, retrospective pronouncements such as these reveal something of how "different signs and symptoms were given sta-tus and significance by different writers at different historical periods."[70] The case of Hildegard is a prime illustration of how early twentieth-century clinicians seized on the promise of aura to deliver a tangible sense of medical certainty. When their patients could say "I see that!" their migraine could be diagnosed quickly and easily, regardless of the other symptoms they might experience. The culturally, socially, and medically elevated status of migraine aura emerging from the late nineteenth and early twentieth centuries would continue to shape ideas about migraine and clinical research throughout the remainder of the twentieth century.

That Hildegard's and Conway's migraines have become historical fact illustrates an interesting paradox: historical cases or diagnoses can gain authority the more they become detached from the contexts and beliefs that were needed to support and verify the diagnosis in the first place.[71] As they have become established instances of neuromythology, Hildegard and Conway have imbued modern medical concepts with a long historical provenance, giving the impression that there is something permanent and essentially neurological about the disease of migraine. The embrace by professionals of figureheads such as Willis, Conway, and Hildegard needs to be seen as part of a wider process of claiming political and medical authority for neurology.[72] Hildegard of Bingen, Anne Conway, and trepanation are not just episodes in the history of migraine. Rather, they can be seen as significant stories working to confirm twentieth-century medical knowledge as the pinnacle of a much longer history of progress, rationalism, and enlightenment. It is no coincidence that all of these accounts have their origins in the early twentieth century, a moment characterized by profound professional disagreement and diagnostic uncertainty about migraine's identity.

CHAPTER EIGHT

"Happy Hunting Ground"

*Conceptual Fragmentation and Experimentation
in the Twentieth Century*

The Nurse with a Hole in Her Skull, 1936

In 1936, Alfred Goltman, a physician from Tennessee, reported on one of his cases in the prominent medical journal *Allergy*. The patient was a twenty-six-year-old woman with a history of headaches, nausea, and vomiting since childhood. Goltman believed the observations he had made on this patient helped reveal the pathological physiology of migraine. He had first met the woman, a registered nurse, in 1931. He recorded that for as long as she could remember, she had experienced "typical migrainous attacks." A languid feeling warned of the attack's approach before pain, beginning over her right eye, gradually radiated backward until it covered her whole head. The headache would last between one and three days, and, as the pain reached its height, she would vomit. Goltman paid little attention to her family history, but he did note his patient's observation that eating wheat consistently produced an attack. Although wheat had proven to be the principal offending allergen, Goltman's tests also suggested she was sensitive to milk, cheese, seafood, some nuts, fruits and vegetables, feathers, and dust. Measuring her blood count, urine, nitrogen level, blood calcium, and spinal fluid, Goltman found them all to be normal.

Goltman did make one peculiar observation: the nurse had a depression in the left frontal region of her skull. The area, an inch in diameter, also contained a marked concentration of blood vessels. The woman's history revealed that four years before meeting Goltman, she had been admitted to the Memphis Baptist Hospital's neurosurgical service under the care of neurosurgeon Dr. Raphael Eustace Semmes. Semmes was the first neurosurgeon in that city, having been trained at Harvard University by Dr. Harvey Cushing, an American, often known as the father of modern neurosurgery (and, incidentally, the man responsible for suggesting that migraine had been Anne Conway's problem, as we discussed in the previous chapter). In Memphis, Semmes had performed a "craniocerebral exploration" through a burr hole, a small circular opening made in the woman's skull, while she was experiencing a severe headache. As was his usual practice, he performed the operation under local anesthetic. He opened the dura—the thick membrane surrounding the brain and spinal cord—and "a quantity of fluid escaped under increased pressure." Semmes found no evidence of a tumor.[1]

Semmes's procedure drew on decades of excitement about the possibilities of discovering the localization of cerebral function and, related to this, the development of neurological surgery. In the late nineteenth century, British, American, French, and German surgeons competed to open up skulls to treat cranial blood clots, abscesses, tumors, epilepsy, and mental illness, particularly when these had been caused by trauma. Their investigations were aided by technological developments, such as anatomical staining and electrical stimulation, and an enthusiasm for experimenting, using animal studies.[2] Between the 1890s and the 1920s, some surgeons believed brain surgery could cure inherited criminal tendencies and remake a person's social identity by altering their character. Following this theory, some surgeons operated on children who were referred to them by juvenile courts, in an attempt to release pressure on the brain, a procedure with a mortality rate of 42 percent, according to one sample. By the 1930s, the trend of intervening surgically to alter human behavior headed toward its peak with the development of frontal lobotomy as a treatment for mental illness.[3] Semmes's surgical procedure— drilling a hole in the skull of a nurse while she experienced a migraine— marks a moment between what now appear to be two very troubling eras in experimental neuro- and psychosurgery. It is easy to be horrified today by the apparent recklessness and cruelty of lobotomy and procedures related to it, but, at the time, the risks of such surgical interventions were not only accepted in the mainstream—by both patients and physicians— but they were also popular. There were few effective treatments for neurological and psychiatric disorders, and surgery often seemed to work, in a sense, by beneficially changing the patient's personality and restoring their productivity.[4]

Semmes's patient survived the surgery, but her migraine headaches did not stop. When Goltman later observed her healed head, he noticed something interesting: during her headaches, the definite depression that had been left by the skin healing over the hole in her skull began to fill up, "gradually assuming the appearance of a tumor." The bulge was not tender, nor did it appear as if brain tissue was "protruding through the skull opening." As the migraine attack ended, the swelling would recede and return to a concavity. For Goltman, this added support to the theory, first proposed during the nineteenth century, that migraine headache must be vascular in origin and characterized by dilation of the blood vessels during the attack. Goltman's paper would prove to be influential in the emergence of vascular explanations for the mechanism of migraine during the 1930s, but the combination of experimental surgery, allergic theories, and observations of the brain and vascular system featured in Goltman's paper illustrates how vascular ideas jostled for position among other theories as the international field of migraine research fragmented in the early decades of the twentieth century.

This chapter examines that period's range of medical theories about migraine's causes, symptoms, and definitions. It traces the emergence of the idea that migraine affected not just a particular type of person, based on their gender and social status (as had been common from the late nineteenth century), but a particular type of personality. These debates occurred alongside, as part of, and, in some cases, in opposition to endeavors to find effective treatments. Semmes's procedure on the young woman, and Goltman's later observations about her case, illustrate how migraine came to be seen as potentially fruitful—not to mention frustrating—for a variety of medical specialties in the twentieth century. Ultimately, migraine would be claimed by neurology.

Happy Hunting Ground

In the late nineteenth century, physicians tended to fall into one of two camps—supporting either vascular or nerve-storm theories of migraine—as represented broadly by the ideas of British doctors Peter W. Latham and Edward Liveing, respectively. By the early 1930s, as British neurologists Macdonald Critchley and Fergus Ferguson commented, the condition had become "the happy hunting ground of the theorist . . . attacked by representatives of all branches of medicine."[5] As we saw in the previous chapter, by the early twentieth century, physicians were pessimistic about treatments and disagreed wildly on how to classify and diagnose migraine. In part we can identify the emergence of this situation as early as 1888, in William Gowers's misgivings about either explanation in his *Manual of Diseases of the Nervous System*. In his now classic 1933 textbook of clinical neurology, *Diseases of the Nervous System*, Walter Russell Brain was similarly equivocal, noting that migraine's etiology was a "matter of speculation." For Brain, the most plausible explanation (though he was careful to qualify that this was still hypothetical) was that migraine was due to "arterial spasm followed by dilatation occurring within the distribution of the common carotid artery."[6]

Two decades later, in 1955, Massachusetts physician John R. Graham observed that the field of migraine research had advanced little in two decades. Graham, the founder of the Headache Research Center at Faulkner Hospital in Boston, was becoming an extremely influential figure in migraine research by the 1940s. He was also fond of a good analogy. For him, the best way to represent this professional impasse was with an updated version of the parable of the blind men and the elephant. A cartoon illustrating this appeared as the frontispiece to his little book on the treatment of migraine (fig. 8.1). The original parable came from India, about a group of men who each tried to describe an elephant based on partial knowledge, coming to blows as they disagreed about the others' experience. Graham's version of the fable showed the "ordinary sick headache" elephant surrounded by specialists in white lab coats: a neurologist, a psychiatrist, an allergist, an endocrinologist, an internist, and an ophthalmologist. Each of the men was pulling on a different bit of the elephant. The endocrinologist tugged on the ears, labeled menstrual migraine; the allergist hugged a front leg, designated as cyclical vomiting. The psychiatrist (swinging from a tusk) and the neurologist (peering into the trunk) both appeared to be attempting to tackle classic migraine (migraine with aura). Graham saw the fable as epitomizing the medical profession's attempts to grasp migraine's true nature in the first half of the twentieth century. Each of the elephant's "interesting appendages" had its characteristics, but how these parts were related to migraine as a whole, or shared common physiological rules, remained a mystery. Graham then presented a long list of problems hampering research into migraine pathology and therapies. These included trigger factors, which varied between patients, and observations that migraine often spontaneously remitted or worsened in relation to changing life situations, weather, illness, holidays, or work, "with the result that concurrent medical therapy may receive credit or blame that is not its due." Migraine was notorious for apparently responding to new medicines, and it was greatly influenced by doctor-patient relationships and the placebo effect. Graham felt that trials were being either inadequately carried out or reported. Finally, there was still confusion and disagreement about which headaches should even be included within the diagnosis of migraine.[7]

Before they could determine the shape of the elephant, it seemed, doctors first needed to agree as to which animal they were going to work on. At this

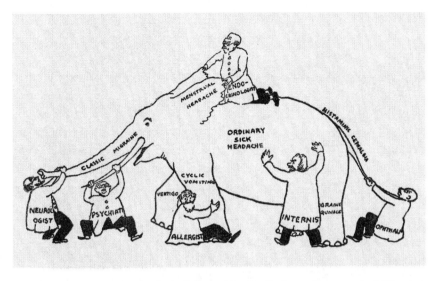

Fig. 8.1. "Ordinary Sick Headache," from John R. Graham, *Treatment of Migraine*, 1956. Courtesy of the Wellcome Library, London, licensed under CC-BY

point, there had been an important shift in the geography of medical authority. Whereas, in the nineteenth century, the main contributions to theories of migraine had come from Europe, by the early twentieth century, many of the most influential researchers in allergy, psychology, and vasculature would be based in the United States.

From Toxins to Allergy

By the turn of the twentieth century, approaches to migraine had embraced theories about uric acid, visual defects, uterine and menstrual disorders, eyestrain, teeth caries, adenoid growths in the pharynx, and abnormalities of the nose.[8] In 1902, J. M. Aikin explained how toxins could be accommodated within Liveing's theory of nerve-storms. The nerve cells, "bathed in their life current," held out against toxins until they were overcome, at which point an explosion—or nerve-storm—occurred. For Aikin, these ideas showed that recent germ theories of disease could also be applied to organisms originating from within the body, which produced disease when they accumulated beyond the body's ability to cope. Aikin proposed treatments to eliminate toxins and restore the processes of digestion through enemas, irrigation, and hot water taken by mouth.[9] Thus it was not much of a leap from seeing migraine as a result of sensitivity to, or poisoning by, toxins in the body to including it within a new and exciting concept of disease, one gaining a great deal of attention in the early twentieth century—allergy. Moreover, a language based on this idea of sensitivity continued a way of thinking about migraine in relation to nerves, a concept that had emerged in the eighteenth century. In 1906, Austrian pediatrician Clemens von Pirquet had coined the term "allergy" to describe any form of altered biological reactivity. Allergens—including insect stings, pollens, and strawberries—were foreign substances that provoked an immune reaction once they were introduced into a hypersensitive body.[10] During the 1910s, French doctors discussed possibilities for developing desensitizing therapies for a whole range of chronic conditions appearing to originate in hypersensitivity and anaphylaxis, such as arthritis, rheumatism, asthma, and migraine. Factors suggesting migraine might have its origins in allergy included its periodicity, the clear influence of heredity, its early onset in children, and the absence of discernible pathological changes in the body.[11]

George Bray, who worked in the allergy clinic at Great Ormond Street Children's Hospital in London, set out the state of allergy knowledge relating to migraine in 1931. He explained that many migrainous cases also had positive skin tests, often displaying multisensitivity to foods such as wheat, milk, fish, eggs, chocolate, beans, and meats, as well as to inhalants such as feathers and animal hair. Bray suggested that many cases of migraine could be treated solely on an allergic basis.[12] In 1934, influential American allergist Warren T. Vaughan declared that, by using allergic treatment alone, he had helped 50 percent of his headache cases, most of which were migrainous. He was hopeful that future allergic approaches—that is, those advocating the avoidance of particular foods—would provide relief in up to 70 percent of these cases.[13] This was the approach that Goltman had taken with the nurse whose problem opened this chapter, and it seems to have changed very little since the late nineteenth century, when Alexander Haig claimed he had cured his children of migraine by changing their diets. As Matthew Smith has argued, food allergists "were inclined to suspect food allergy as the cause of every chronic health problem encountered in the clinic."[14] Referring to Critchley's happy hunting ground quote, a Danish doctor reflected on how allergists liked to give the impression that they had "captured the prey" of migraine. Nonetheless, by the 1950s, findings of a similar incidence of migraine among allergic and nonallergic persons, and little evidence of a hereditary relationship between it and asthma, were beginning to undermine allergic theories in migraine research, although the significance of food in precipitating migraine attacks was undeniable.[15] The focus on foods and allergy illustrates how Liveing's notion of a nerve-storm, decades after *On Megrim* was published, continued to shape the debate by taking it beyond a strictly neural explanatory framework.

In a symposium on migraine held in London in 1963, Vera Walker, a consultant at the Oxford Eye Hospital clinic, described the "continuous stream" of patients with inflammatory conditions who came through the door, of whom at least half had headaches of some sort. Walker recalled that she had begun to take migraine more seriously after discovering Erich Urbach's treatise on allergic diseases, published in 1944. She had become fascinated, to the extent that she "closed the clinic for a month and read everything I could find on the subject of migraine." In 1944, Urbach and Philip M. Gottlieb published *Allergy*, nearly a thousand pages in length. They described migraine as a "symptom complex" and emphasized the importance of eliminating any organic disease before investigating hypersensitivity to foods like wheat and chocolate, or inhaled allergens, such as roses, violets, perfumes, turpentine, naphthalene, and tar. Urbach and Gottlieb proposed that if problem foods couldn't be eliminated, then "deallergization" might be tried. This involved giving the patient minute quantities of the sensitizing foods at first, before gradually increasing the amounts. Walker had learned to suspect an allergy to common foods when a patient reported that their migraine occurred in a definite cycle over the course of days or weeks. "The body can tolerate wheat, milk, eggs, and so on for just so long and no longer," she explained. This time interval could be shortened if some physical shock or nervous tension intervened to precipitate an attack. Walker believed that around half of her migraine patients could be helped by cutting out certain foods, most commonly wheat, cow's milk, cheese, tomatoes, chocolate, fish, and shellfish.[16] In 1962, Macdonald Critchley also talked about migraine as something that built up or became due, to be triggered, for example, by eating chocolate. Critchley recalled Emile du Bois-Reymond's observation from 1860, when, "for some time after an attack, I may expose myself with impunity to certain influences which before would infallibly have induced a seizure."[17]

Endocrine Research

Allergy wasn't the only early twentieth-century discovery that seemed applicable to migraine. In 1905, British physiologist Ernest Starling had given the name "hormone" to the internally secreted compounds produced in glands, including the pituitary, ovaries, and testes, that were carried around the body in the blood. As Chandak Sengoopta notes, these hormones added weight to the notion of a body regulated by chemicals, rather than the nervous system, and a range of glands maintained hormonal balance, in order for the body to function properly.[18] In 1919, Irving H. Pardee, a physician in the US Army, proposed that "a frontal headache which does not yield to the usual remedies" was one of the earliest symptoms of a malfunctioning pituitary gland.[19] By the 1920s, Sengoopta states, "the glands were seen to possess virtually miraculous powers, not simply over the narrowly sexual aspects of life or behaviours, but over the entire body and mind." With respect to migraine, one theory was that temporary enlargement of the pituitary, rather than hormones per se, put pressure on the cavernous sinuses and caused migraine's distinctive visual and optic disturbances. The hereditary nature of migraine could be explained by an unusually small sella turcica (the depression in the bone in which the pituitary gland is positioned), making a person particularly sensitive to the gland's swelling.[20] In the 1930s, researchers discovered that migraine attacks were preceded by an increased concentration of prolan (a hormone produced in the pituitary that stimulated ovarian follicles) in the urine, and that they could induce headaches by injecting this substance.[21] The authors of one study went so far as to propose that a headache so frequently associated with women's reproductive cycles should be given an endocrine classification.[22]

The availability of a huge range of standardized pure and synthetic hormonal preparations, some of which could be bought in drugstores without a prescription, offered even general practitioners who were interested in migraine an experimental access to the exciting new field of endocrinology. Extracts could either be used individually or in combination, in doses that were entirely up to the clinician to determine. It was completely logical to take a hormone—such as the crystallized ovarian extract theelin, which had been prepared with the restoration of normal sexual function or the treatment of amenorrhea in mind—and apply it to migraine, a disorder that was clearly associated with women's menstrual cycles, or whose symptoms might be explained by a physiological problem located in and around the pituitary.[23]

The possibilities for hormonal experimentation were so broad that Critchley and Ferguson warned of some "pluriglandular therapists" who had brought endocrine therapies into disrepute by being neither "discrete [n]or scientific" in their claims and their use of hormonal products for treating migraine. Critchley and Ferguson were unconvinced by the theory of a swollen pituitary pressing against the sella turcica and observed that "almost all the endocrine organs have been blamed at one time or another for attacks of migraine," but they did accept that practical and theoretical results suggested endocrine therapies were worth considering for treating menstrual migraine.[24] For instance, E. F. Hartung had recommended using a combination of "anterior and posterior lobe pituitary extract," "whole-gland extract" and "whole powdered gland" in migraine. Other researchers experimented with placental hormone or ovarian follicular hormone (theelin). Critchley and Ferguson recommended theelin and thyroid among a range of treatments that could be administered between attacks.[25] Later researchers proposed that the administration of emmenin (human placental extract) or progesterone might terminate and even prevent attacks.[26] In menstrual migraine, Urbach suggested hormonal substitution therapy, including ovarian, corpus luteum, or pituitary extracts.[27]

California doctor William Moffat described in detail his method for prescribing gonadotropic factor, extracted from the urine of pregnant women (follutein), in cases where migraine was associated with menstruation, a technique he had developed over two years and claimed had worked in all of the seventeen cases of menstrual migraine he had treated. Women would be given a small dose (two to six rat units) between five and seven days after the onset of the menstrual period. The dose was gradually increased over the next ten days, then rapidly increased to a maximum (between 50 and 125 units) on the fourteenth day. Moffat did not know why the gonadotropic factor would work, proposing that it either corrected a previously existing hypofunction, or, giving credence to allergic theories, that the increasing amounts of the preparation desensitized patients and prevented attacks.[28]

Degeneration

In his work on allergy, Urbach quipped that there was only one truly effective prophylactic for migraine: "to persuade an individual suffering from migraine not to marry anyone suffering from the same affliction, or at least not to have any children." Since migraine patients, however, were "quite often talented and highly intelligent personalities," Urbach suggested that this advice would not serve the interests of the community.[29] His statement may have been intended lightheartedly, but it illustrates the continuing importance of a theme that first emerged in chapter 6, when discussions about the relationship between migraine and epilepsy, and the obvious significance of heredity, found migraine a place at the margins of discussions about physical, mental, and social degeneracy. In 1909, in a paper for the *Eugenics Review*, physician and prominent eugenicist Alfred Tredgold had taken long-held ideas about the heredity of nervous disorders a step further.[30] Tredgold warned of the cumulative degeneration that could lead to mental deficiency over subsequent generations.

At first, he argued, the mental change might present itself as migraine or mild epilepsy; later generations might develop insanity or dementia. Over time, the degeneration would become structural, rather than just functional. Eventually, it would produce "actual defect of mind structure—amentia or mental deficiency."[31] For Tredgold, it was vitally important to spot people with "defects" such as migraine, which were at the mild end of the spectrum, to prevent degeneration from progressing far enough over time to impede an entire nation's strength. As Mark Jackson explains, "It was this focus on the degenerative danger of defectives, together with the use of family pedigrees to chart neuropathic constitutions, that linked medical models of feeble mindedness to eugenics, both as a scientific analysis of hereditary difference and as a professional middle-class programme of social and political reform concerned primarily with racial purity and national efficiency."[32] Warnings such as Tredgold's were not just the work of a marginal fringe. In 1913, Britain passed the Mental Deficiency Act, which allowed for the institutionalization of "mental defectives." Ultimately, the eugenicists believed, "some human life was of more value—to the state, the nation, the race, future generations—than other human life."[33] In this light, Urbach's casual comment about breeding takes on a disconcerting significance.

In 1927, British psychologist and epidemiologist Francis Graham Crookshank (a "brilliantly clever, but unstable" man) explained that migrainous men were "thinking introverts" (a phrase he borrowed from psychoanalyst Carl Jung), generally of robust physique, energetic, industrious, and from long-lived families, but with "a certain organ-inferiority" that manifested as facial asymmetry, deviation of the nasal septum, and dental irregularities.[34] The significance of all this, Crookshank suggested, was that "under strain and stress," it was men with these kinds of congenital and acquired inferiorities who had become "functionally blind, deaf, or dumb" during the First World War. Crookshank saw the migrainous brain storm as a "defence and flight and excuse mechanism," analogous to the reactions of men faced with physical danger. Yet it was the psychology of the migrainous person that was most problematic. These were people whose mental state was dominated by repressed rage and humiliation. Sexually jealous as children and maladjusted as adults, such individuals were deeply unhappy, plagued by the need to assert their superiority, not least over the opposite sex. Turned inward, this emotional repression formed the basis of a migraine brain storm. Thus, Crookshank believed, the physician's role was to help a young adult patient—whose life was still before him—"strip himself of his cloak of make-believe" so he could "work out his own salvation."[35] Crookshank believed he was offering a metaphysical solution to a problem that science could not solve: curing bodily disorder by adjusting the unconscious mind. Crookshank's ideas about the unconscious state of a migrainous person were influenced by the theories of continental psychoanalysts Carl Jung, Sigmund Freud, and, particularly, Alfred Adler, with his work on the inferiority complex. Like many other British doctors, Crookshank took what Tracey Loughran has identified as "a magpie approach," selecting those aspects of continental psychology that seemed most useful.[36]

Freud himself, as has often been noted, had migraine, which he considered to be a tyrant to be rebelled against.[37] In a letter to his wife in 1885, he blamed an attack of migraine on the tartar sauce he had for lunch. He "took some cocaine, watched the migraine vanish at once," and went on writing.[38] We can see in Crookshank's book how a clumsy borrowing of psychoanalytical theories added a new layer to existing understandings of the role of stress and emotions in migraine, but it also shows how the experiences of war had a profound effect on how neurologists, psychiatrists, psychologists, and physiologists understood the relations between mind and body.[39] The postwar context that informed Crookshank's concepts, as well as decades of discussion about migraine as a potential gateway to hereditary degeneration (an association combated by the repeated insistence of many physicians that migraine was a disease of intellect), provide more pieces in the puzzle of how and why migraine's legitimacy became eroded. By drawing on ideas about trauma and neurosis that had informed doctors' responses to the mental and nervous disorders seen in returning soldiers during the First World War, Crookshank was questioning the moral and mental strength of people with migraine.

Migraine Personality

Alongside allergic and hormonal theories, ideas about migraine and personality gained traction during the 1920s and 1930s, particularly in North America.[40] One of the most influential proponents of the concept of a migraine personality was American physician and popular health columnist Walter Alvarez. Much of the discussion about migraine personality took on a very negative tone, but in a self-help book published in 1952, Alvarez presented migraine as a confirmation of his readers' intellectual superiority. Migraine was a plague, perhaps, but at least it was one of "wide-awake, attractive, and well-educated persons." For Alvarez, the typical migraine patient was female, and her headache was only half of the problem. These women had a distinct personality and appearance, so much so that Alvarez claimed one of them only had to enter the room for him to suspect her trouble. His description was designed to flatter: "such a nice trim figure, such a bright, eager, and intelligent face."[41] When writing for a professional audience, however, Alvarez was less complimentary, describing the women as tense, perfectionist, hypersensitive, easily fatigued, and often depressed or disconnected. Although, in most ways, she would be "decidedly feminine and sexually attractive," there was a masculine element to her nature, "which causes her to act independently and to think dispassionately much as does an able businessman." Many migrainous persons were also allergic, which Alvarez posited as being part of their exaggerated sensitivity in all areas of their lives. In a section that could have been lifted straight out of the nineteenth century, Alvarez explained that many women with migraine had inherited not just a nervous predisposition, but a "frail and sickly body too weak to stand up to the strains of life." While Alvarez did not suggest any outwardly visible physiological inferiority, he did note that these women often had "defective and poorly functioning pelvic organs," dysmenorrhea, and "severe monthly storms."[42]

In 1948, neurologist Harold G. Wolff published *Headache and Other Head Pain*, which would undoubtedly become the most influential study of migraine in the twentieth century. If the previous decades had been characterized by disagreement and fragmentation, Wolff's vascular research galvanized the professional headache community, while his ideas about the "psychobiologic constellation" of migraine also played an important role in cementing assumptions about personality. Wolff collated his observations from a study of forty-six subjects with migraine and found that certain features occurred "with striking frequency." As children, more than half of the migraine patients had been "delicate," shy, withdrawn, and obedient to the desires of their parents. "They were commonly sober, polite, well-mannered children who did their school work conscientiously." But there was another side to this docility; they could be unusually stubborn, or inflexible in certain situations. Overall, Wolff thought, migrainous children were sensitive, but generally trustworthy, energetic, and respected, with the result that they were given responsibilities and special privileges at an early age. By adulthood, their personality traits became distinctive. Tension was an "emotional state common to all," and nine-tenths of the subjects were "unusually ambitious and preoccupied with achievement and success." These were conscientious and hardworking people, perfectionist and exacting. They needed order, and they appeared tireless to others. Their personalities made interacting with others difficult. They were unable to delegate and became inflexible, impatient, and resentful. Although courteous, graceful, and charming, there was little warmth; the migrainous person was cold, aloof, detached. Nonetheless, there were contradictions in Wolff's migraine personality portrait. On the one hand, he observed that these people dressed well, if conservatively, and the women "sometimes sacrificed a degree of attractiveness for austerity or severe neatness," but others, despite having orderly habits of work, were "indifferent about their personal appearance and households."[43] Wolff's diagnosis of the migraine personality was not as overtly gendered as Alvarez's, except in the realm of sex. Among the men, sexual activity was "adequate," but four-fifths of the women expressed sexual dissatisfaction and rarely obtained orgasm. For these women, sex was "at best, a reasonable marital duty."

Wolff described migraine attacks as the result of a failure to adapt to situations in the external environment, such as weekends or vacations, or to an internal bodily state. For "the perfectionist, driving woman," migraine would attack when she refused to acknowledge flagging energy and attempted to perform in her usual manner. Her "essential psychobiologic rigidity" prevented her from making suitable adjustment to changes in her "internal environment."[44] No single characteristic, however, defined the person liable to migraine. Wolff identified a "multiplicity of personality features, life situations, and emotional reactions" as being of importance. He listed so many characteristics that almost anyone might recognize themselves or others as a migraineur.

Wolff's colleague, John Graham, (the author of the elephant parable with which we started this chapter) argued that patients who suffered most from migraine tended to have "a personality that seeks and creates stress and a physiology that handles it poorly." These patients didn't just react over time to an accumulation of stress, they actively sought it out, and even created it. In this statement, we can see how migraine's relationship to stress had evolved from a physiological and hereditary disposition in the nineteenth century to a psychological failing in the twentieth. Accordingly, in addition to the usual prescriptions aimed at restoring and fortifying the nervous body, Graham proposed that treatment needed to be behavioral, by "teaching the patient new attitudes that make it unnecessary to create stresses and easier to withstand those that cannot be avoided."[45] Graham didn't directly discuss the gendered demographics of migraine, but out of thirty illustrative examples in his book, twenty-eight were women. He suspected one forty-year-old woman's story to be "somewhat exaggerated," until a visit to her home verified not only "the prostrating nature of her attacks, but . . . the influence of a schizophrenic mother and a poverty-stricken life on 'the welfare.'"[46] Graham described a fifty-four-year-old single woman, who was a music teacher and church organist, as rushing and tired, frequently missing meals. It took a conversation with the doctor for her to realize "she was an overly ambitious person who tried to fulfill with too much perfection the requirements of her various jobs." In Graham's examples, migraine appears as a physical and psychological manifestation of the pressures of modern society. A plethora of failings included poor diet; irregular mealtimes; morning deadlines and overcrowded schedules; late awakenings on weekends and holidays, a lack of breaks, failure to take proper vacations or to "get away from their children periodically"; excessive participation in community and church activities; overanxiety about guests, shopping, and vacations; long car journeys; and "acting as chairman (because nobody else will accept)." Migraine patients were particularly unable to delegate, Graham suggested, and "do it all themselves." Evoking once more the nineteenth-century idea of migraine as a nervous storm, or explosion, Graham described all of these failings and deviations from a healthy life as "fuses to the migraine bomb."[47] Education was the most important therapy, and the family physician—the target audience for Graham's book—was the best person for this job. By the late 1960s, it was clear that a major weakness of nearly all the personality studies was that they made no attempt to compare migraine patients with any other group, and they failed to recognize the inherent biases of the self-selecting groups of patients who had sought help from clinics—the population on which the studies were based—rather than representative population samples. Indeed, some physicians were dismissive of the whole genre. "A great deal of nonsense has been written about the lifestyle of migraine sufferers, their personality, attitudes, ambitions, and frustrations," J. B. Foster declared in 1975.[48] As Macdonald Critchley looked back over his career, he admitted that while he had viewed the growth in psychological literature as alarming, later, more nuanced work had been valuable in showing how psychological factors were important as aggravating, rather than causative, factors.[49]

Ergotamine

In addition to their ideas about personality, Harold Wolff and John Graham were key figures in a paradigm shift in understanding the physiological mechanism of migraine. In 1938, a decade before the publication of *Headache and Other Head Pain*, they had published the results of a study that would change the field profoundly, demonstrating unequivocally that the drug ergotamine had a dramatic effect in treating migraine pain, and that migraine, therefore, had a distinct somatic basis. Perhaps more importantly, they were able to show why ergotamine was so effective.[50] Physiological explanations for the effects of drugs were not incompatible with psychological theories of migraine. Wolff had learned from Adolf Meyer (the psychiatrist responsible for the idea of psychobiology) that psyche, personality, and stress could contribute to physical disease. If personality could be the cause of migraine, then vascular disturbance was the mechanism.[51]

Ergotamine was the only specific drug available for migraine at the time of Graham and Wolff's experiment. Ergot of rye—a common crop disease caused by the fungus *Claviceps purpurea*, in which small, purple-black, elongated ergots replace the grain in the heads of rye and other grasses—had long been known for its ability to stimulate the uterus during childbirth.[52] In 1868, Edward Woakes had recommended the use of ergot extract for migraine, because of its vasodilating effects. By the early 1930s, physicians were regularly reporting on trials of its administration, effects, and complications in medical journals, claiming an efficacy of up to 90 percent.[53] In their study, Graham and Wolff undertook experiments on sixteen subjects over the course of thirty-two migraine attacks. They placed tambours—tiny, drumlike instruments—that could sense the patients' arteries through the skin and attached mirrors to these diaphragms. Rigging up a system of lamps that would throw a beam of light onto the mirror and into the slit of a camera, they were able to record pulsations from the arteries onto a piece of moving bromide paper. They recorded blood pressure at the same time, and the patients—who spent the duration of the experiment "reclining comfortably on a couch"—reported the intensity of their headache. The researchers made initial observations, as controls, before injecting the patients with ergotamine tartrate (Gynergen), produced by the Sandoz chemical company.

One graph from Graham and Wolff's article stood out.[54] It showed unequivocally how the pulsations of the temporal arteries dropped precipitously, either immediately or within a few minutes, after an injection of ergotamine. In ten minutes, the patient reported that the headache had gone. This graph, however, represented only one patient; by no means all responded so dramatically. A second graph showed a much weaker response: a gradual decrease in pain over an hour, accompanied by a similarly gradual overall decrease in pulsation amplitude. In two cases, the pulsations initially decreased and then increased after the administration of ergotamine. In three more, the pulsations increased. Overall, Wolff and Graham reported that across thirty-four patients, the average reduction in pulsations due to ergotamine tartrate was 52 percent. They also used before-and-after photographs of the forehead of one of their male patients to illustrate the visible constriction of the superficial temporal vessels. They concluded that the most acceptable explanation for ergotamine's ability to end migraine headache was that its vasoconstricting action narrowed the "painfully stretched and dilated" cranial arterial walls, supporting the theory that the pain was due to the distension of these arteries.[55] If psychiatric approaches were designed to prevent the attack from happening in the first place, ergotamine seemed to be the answer once an attack was underway.

British pharmaceutical company Burroughs Wellcome considered developing a new ergot-based drug for migraine in 1948, in response to Sandoz's creation of a product combining ergometrine and caffeine, which promised excellent results.[56] Ergometrine was touted as being even more effective for migraine than ergotamine, and, as one correspondent to the *British Medical Journal* noted, it claimed to avoid the "serious toxic effects" of ergotamine. Moreover, ergometrine could be given by mouth, rather than by injection.[57] In an archival folder of Wellcome Burrough's "developmental rejects," a memorandum reveals discussions about the proposed new product. If caffeine could increase the anti-migraine action of ergometrine, the memo suggested, the combination of ergometrine and caffeine had the potential to be more effective than ergotamine, and have the advantage of considerably greater safety and freedom from side-effects."[58] The proposal seemed promising. "This is interesting—it has possibilities," a scrawled note suggested. Within a month, the Wellcome Chemical Works had been instructed to produce one thousand compressed tablets, to be subjected to a clinical trial. While this particular process appears to have gone no further, Wellcome Burroughs' breakthrough in the migraine market would come in 1956, in the shape of sugar-coated Migril tablets. Migril combined ergotamine with caffeine and cyclizine, a fast-acting antiemetic that prevented nausea, a major side effect of ergot derivatives. Migril's power to avert migraine, if taken as soon as premonitory signs were noticed, gave it an edge over its competitors, notably Sandoz's Cafergot-Q tablets, which promised only "quicker relief" and did not contain cyclizine. Migril was a huge success. By 1961, Migril imitations were available in at least ten countries.[59] By 1967, advertisements in the *British Medical Journal* claimed that over two million migraine attacks per year were being treated with the new drug.

Early marketing campaigns, aimed at physicians, pitched Migril as "today's master plan against migraine." Leaflets emphasized the importance of cyclizine hydrochloride as a modern breakthrough, making ergotamine bearable in a larger, "truly effective" dose. Migril promised "3D relief": dispelling headache, defeating nausea, and dispersing visual disturbances. For British customers, Migril was available in tablets, while the European market preferred injections. For doctors—ever attentive to their patients' busy professional lives—Migril promised "insurance" with a product that could be taken "anywhere, at any time."[60] The literature implied that simply carrying dosages of Migril improved a patient's life, through the confidence that came from knowing effective "counter-measures" are "now in their hands." Brochures represented men as ballet dancers and jockeys—professions requiring skill, precision, and strength. By 1961, Migril promised to "master" migraine. The imagery was of professional male masters: the hunt master, circus master, schoolmaster, and degree holder (fig. 8.2). These patients could now view their aura not as a threat, but as "a call to prompt and effective action." The brochures depicted men functioning at a high professional level at all times. Their suffering is invisible, internalized, and their professional personas do not betray the inner experiences that require mastering.

Women, on the other hand, were portrayed as sufferers, with their head in their hands, even in leaflets that otherwise used the same language of mastery. When women weren't being shown in pain, they were portrayed as "cured," smiling and able to go on with their colorful social lives. One ad pictured "Mrs. Janice Everett, age 41. Married. Three children. Employed as a bank clerk." Mrs. Everett, in a brightly colored top, getting out of her car, was, of course, smiling (fig. 8.3). In one undated bilingual ad for the South African market, a white woman was shown as half of the doctor's problem: "Migraine is two headaches . . . your patient's and yours" (fig. 8.4). The Migril ads drew on, and perpetuated, highly gendered stereotypes that had emerged about migraine over the preceding century.

We might see the gendered nature of the Migril ads in the context of other postwar pills, like diazepam (Valium), that came to be seen as "mother's little helpers." As David Herzberg has shown for the case of Prozac, advertising for Migril utilized a language of modernity, consumerism, and self-fulfillment, enabling those who took the drug to juggle their modern professional, social, and family lives.[61] There were, however, important differences in how men and women were portrayed. While men appeared nearly as often as women in the brochures' pictures, they were never depicted either with, or as, a problem. They were independent masters, whose engagements with medical prac-

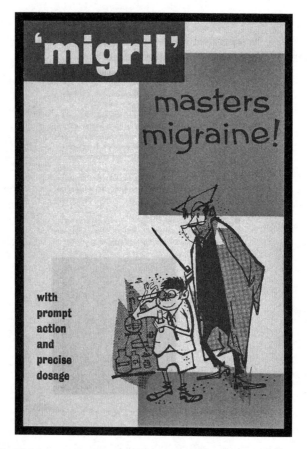

Fig. 8.2. "*Migril" Masters Migraine!*, Wellcome Burroughs promotional leaflet for migril, 1961, WF/M/PL/199, folder 2. Courtesy of the Wellcome Library, London, licensed under CC-BY

titioners could be seen almost as a professional transaction, procuring insurance and confidence. Women, on the other hand, needed help.

While twenty-first-century marketing materials overwhelmingly portray women, in the 1960s, men were also displayed prominently in the pharmaceutical literature, albeit always as professionals, and always in control of their bodies.[62] All they needed was a little pill-shaped confidence. By 1966, Wellcome Burroughs had updated their approach to marketing Migril, emphasizing speed in addition to mastery. Partly this was a way to help physicians educate their patients. The sooner Migril was taken, the "greater and quicker is the relief of pain," but it also tapped into a lucrative market. Begin-

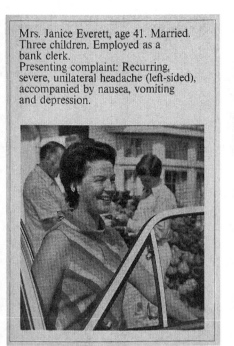

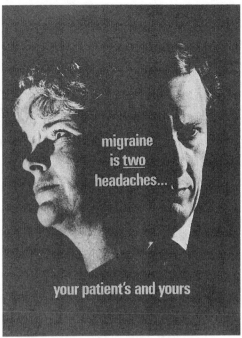

Fig. 8.3. (left) "Mrs. Janice Everett, age 41," Wellcome Burroughs promotional leaflet for migril, 1969, WF/M/PL/199, folder 4. Courtesy of the Wellcome Library, London, licensed under CC-BY. *Fig. 8.4. (right) Migraine Is Two Headaches*, Wellcome Burroughs promotional leaflet for migril, South Africa, undated, WF/M/PL/199, folder 6. Courtesy of the Wellcome Library, London, licensed under CC-BY

ning in 1968, the advertisements featured a countdown, from "ten" to "stop." The patient described in this campaign was explicitly coded male, gaining protection against "all the symptoms" of migraine, his "confidence restored by the rapidity of effect."[63] It is no coincidence that the idea of the countdown came in the same year that Stanley Kubrick's film *2001: A Space Odyssey* was released. Billed as "a countdown to tomorrow, a roadmap to human destiny," and the "masterwork" of its director, the excitement surrounding this futuristic film tapped into the cultural enthusiasm for space and its exploration. The 1960s had also seen a highly publicized competition to break the land speed record. Speed, modernity, and mastery reflected everything Burroughs Wellcome wanted ergotamine to represent.

The effectiveness of ergot had been widely accepted since the late nineteenth century, but clinical trials conducted in the 1960s gave surprisingly equivocal results. One double-blind controlled trial, conducted on eighty-eight women and published in the *British Medical Journal* in 1970, suggested ergot was hardly more effective than a placebo. Moreover, the authors found that ergot seemed to aggravate a migraine attack significantly more often than the placebo, and one woman withdrew from the trial because ergotamine made her feel so giddy.[64] Patients' responses to and tolerance for ergotamine were highly variable, whether the drug was given by mouth, injection, or suppository. Overdoses of the drug could result in vomiting, numbness, tingling, and painful cramps, particularly when it was injected. Concern was also growing about the toxic side effects of ergotamine, especially ergotism, a rare but potentially serious condition with symptoms that included convulsions and miscarriage. Ergotamine combined with caffeine was supposedly better absorbed, but the stimulant effect of caffeine might stop patients from sleeping, which was, in itself, often a natural way to end attacks. Other researchers were worried about ergotamine-induced headaches. After prolonged periods of taking ergotamine, the nausea and vomiting of migraine would be absent, but the headache would remain. Further studies reported that ergotamine overuse resulted in constant nausea for between a third and half of the patients. Ergot was dangerous for patients with known vascular disease, liver disease, or pregnancy, and, when taken too frequently, tended to exacerbate the development of the next attack.[65]

In 1956, John Graham had implied that problems of compliance with treatment regimes represented a psychological failing on the part of the patient. In one of his examples, using language highly suggestive of an unhealthy emotional relationship, he described trying to divorce a woman from her ergot with the help of the opioid Demerol and sedatives. Further research on ergot now made it seem much more likely that this was a problem inherent in the drug.[66] In Oxford, Vera Walker was experiencing similar difficulties with patients in her clinic. "The most difficult patients of all are those who report that they have been taking Cafergot, Migril, or Orgraine every 36–48 hours and cannot do without it," she explained. In many cases, migraine drugs appeared to be having a toxic effect. In Walker's experience, the only treatment that worked was similar to one given to chronic alcoholics: a very gradual withdrawal, accompanied by moral support from the physician.[67]

Although ergotamine could be very effective, Jes Olesen remembers that doctors "didn't quite know how to use it." Ergotamine was clearly important, and its action must relate in some way to migraine's pathological physiology, because it had no general sedative or analgesic qualities, but it was a "dirty" drug. It worked on too many receptors and, thus, its mechanisms could not be used as a way to understand migraine.[68] In 1970, Joseph "Nat" Blau, consultant physician to the National Hospital for Nervous Diseases in London, suggested that if physicians were asked about the drugs they personally took for migraine, it would not include ergot: "They usually admit to taking only a simple analgesic."[69] For all its problems, until the 1980s, ergotamine nonetheless remained the only treatment that *really* worked against migraine attacks, but, compared with specific drugs for other diseases, such as vitamin B12 for anemia or digitalis for heart failure, it simply was not good enough. It frequently failed to relieve attacks, and it did not work for all patients.

There were alternatives, however. Many practitioners continued to use Gowers' mixture, although its pharmacology was not understood.[70] Among the mixture's ingredients, nitroglycerin (which had been William Gowers's drug of choice), amyl nitrite, and histamine all dilated the blood vessels, though this result could be accompanied by unpleasant, even dangerous effects for the patient (as we saw in chapter 5). The promotion of histamine therapy grew out of observations that histamine headache and migraine might be related through a similar vascular physiology. In clinical use, however, it required juggling doses, repeating injections, and even ordering hospitalization, although there seemed to be some evidence that antihistamine might work for some people.[71] At the City Migraine Clinic in London, Marcia Wilkinson reported that sedatives and tranquilizers were often effective if the patient was then able to sleep, a process that commonly ended an attack.[72] Graham shrugged off vitamins as "harmless and a possibly useful adjunct," and he dismissed those who claimed to be able to cure migraine with surgery, comparing them to "the gardener who cuts off the tops of the weeds rather than pull them up by the roots. Sometimes the noxious plants grow again in their original site, and at other times they sprout up again with renewed vigor in new locations."[73] One of the most ardent advocates of combining hormonal and allergic therapies for migraine was British doctor Neville Leyton, at the Putney Migraine Clinic, which opened in February 1950. From the start, the clinic focused on preventive therapy for migraine, rather than acute treatment. In describing the clinic's ethos, E. Harvey Sutherland explained that at Putney, they considered it wrong to send a migraine patient to a neurologist, when "a large number, if not all, of migraine sufferers have some imbalance of the hormones circulating in the body at certain times."[74] The clinic's doctors prescribed hormones to maintain a normal balance in the body and injected or orally administered desensitizing agents. While it might take many months to try the whole range of products, "by far the majority of individuals who have attended the Migraine Clinic at Putney show very definite improvement," Sutherland claimed. He was highly critical of a medical profession that had been taught migraine was unimportant and untreatable, except with sedatives and ergotamine, as well as of researchers who seemed more interested in the theoretical aspects of headache production than the relief of individuals. "It should seem far more important to patients in general that they should be relieved of their headache than to know just why, scientifically, that headache occurs," he wrote.[75]

Methysergide (later to be marketed as Deseril or Sansert) had been synthesized from lysergic acid (from which LSD is derived) and initially promised "remarkable" results in migraine prophylaxis when its use was introduced by Italian neurologist Federigo Sicuteri in 1959. Most importantly, while ergot had only ever been helpful in ending an attack in progress, methysergide worked as a prophylactic, showing that migraine's cause, as well as its mechanism, must be somatic.[76] The introduction of this drug fundamentally affected how doctors saw their migraine patients, signaling the beginning of the psychological framework's demise. Neil Raskin, an American physician, recalls being quite astonished at how methysergide changed the profession's thinking about the nature of migraine. "Prior to that time, and all through the [19]40s and 50s, migraine was thought to be predominantly psychosomatic," he remembers. "I think back to all those patients that I had sent to psychiatric consultants. . . . Suddenly, patients could take a few tablets of methysergide and within a week they were headache free. No change in their internal milieu. Cured." Even more than ergot had done, methysergide legitimized vascular theories of headache, transforming a psychosocial problem into a scientific one.[77] Unfortunately, unless the drug was used under strict medical supervision, it could produce serious side effects, including nausea, vomiting, diarrhea, insomnia, hallucinations, and retroperitoneal fibrosis, a rare inflammatory disorder affecting the lining of the abdominal cavity. Between the 1960s and the end of the century, tricyclic antidepressants, antiepileptics, beta-blockers, and calcium channel blockers had varying degrees of success in migraine prophylaxis. Nevertheless, some physicians believed a cure-all wonder drug would simply never be found.[78]

Serotonin

The serum vasoconstrictor serotonin (5-hydroxytryptamine, or 5-HT) is one of the most remarkable chemicals in the human body. It is a monoamine neurotransmitter (others include dopamine, noradrenaline, and histamine),

a chemical messenger that performs a fundamental role in the normal functioning of the nervous system. Around 90 percent of the human body's serotonin is found in the gastrointestinal tract, where it regulates intestinal movement. In addition, 5-HT is stored in blood platelets and synthesized in the
central nervous system. It regulates sleep, appetite, and body weight, and it
is a clotting factor in healing processes. Serotonin affects a person's ability to
withstand pain by physically suppressing pain signals. It is linked to mood,
and low levels of serotonin are thought to play a role in some mental health
disorders, such as depression, aggression, obsessive behaviors, anxiety, and
alcoholism.

Serotonin had been named in 1948 by researchers Maurice M. Rapport,
Arda Green, and Irvine Page at the Cleveland Clinic, who were working on a
newly discovered blood contaminant.[79] In 1953, biochemist Betty Mack Twarog
demonstrated the presence of 5-HT in the brains of mammals. Soon, hundreds of papers on serotonin were being published each year. It was clear that
serotonin produced an "almost bewildering array" of antidiuretic, vasoactive,
psychological, neurological, and gastrointestinal effects throughout the body.[80]
For migraine researchers, the possible links between serotonin and migraine
were striking, particularly once Wolff and his colleagues had demonstrated
that injections of serotonin could produce migrainelike symptoms.[81]

The effectiveness of methysergide, which simulated the effect of serotonin
on vascular receptors, strengthened the theory that serotonin must be intimately involved in the biochemical process of migraine headache.[82] Although
the drug itself had proven to be problematic, neurologists were convinced
that 5-HT played an important role in migraine. In 1961, three researchers
from Florence, Italy, drew attention to an increased excretion in urine, during
migraine attacks, of 5-hydroxyindoleacetic acid (5-HIAA), a byproduct of serotonin metabolization. Four years later, the Australian-based group of Don
Curran, Anthony Hinterberger, and James Lance, working in what had been
a "rundown fever hospital" at the University of New South Wales, reported a
fall in blood plasma levels of serotonin during migraine headaches. Lance
observed that this happened in over 85 percent of their patients.[83] In 1975,
Michael Anthony and James Lance proposed that migraine was a "low-sero-
tonin syndrome," caused by some factor in the blood that would lead to a
"sudden discharge" of serotonin from storage sites in the body, including the
platelets. Edda Hanington's work on tyramine had been particularly suggestive. In 1967, Hanington (who was, at the time, assistant director of the Wellcome Trust in London) had first suggested that a sensitive, localized vascular

response to tyramine (an amino acid derivative thought to be naturally present in many of the common foods implicated in migraine attacks, particularly cheese), might explain some attacks of migraine.[84] By 1981, Hanington and her team were very confident that abnormal platelet behavior (precipitated by stress, hypoglycemia, or dietary or hormonal factors) was inextricably linked with migraine and argued that the disease should be considered a common blood disorder.[85]

Anthony and Lance thought an increase of serotonin in the blood could produce constriction of the intracranial vessels, accounting for mood changes and other neurological phenomena that preceded the headache. As the released serotonin was then excreted or metabolized, its levels in the blood would fall rapidly, causing the vessels in the scalp to dilate and the capillaries in the skin to constrict. Fluctuations in plasma serotonin could also cause nausea and vomiting. As plasma serotonin levels increased, relief would follow.[86] So where did the serotonin go? Some of it would be metabolized as 5-HIAA, as Federigo Sicuteri and colleagues had observed in 1961, while another portion would be excreted unchanged in the urine. Anthony and Lance's theories about the ability of serotonin to simultaneously dilate some blood vessels and constrict others potentially answered one of the major issues Graham and Wolff's earlier work had not addressed: if migraine pain was due to vasodilation, how was one to account for the distinctive pale appearance of many migraine patients during their attacks?[87]

John Cumings emphasized the need for researchers to focus their attention on serotonin. If the cause of the mode of serotonin release and its incorporation into blood platelets could be found, and if researchers could learn how these were controlled, "one would have taken a few steps towards discovering the origin of migraine," he predicted.[88] From the early 1970s, by taking Wolff's observations about distended temporal arteries and Lance's work on 5-HT antagonists as a basis, Patrick Humphrey and his team at the Glaxo pharmaceutical company focused on the pharmacology of methysergide, in order to find out what was unique about its efficacy in migraine. Having identified a new atypical serotonin receptor type (now known as 5-HT$_{1B}$), localized in cranial blood vessels, Humphrey and his colleagues worked to develop a new drug that would specifically target this receptor.[89]

That drug was sumatriptan, synthesized and patented in 1984. Initial trials proved that it was a highly effective and well-tolerated rescue treatment for migraine patients with and without aura. Marketed as Imitrex, sumatriptan became available in Holland, Britain, New Zealand, Sweden, Luxembourg, and Portugal in 1991, and a further twenty-five countries by 1993.[90] By the end of the 1990s, there were seven triptans on the global market. For physicians, the results of this drug, the first to be developed specifically for the treatment of acute migraine attacks, appeared to be miraculous. Within minutes, patients' headaches, disability, nausea, and photophobia were significantly reduced.[91] Sumatriptan aborted migraine in half of the patients, and reduced pain in 70 percent. Nevertheless, there were certain concerns about its safety. In 1995, the American magazine *Mother Jones* ran an article by investigative reporter Nicholas Regush, titled "Migrainekiller," reporting the case of Dianne Riley, who had died after being injected with a six-milligram dose of Imitrex. Two months later, her family filed a lawsuit against Glaxo (by then the world's largest pharmaceutical company after its purchase of Wellcome), accusing it of downplaying evidence that the drug could have serious cardiac effects in patients with undiagnosed heart conditions, as well as failing both to label the drug properly to warn doctors of the risks to patients, and to indicate what they should do in case of a negative reaction. The article went on to discuss concerns that Imitrex might have long-term effects on heart vessels, increasing the risk of stroke.[92] Humphrey was well aware of these worries. Ensuring the safety of the drug through studies and emphasizing the importance of diagnosis to physicians was imperative; the possible cardiovascular risks were his "biggest worry for a number of years."[93]

The Neurological Turn

While serotonin was changing how researchers approached pharmacological developments regarding migraine, equally significant changes in classification were taking place. In 1962, the American Ad Hoc Committee on Classification of Headache, chaired by Arnold P. Friedman, MD, and including among its panel members John R. Graham and Harold G. Wolff, had proposed a new classification for headaches. The divisions were based on pain mechanisms and rested on experimental and clinical data, "together with reasonable inference." The committee hoped their classification, although admittedly incomplete, could serve as a diagnostic framework in clinical practice to ensure that patients received proper treatment. While Friedman was a prominent neurologist, the influence of Graham and Wolff's vascular theories on the classification was clear. The committee proposed fifteen categories of headache, of which the first, vascular headache of migrainous type, included five subcategories: classical migraine, common migraine, cluster headache, hemiplegic and ophthalmoplegic migraine, and, finally, lower-half headache. Although the classification was widely used in the years to come, in retrospect Jes Olesen has described it as "completely non-operational." The inclusion of ambiguous words such as "usually" and "commonly" meant that "you could diagnose any kind of headache as migraine according to those criteria if you wanted to."[94]

We might see the ad hoc classification as marking the end of a theoretical era, rather than the beginning of a clinical one. By the 1970s, it seemed increasingly likely that neurological, rather than vascular, processes might be the primary cause of migraine. In America, a new generation of neurologists took over the leadership of the American Association for the Study of Headache, in an effort to transform the field scientifically.[95] In *The Headache and Migraine Handbook*, a guide designed to help members of the general public understand migraine, Nat Blau described how he came to believe "we had been barking up the wrong tree by concentrating on blood vessels alone."[96] He imagined migraine as a symphony with up to five movements: prodrome, aura, headache and other symptoms (the essence of migraine), resolution of headache, and postdrome, or the hangover. Other neurological symptoms of migraine besides aura included photophobia, phonophobia, general irritability, hypersensitivity to vibration and smells, poor concentration, sleepiness, yawning, and even increased libido. Sleep also played a role. This symphony included the entire process of the migraine attack, rather than simply the parts that could be explained by the vascular hypothesis.[97]

In an important paper published in *The Lancet* in 1981, Danish researcher Jes Olesen and colleagues demonstrated that there was no measurable alteration in cerebral blood flow during migraine without aura. This contrasted with classical migraine (migraine with aura), in which they found a wave of diminished blood flow spreading across the brain at approximately two millimeters per minute, a speed that correlated with Leão's theory of cortical spreading depression.[98] Their findings about cerebral blood flow not only undermined a key tenet of the vascular hypothesis, but also posed a significant conceptual challenge for the field by reigniting a fundamental debate about whether migraine was more than one disorder. Olesen and colleagues concluded that the two forms of migraine (classical and common) might have a different pathophysiology.[99] At the City of London Migraine Clinic, Marcia Wilkinson and her team had a number of issues with Olesen's study, not least that it relied on patients whose headaches had been induced with red wine.

Wilkinson argued that comparing spontaneous classical migraine with red wine–induced common migraine was not necessarily valid.[100] Nor did the results account for patients who experienced both classical and common migraine, as Wilkinson herself did. Partly on the basis of the blood flow results, Dewey K. Ziegler proposed that migraine should be thought of as "not one, two, or three illnesses, but several, even a multitude."[101] The ongoing debates about classification also precluded any possibility of accurately understanding migraine at the population level. Into the 1970s, researchers were pointing out that it was not possible to determine migraine prevalence without solving the "important problem" of an accurate definition of migraine, a difficulty that had been raised periodically since the 1930s. In 1975, W. E. Waters and P. J. O' Connor estimated that migraine prevalence in women was roughly twice that of men.[102] In 1980, a community study by researchers in Jerusalem estimated a prevalence of three to one, with an overall prevalence of 10 percent.[103]

The International Headache Society (founded in 1981) published its first *International Classification of Headache Disorders* (*ICHD-1*) in 1988. This was the result of three years' work, with the contributions of twelve subcommittees, and it was the first substantial headache classification to include operational diagnostic criteria. The committee, chaired by Olesen, recognized that there would inevitably be mistakes discovered only through use, but they expressed their hope that the classification would nevertheless inform clinical practice and stimulate interest and research to improve the classification, as well as increase the understanding of headache epidemiology.[104] The committee classified headache into four primary headache groups: migraine (within which, migraine with and without aura were considered to be different types), tension-type headache, cluster headache, and other headaches. Over the following years, *ICHD-1* was accepted widely and translated into more than twenty languages. In the 1990s, the emergence of triptans as a revolutionary new treatment for acute migraine attacks was an important—and successful —early test for these new diagnostic criteria. When combined with the new *ICHD* classification, researchers could follow up with patients much more effectively. For Anne MacGregor, this coincidence is "really incredible."[105] The *ICHD* criteria meant that, for the first time, researchers were able to produce prevalence studies based on internationally accepted and clinically useful criteria. In 1995, the first prevalence study of specific headache types in a general population finally confirmed that women were three times as likely to experience migraine in their lifetime as men.[106]

Conclusion

The twentieth century witnessed the rise and fall of toxic, ocular, allergic, psychological, and vascular theories of migraine. Of all these ideas, the vascular model had proven to be the most enduring, until, by the 1990s, neurobiological explanations of migraine gained the upper hand. Perhaps most significantly, functional magnetic resonance imaging of blood vessels revealed that there was no relationship between the pain of migraine attacks in migraine without aura and abnormal cerebral blood flow. The discovery of serotonin, and drugs that could target its receptors in the brain, was a game changer in the search for effective treatment. The success of triptans that followed had a number of consequences for industrial and academic research on migraine, not all of which were necessarily positive. On a practical level, there was a dramatic effect on the flow of patients to headache and migraine clinics. Anne MacGregor remembers that the "brilliance" of sumatriptan "killed off research on acute patients. . . . Why on earth would they want to not take their triptan, to come along, and be involved in clinical trials when they would then be throwing up in a taxi on the way there?"[107] Triptans also made the pharmaceutical industry reluctant to continue funding research into new drugs because, as Jes Olesen has commented, "people feel that the triptans solve all problems." Then there was the re-ignition of a debate about drug responsiveness and classification. In 1967, Macdonald Critchley had proposed that responsiveness to ergotamine could be considered diagnostic for migraine.[108] The same question came up with triptans. Olesen emphatically rejected any proposal that drug response might be a useful factor in developing a classification, explaining that it would prevent the possibility of testing new drugs.[109] It was clear, however, that while the development of oral triptans represented a real therapeutic breakthrough, as well as a paradigm shift for research, problems related to migraine had not all been solved. A large proportion of patients did not respond to oral triptans, and how they worked remained unclear. Were they acting as a vasoconstrictor on intracranial blood vessels, or acting directly on the neurons in the trigeminal nervous system?[110]

In a 2011 commentary entitled "The Vascular Theory of Migraine—a Great Story Wrecked by the Facts," Peter Goadsby declared that the triumph of neurology in putting migraine "back into the brain," combined with the development of drugs having neuronal, rather than vascular targets, is a victory for patients, freeing them from "any potentially vascular complications of antimigraine therapeutics in the future." Goadsby presented the vascular theory as a block to medical progress and saw its demise as "ushering a new era."[111] What is striking, however, is how closely this rhetoric of reclaiming migraine for neurology and the brain mirrored discussions from almost a century earlier, proclaiming the triumph of neurosis over biliousness that we saw in chapter 4. Even as migraine has been put back into the supposedly gender-neutral brain, it carries the baggage of history with it.

In particular, the ongoing fascination with, and emphasis on, visual aura has had profound implications for research. The key question of whether the two main types of migraine (with and without aura) are essentially different things remains unanswered. Edda Hanington commented that much of the research published on migraine—including her own on platelet disorder—was based only on subjects who had migraine *with* aura, because it was easy to diagnose accurately. If Hanington's point is relevant to the field as a whole, then it is clear that data obtained from only one group of patients cannot represent the overall migraine population. In particular, it will tend to exclude women whose migraine is related to the menstrual cycle, who may experience the greatest levels of pain, and who form the majority of individuals with the disorder.[112] We simply don't know the extent to which a focus on the recruitment of patients with migraine aura may have skewed the scientific data.

CHAPTER NINE

"If I Could Harness Pain"

The Migraine Art Competitions, 1980–1987

A Woman in the Kitchen, 1981

An ordinary suburban kitchen, early 1980s (fig. 9.1).[1] Sunlight streams through the windows onto a chaotic scene. Crockery and dirty saucepans pile up around the sink. A kitten plays in the milk spilling from an upturned tumbler by the sink, and a mop lies abandoned on the floor next to the puddle. Vegetables on the counter lie waiting to be chopped. Laundry tumbles out of a washing machine. In the shade of the cupboard, a woman sits on the floor, her head in her hands, apparently overwhelmed by the detritus of daily life. Executed in watercolor, this work of art is vividly evocative of the everyday effects of migraine. Apart from the details of a normal routine gone awry, the diagonal lines of light and shade, the drape of the curtains, and the angle of the open cupboard door all hint at the disorientating zigzag of a migraine aura. "I was seeking to portray the futility and despair of trying to cope," the artist of this picture later commented. "Attempting to maintain a normal routine for the family with faulty vision, clumsiness, and pain that clouds all coherent and rational thought can only end in one result: chaos."[2]

The painting of the woman in her kitchen is one of around nine hundred original artworks submitted by members of the public to four international art competitions, held between 1980 and 1987. The competitions were run by the British Migraine Association (known as Migraine Action since 1997) and sponsored by the pharmaceutical company Boehringer Ingelheim. The collection of nearly six hundred pieces that remains is a unique and remarkable archive.[3] Ranging from simple line drawings on cheap file paper to detailed and intricate pieces of art employing diverse techniques—including oil, water-

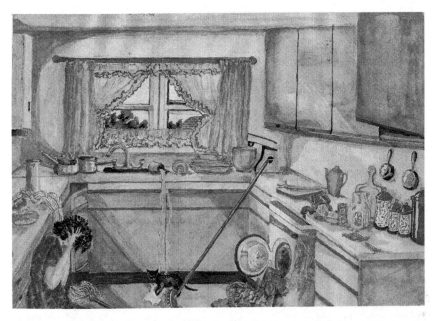

Fig. 9.1. Untitled artwork, submitted to the Third Migraine Art Competition, 1981, image 14. Courtesy of Migraine Action via the Wellcome Collection, licensed under CC-BY

color, collage, and airbrush—the collection represents the work of around 450 artists, of whom three-quarters were women, and one in ten were children age sixteen and under. The vast majority of these individuals had no artistic background. Together, the pieces form a powerful and, at times, deeply uncomfortable witness to the intense pain and disruption of migraine, an experience beyond the scope of much of the scientific literature. This chapter is about the migraine art collection, the creation of which arose out of a particular constellation of factors. These include an emerging sense of identity and advocacy among migraine patients, increasing pharmaceutical interest in the condition, a recognition of the value of art as a tool for communication and therapy within the physician-patient encounter, and the idea that migraine was part of the identity of a migraineur. The collection reflects the increasing visibility of migraine, and people with migraine, in public discourse, even as it reveals the disjuncture between lived experiences of pain and the priorities of the pharmaceutical industry and medical profession. Finally, the artwork represents the experience of migraine as medical knowledge was on the cusp of a new neurological and pharmaceutical era.

The Context

The British Migraine Association, the first organization founded to officially represent people with migraine, had been formed in March 1958 by Peter Wilson, an employee of the City Council in Bournemouth, a large town on the southern English coast. He had experienced migraine from the age of twelve. The association had a somewhat modest beginning. Wilson placed an advertisement in the local newspaper, the *Bournemouth Evening Echo*, inviting anyone with migraine to attend a meeting. Ten people came, and each contributed £10. Within a year, the association had more than a thousand members. An advertisement in the popular magazine *Woman's Own* boosted recruitment, and in 1960, a further two thousand people joined. Initially, the association sent its members a single-page newsletter, with details of free migraine clinics at four hospitals, but its founders soon began to envisage a greater role for it and organized the first of what would become biennial research symposia held in London.[4] The early success of the British Migraine Association reflected a very real sense that the medical and political establishments were uninterested in migraine and dismissive of its sufferers. Writer Pamela Hansford Johnson, Baroness Snow, who became president of the British Migraine Association in 1961, remembers the response of the people around her when she had her own first attack, at the age of eleven, "in the days when people said that little girls could not have headaches."[5] In her 1959 novel, *The Humbler Creation*, she had described "a migraine attack in all its repulsiveness." After the book's publication, she had been surprised to receive a flood of letters saying "This is me." Johnson believed her writing had attracted so much interest because she had managed to express "the personal humiliation of the complaint." This humiliation, she explained, resulted from the continuing influence of psychosomatic theories, which made people feel as if they ought to be able to control their nervous nature, ridding themselves of migraine by an act of sheer will.

In 1960, the British government was asked to urgently investigate the dearth of support available for people with migraine. In a House of Commons debate, a Member of Parliament (MP) for Glasgow, Mr. Jon Rankin, reminded his audience that in 1954, the British government had told people with migraine to "cheer up," because a lot of research was in progress. Yet in 1960, "nothing appears to be happening." Referring to the work Neville Leyton was doing with hormonal and allergic therapies at the Putney Clinic, Rankin commented that migraine only seemed to be being cured by "private benevolence,"

not "public munificence." He could not understand why, despite Leyton's success at Putney, the doctor was not being admitted to the "magic circle" of the
National Health Service (NHS). Another MP, Richard Harris, argued that
specialist treatment clinics should be established within the NHS. In response,
Edith Pitt, Parliamentary Secretary to the Ministry of Health, explained that
the government had no authority to tell doctors which treatments to use, nor
to advise them on research matters. This was the responsibility of the Medical Research Council. The problem, she tactfully suggested, was that Leyton
seemed not to have persuaded the majority of doctors that they should copy
his therapeutic approach.[6] Apart from illustrating the extent to which hormonal and allergic approaches to migraine remained peripheral to standard
prescriptions of sedatives and ergotamine, the debate in the British Parliament illustrates how migraine advocates were seeking to establish services
that would address their needs within a new nationalized health system that
was still establishing the boundaries of its service. At the same time, there was
a palpable sense of limbo, since ongoing research into vascular and sensory
mechanisms seemed to have stalled, rather than delivering tangible results to
benefit patients.

In America, Keith Wailoo has also identified this as a time of transition, as
earlier high mortality rates from infectious diseases entered "a new era when
a host of chronic degenerative ailments became society's chief burden." The
postwar pharmaceutical industry offered "a powerful new armamentarium"
of sedatives and tranquilizers, pain relief for "a rising tide of crippling arthritis pain, migraines, back pain, cancer-related pain, and unspecified subjective
pains."[7] On both sides of the Atlantic, the post–World War II period raised
urgent questions about the role of government in the delivery of relief, the
regulation of research and industry, and the means to determine what constituted true pain, worthy of attention and resources. Wailoo suggests we might
see the 1960s and 1970s as being characterized by the "slow expansion of a
bureaucracy of relief."[8]

By the early 1960s, the implicit compact in Britain, which had seen its
citizens accept that government and the medical profession would deliver
healthcare on their behalf, was beginning to weaken. Patients began to expect
higher standards and greater accountability, and clinicians started to involve
their patients more in primary care.[9] In 1962, neurologist Macdonald Critchley
pleaded for colleagues to establish migraine and headache clinics. He promised that family doctors would welcome places where they could send difficult-
to-diagnose patients, who would be "profoundly gratified" to be taken seriously

and sympathetically handled. For neurologists, there would also be a payoff. Clinics would create hubs of potential subjects for research, afford a peep into the ecology and natural behavior of this "tantalizing but fascinating disorder," and present enhanced opportunities for assessing drug therapy.[10] The migraine clinic Marcia Wilkinson founded at the Elizabeth Garrett Anderson Hospital took a particularly innovative approach to welcoming patients who were in the throes of an attack. For London's workers, Wilkinson's clinic offered a couch, analgesic treatments, and antiemetic tablets, instead of a painful commute home. There was even an ambulance that could collect people and bring them to the clinic.[11] In its first four years, eight thousand people were treated, of whom a quarter arrived during an attack. In setting up the clinic, Wilkinson had taken inspiration from Elizabeth Garrett Anderson's 1870 MD thesis on migraine, which showed a profound understanding of migraine in combination with sound practical advice, emphasizing the well-being of the patient through nutrition, regular meals and habits, rest, "and great quantities of hot tea."[12] While Garrett Anderson's work had been ignored by her Victorian contemporaries, a century later, Wilkinson's approach gained great respect from her colleagues. Patrick Humphrey, who, as director of the Glaxo Company's Division of Pharmacology, would be instrumental in the development of the triptan class of drugs, recalls that it was Wilkinson who had made him realize the need for new, effective migraine medicines.[13]

By 1967, there were eleven migraine clinics in Britain. Most were in the southeast, including four in London, but patients could also access specialist help in Birmingham, Stoke-on-Trent, Newcastle, and Edinburgh.[14] The clinics established in the 1960s and 1970s acted as important hubs, linking patient advocacy and focused treatment with pathological investigation and pharmaceutical development. They offered patients a range of established medications, including methysergide, ergotamine, sedatives, and hormone therapies, but they were also at the forefront of new approaches. Researchers affiliated with the clinics found that the patients who came there were often willing volunteers for double-blind trials to test new drugs and to investigate theories regarding migraine mechanisms. The papers that came out of these settings made public some of the most significant advances in late twentieth-century migraine knowledge, particularly the shift from a vascular to a neurological framework for understanding this disorder. For example, Dr. Edda Hanington's early reports on tyramine headache in the late 1960s came from interviews with 160 patients at the Elizabeth Garrett Anderson Hospital and demonstrated a clear relationship between diet and migraine attacks.[15] The British

Migraine Association had aided Hanington's research by circulating a questionnaire about dietary factors to all subscribers of *Migraine News*. The responses of 240 members helped confirm Hanington's ideas about the role of tyramine, which would be so important to the development of the blood platelet theory of migraine in the 1970s.[16]

Clinics were also opened in other countries. At the Copenhagen Acute Headache Clinic, Jes Olesen and his colleagues researched changes in cerebral blood flow during migraine attacks.[17] In Houston, Texas, Ninan T. Mathew's research with eighty clinic patients led to an early recognition that episodic migraine might transform into more chronic manifestations and daily headaches through factors such as stress, excessive use of medication, hypertension, and adverse life events.[18] Publications based on research with patients from specialist clinics included topics as diverse as therapeutic experimentation with drugs (including clonidine and aspirin), the treatment of pain-trigger areas in the scalp and neck, measurements of serotonin levels in and between attacks, psychological aspects, weather, outcomes of pregnancy for women with migraine, prodromal symptoms, and cerebral blood flow.[19]

This period is also notable for being the moment when the idea of the "migraineur" was at its most prominent, in both academic and popular use. The term seems to date from 1936. In an article on "Allergy as a Factor in Headache," C. L. Hartsock and F. J. McGurl outlined an intensive dietary regimen for what they called the "true migraineur." In his 1957 novel, *The Last Angry Man*, American writer and journalist Gerald Green reflected the dominant psychological theories of the day by making the protagonist, Dr. Sam Abelman, a typical migraineur, who was "bothered by details, worrisome, demanding perfection in yourself, which is understandable, and in others, which is very dangerous."[20] In the mid-1960s, use of this term began to increase, and rapidly did so since the 1970s. Two significant publications help explain this burgeoning sense of migraine as identity. The first was Joan Didion's 1968 essay, "In Bed," in which she describes her relationship with an "uninvited friend." Migraine had been central to Didion's life from her first experience, at age eight. "Three, four, sometimes five times a month, I spend the day in bed with a migraine headache, insensible to the world around me," the essay began. Without drugs, Didion could function "perhaps one day in four." As a teenager, Didion thought she could deny migraine's existence, ignore it, fight it, and it would go away. Spending one or two days a week in bed, "unconscious with pain," when there was nothing wrong with her, had seemed "a shameful secret, evidence not merely of some chemical inferiority but of all my bad

attitudes, unpleasant tempers, wrongthink." Everyone knew, she explains—
in a reference to the psychological paradigms that dominated medical and
popular understandings at the time—that migraine headaches were either
imaginary or self-inflicted. So she persisted, wishing "only for a neurosurgeon who would do a lobotomy on house call."[21] If Didion's work highlighted
the effects of migraine on everyday life, Oliver Sacks's *Migraine* made the idea
of the migraineur into a best seller. Sacks reflected on the romantic view of
the characteristics of male and female migraineurs in the work of writers such
as Walter Alvarez (and the contrast with how people with epilepsy were seen
in terms of having a hereditary taint, or a constitutional stigmata). A migraineur, then, was not just someone who experienced migraine, but a person
whose physical appearance, comportment, social interactions, and intelligence
were all shaped by, even defined by, their neurological makeup.[22] Quoting
both Didion and Sacks in an article for the *Washington Post* in 1986, Pamela
Margoshes asked for an end to prevailing stereotypes of migraine sufferers as
"weak, perennially petulant, hyperventilating, overwrought nellies whose
blood vessels dilate at the drop of a hat. Because the old myths are simply not
true. Migraine is not a personality disorder. It's a neurological tornado, a force
of nature."[23]

Finally, it is important to note the significance of art therapy and "outsider
art." In institutional settings, health professionals saw the allocation of time
to creative activities as a way to occupy patients, but further interpretation
of this artwork offered an opportunity to gain access into the minds of those
patients. Alexander Weatherson, chair of the British Association of Art Therapists, described how art therapy could give patients a voice by allowing them
to express their fears and struggles, as well as being a creative way to appeal
for help, understanding, and sympathy.[24] By the early 1970s, some researchers
were also becoming interested in art as an insight into the more subjective,
lived experience of migraine, particularly when the patients were children. A
study published in the journal *Neurology* in 1973 reported the results of en-
couraging children to draw what they saw or felt during a migraine attack. As
well as representing their experiences of scotoma and other visual phenomena, one child depicted how other people appeared unusually small, while
another drew a room, with her mother being upside down. A girl created an
image of herself lying on a railroad track as the train passed over her. For the
article's authors, this variety of experiences was the most remarkable aspect
of their experiment.[25]

The idea of outsider art was closely related to the art therapy movement. First used in 1972, the term describes art created by self-taught artists, including patients with mental illness and autism, as well as art that was simply unconventional and idiosyncratic, ignoring tradition or cultural influences. One of the originators of the term, Roger Cardinal, proposes that outsider art "offers its audience a thrilling visual experience . . . an art of unexpected and often bewildering distinctiveness" that reveals "private worlds . . . so remote from our normal experience as to appear alien and rebarbative." Discussing drawings by artists with autism, Cardinal is less interested in the images as scientific documents revealing signs of disease or psychic distortion than in simply accepting, and respecting, these creative outputs as art in and of itself.[26]

By the 1970s, art had become widely accepted as a legitimate, and often revealing, expression of the experiences and effects of illness on ordinary people's lives.[27] Migraine researchers' belief that art could provide a view into the (mal)functioning of the brain itself echoed the discussions of a century earlier, when men of science extolled the virtues of Hubert Airy's veritable photograph of a morbid process in the brain. While earlier discussions had excluded anyone who could not be relied on to represent their aura objectively, unsullied by the inconvenient intrusion of pain, by the late twentieth century, patients were more often being seen as active participants who could make an effective contribution to migraine understanding. This emerging context of cooperation, awareness of (and interest in) the effects of migraine on patients' lives, and a knowledge exchange between patients, charities, clinical researchers, and pharmaceutical companies was important in improving research, but it also lay behind the idea for the art competition and helps explain its success.

The Competition

In 1973, Derek Robinson, a marketing executive from the pharmaceutical company Boehringer Ingelheim, had been searching for images for educational and advertising material to help promote a new clonidine drug for migraine, called Dixarit.[28] Robinson met Kenneth Hay, a general practitioner from Birmingham, England, whose patient, an art teacher, had explained her migraines to him through sketches.[29] Inspired by the idea that more people might make migraine art as a way to communicate their experiences, Dr. Hay introduced Jean Butter to Robinson, who saw the potential her images had for marketing his company's products. In 1979, the British Migraine Association agreed to cosponsor a public art competition, and the first call for entries was sent out in the charity organization's *Migraine Newsletter* in August 1980.[30]

The instructions to entrants for the first competition were very specific: they must be migraine sufferers themselves and should draw or paint either their own impressions of one of the forms of visual disturbance that heralded a classical migraine attack or illustrate the effect of migraine on their lives. Pain was not mentioned. Peter Wilson, representing the aims of the British Migraine Association, hoped to attract entrants with artistic skills, as well as welcoming "natural, even primitive" depictions of the most dramatic aspects of migraine, in order to emphasize its separation from common headaches.[31] The competition was a huge success, attracting more than three hundred entries over the nine months when it was advertised. A panel of judges—including, Dr. Nat Blau (secretary to the Medical Advisory Panel of the Migraine Trust and joint honorary director of the City of London Migraine Clinic), Jon Liddell (British Migraine Association), Richard Calvocoressi (modern art curator at the Tate Gallery)—were charged with awarding the prizes. Marcia Wilkinson's City of London Migraine Clinic hosted the exhibition from the first competition, with prizes awarded by Dame Vera Lynn.

The winning image, by a professional artist, depicted a rural scene of lush green fields and a dirt road leading to farm buildings on the horizon (fig. 9.2). The impressionistic brushstrokes of the background scene are in stark contrast to the precision of a C-shaped scintillating scotoma that overlays and partially obscures the background, its edges appearing to shimmer and pulsate outward. The artist later explained that his aura began with a small blue dot in the center of his vision, around which would appear a "thin glittering bracelet." Over a twenty-minute period, it would usually break on the left before enlarging away to the right.[32]

With its jagged zigzags, straight lines, and details of blue, red, and yellow, the image closely followed the convention of depicting the type of aura known as scintillating scotoma in a particular way, one that had been established by nineteenth-century men of science and epitomized by Hubert Airy's diagrams. While the detail of the aura is certainly beautiful, it is important to acknowledge the very particular aesthetic tradition continued by this image. The value accorded to the entry (notably, by an all-male judging panel) reflected a century-long tendency to accord the highest status to "accurate," authentic renderings by men of the appearance of stereotypical migraine aura. This was a very narrow and restricted visual language of aura that detached

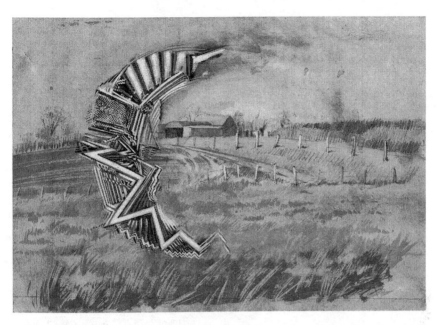

Fig. 9.2. Untitled artwork, submitted to the First Migraine Art Competition (awarded first prize), 1981, image 463. Courtesy of Migraine Action via the Wellcome Collection, licensed under CC-BY

migraine from the failings of the body. The image was scientific, and supposedly objective. We can almost imagine John Herschel and William Gowers nodding their approval.

Representing Pain

As he planned the first migraine art competition in 1980, Peter Wilson had hoped the entries would help highlight the "astronomical human suffering" migraine causes. It seems surprising, therefore, that the organizers of the first competition did not initially anticipate the extent to which entrants would produce pieces of work that not only portrayed aura and the effects of migraine on their lives, but vividly and often brutally represented experiences of extreme pain. Andrew Levy is right when he comments that the most profound impression gained from viewing galleries of migraine art is the repeated violence being done to the head.[33] Even physicians used to dealing with migraine patients every day admitted to finding the migraine artwork difficult to look at. Nat Blau thought the collection was marvelous, but he also added that some images were "like a nail boring through the head."[34]

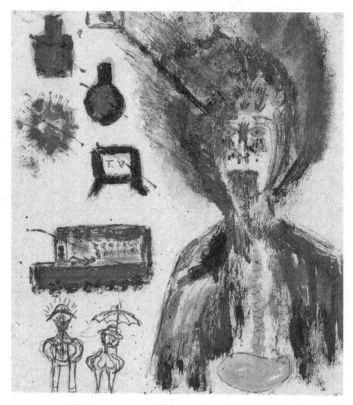

Fig. 9.3. Untitled artwork, submitted to the Second Migraine Art Competition, 1982, image 302. Courtesy of Migraine Action via the Wellcome Collection, licensed under CC-BY

For me, there is one picture that encapsulates the significance of the Migraine Art Collection as a witness to pain (fig. 9.3). Submitted to the second competition in 1982, it is a visceral glimpse inside the body and life of a migraine sufferer. The figure of the woman takes up the right-hand side of the picture. Vigorous brushstrokes in a dark crimson spurt out of the head, arrows bore into the skull, and a spear enters the bloody right eye, while tears fall from the left one. Vomit spills from the mouth, while, inside the body, the stomach and esophagus are picked out in hot, painful red. To the left, a series of crossed-out shapes—bottles (of perfume, or perhaps alcohol), the sun, television, a trip to the theatre—reveal the aspects of normal life she must avoid. The piece might be seen (as can many of the artworks in the Migraine Art Collection) as reflecting and contributing to a genre in which artists, particularly women, have represented their pain, their difficult relationship with medicine, and their feelings about their own damaged, scarred, or deteriorating bodies in often quite shocking and revealing ways.

There are certainly echoes of Frida Kahlo's *Broken Column* (1944) here, a self-portrait in which Kahlo depicted the suffering she endured after a tram accident that left her with multiple fractures of her spine, pelvis, leg, and foot. In *Broken Column*, Kahlo is split open from neck to pelvis, revealing a broken and disintegrating doric column within, her body held together by white straps, representing the steel corset she was forced to wear. The skin of her face and body is impaled by nails, her eyes weeping tears.[35] Art historians have interpreted Kahlo's nails as referencing the Christian iconography of martyrdom, but it seems likely that the many artists who depicted arrows, nails, and drills attacking their heads in their entries to the migraine art competitions were making a much more literal point about the sensation and location of their pain.[36] As I have looked at this piece of migraine art in the context of a wider tradition of self-portraiture, I have been struck by a comment that Ludmilla Jordanova has made in her essay about artist Beth Fisher, who documents the effects of mental illness, cancer, and aging on herself and her family. Jordanova asks us "to look hard at the work itself . . . to perceive its rawness, its fierce, unsettled emotions, its scale, its darkness, its lack of closure, to meditate upon it, but never to lose sight of it as a woman's labour."[37] We should accord the pieces submitted to the Migraine Art Competitions a similar level of respect and dwell on how this body of work provides a profound insight into lives lived with pain, disruption, and the constant presence of an unwelcome force.

These works of migraine art are not easy to look at, and they took courage to make. In his writing on illness narratives, Arthur Frank talks of moral "acts of witness, telling truths that are too often silenced because they speak of what any sane person would rather ignore among life's possible outcomes." Frank has also explained that sick people "must consider it appropriate for private experiences to be represented as public events."[38] These points about appropriateness are highly relevant in this context. Artist John Joseph Brennan (who won the fourth migraine competition with *Migraine Man*), experienced migraine from childhood, and he reflected on how important this sense of legitimacy was for his inclusion of migraine experience in his own creative processes. In art school, he didn't see taking influences from his migraine "as a legitimate means to do good art." Over time, however, it became "a reference, like a support," to which he felt privileged to have access. The clouds, zigzags, and other imagery derived from his migraine experience became part of his own personal visual vocabulary.[39] We shouldn't underestimate how important this validation must have been for entrants unused to publicly expressing their experiences. Many noted on their entry forms or on the back of their pictures that they weren't artists. As Kathy Charmaz argues in her study of chronic illness, "telling anything about illness can mean revealing potentially discrediting information about self." The act of telling (or, in the case of art, showing) strains relationships, risks a loss of control, and raises the potential to be ignored, rejected, or stigmatized.[40]

"Let a sufferer try to describe a pain in his head to a doctor," Virginia Woolf famously suggested, "and language at once runs dry."[41] Yet there is quite definitely a language of pain, and one way (the *only* way, according to David Biro) to convey experiences that resist literal expression is through metaphor.[42] Joanna Bourke has argued that historically, there have been "a set of figurative languages" for representing pain through metaphor. This often includes pain as a monster, companion, or loiterer; a force that cuts, rips, shatters, and burns; an object that hammers, cuts, and squeezes; or, more abstractly, as heat, weight, or color.[43] The Migraine Art Collection is replete with analogies such as these. The artworks depict objects like weights, chains, lightning, flames, drills, hammers, blades on knives, saws, and axes. Again and again, migraine artists have found ways to communicate the sensations they feel in their heads, eyes, necks, and stomachs, such as a nail driven into the side of a head in a flash of jagged white lightning, showing how the "sharp, penetrating . . . pain felt fixed and embedded."[44] One of the most compelling motifs, appearing repeatedly in the collection, is the notion of migraine as an attack by either little people or devils, who often hold pins, hammers, axes, and screws. These attacks could be both physical and sensory. In one image, a little devil drills into the skull, creating a crack through the forehead and over an eye, while his friends lift weights, ring bells, and shine a torch into the woman's eye (fig. 9.4).[45] Devils are featured again in a self-portrait, where they hammer nails into a woman's forehead, eyelids, and temples while she holds her head, shouting in pain.[46] A flock of black, bat-winged characters flit around another head, some turning a screw attached to a clamplike apparatus enclosing the skull, and others using pins, hammers, and knives to inflict a variety of pains on the skull.[47] "It's always waiting," one woman wrote of the flaming monster reaching out with its right hand to grab her throat while holding a dagger in its left.[48]

In 1991, ninety images from the Migraine Art Collection were exhibited in San Francisco in a display entitled *Mosaic Art*. There, the works were viewed by neurologist Oliver Sacks, who incorporated the insights he gained from

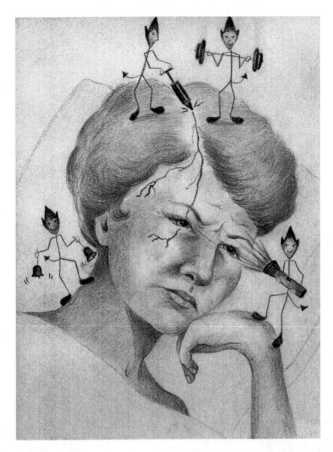

Fig. 9.4. Untitled artwork, submitted to one of the Migraine Art competitions, undated, image 484. Courtesy of Migraine Action via the Wellcome Collection, licensed under CC-BY

seeing the archive into the revised edition of his best-selling book, *Migraine*. Sacks had been particularly struck by the pieces showing cobwebs or nets pinning bodies down, interpreting these as evidence not only of visual, but also of sensory disturbances.[49] It is also true to say that a web can be a powerful metaphor for a sense of isolation and entrapment, particularly when combined with an incessantly ringing telephone,[50] a carving knife and forks taking huge slices from the side of the head (fig. 9.5), or punching hands. Another artist used the idea of being caught in a glass box to indicate how migraine cut her off from normal society (fig. 9.6). "It was a symbol of my reduced world, the restrictions confining me because of my migraine" she explained.[51]

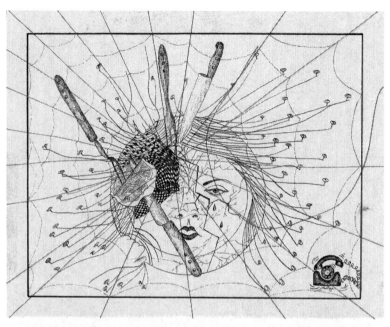

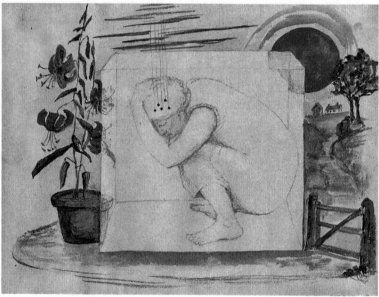

Fig. 9.5. (*top*) Untitled artwork, submitted to the Second Migraine Art Competition, 1983, image 388. Courtesy of Migraine Action via the Wellcome Collection, licensed under CC-BY. *Fig. 9.6.* (*bottom*) Untitled artwork, submitted to the Second Migraine Art Competition, 1983, image 317. Courtesy of Migraine Action via the Wellcome Collection, licensed under CC-BY

In many of the images, the straightforward bluntness of the metaphors is shocking, particularly in the pictures submitted by children, which are some of the most moving, as well as the most difficult to look at. As I've explored this collection, I have often wondered how parents must have felt, after urging their son or daughter to create a picture for the competition, to see the effects of pain, isolation, and unhappiness portrayed through their child's eyes. There is the matter-of-fact brutality with which an eleven-year-old boy depicted a power drill connecting his brain to his eye (fig. 9.7). Children drew themselves being attacked, in one case by a man in a military uniform. A twelve-year-old girl wrote a poignant comment alongside the image of a hammer hitting her skull: "When I have a migran [*sic*] I am continually being sick I never know what to do with myself. Sometimes I feel like killing myself."[52] Loneliness dominates the children's images, showing how acutely aware they are of the life they are already missing. An eight-year-old girl lies on a sofa, hands over her eyes, surrounded by the repeating motif of a clock face.[53] In one picture, awarded first prize in the "under-16" category for the third competition, the chair at the head of the birthday party table is empty, the balloons, presents, and characters in fancy dress waiting for the child who lies in bed. "Please Be Quiet. Do Not Disturb," a flap folded over the image of the sleeping girl requests.[54] In another piece, the same child drew herself looking out from behind the bars of a prison cell, alone except for the spiders, and crying. "If I could harness pain, I could conquer the world," one fifteen-year-old girl wrote on the back of a dark image illustrating her visual disturbance (fig. 9.8). Discos, swimming, school, food, and outdoor activities are all missed because of migraine. The artist who created *Programmed In!* (fig. 1.1), the first image in this book's introduction, submitted another entry, depicting her memories of missing out on maypole dancing as a child, with the zigzag aura above her head drawing our attention to the girl left alone on the grass while her friends played. There is no sentimentality or romanticization of migraine pain in these images. They show that from a young age, people have a shared repertoire of motifs with which to express their experiences of migraine. Metaphors of pain as a weapon, a companion, or an unwanted visitor, or of the body as trapped, split, or disintegrating from the inside out, situate these representations of migraine within a broader body of art and literature that tries to make sense of pain in myriad forms. As we have seen in previous chapters, some of the essential elements of the visual and linguistic repertoire with respect to migraine—boring, hammering, light, noise, fire, and attack—stretch back hundreds, if not thousands of years. Yet the collection also pro-

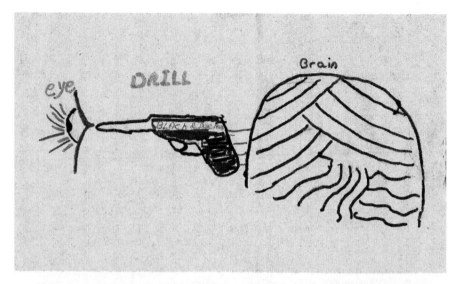

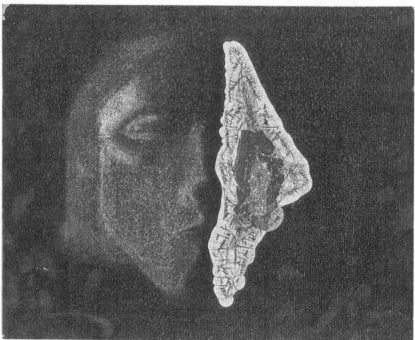

Fig. 9.7. (*top*) Untitled artwork, submitted to the First Migraine Art Competition (under-16 category), 1981, image 427. Courtesy of Migraine Action via the Wellcome Collection, licensed under CC-BY. *Fig. 9.8.* (*bottom*) *The Power of Pain*, submitted to the Third Migraine Art Competition (under-16 category), 1985, image 502. Courtesy of Migraine Action via the Wellcome Collection, licensed under CC-BY

vides important evidence of how experiences of migraine aura and pain are shaped by the social, cultural, and medical contexts of the time in which they were produced.

Migraine Life Histories

Pneumatic drills, ruined shopping trips, the disorientation of navigating in busy public areas, traffic jams, typewriters, and lightbulbs all suggest an amplification of migraine experience in a technologically driven postindustrial society. They provide important evidence of migraine's twentieth-century social history and remind us that however timeless some metaphors might appear to be, the experience of illness is shaped by the conditions of each historical moment. Telephones and televisions are notably recurring themes in the migraine art collection. In *Cause and Effect*, the telephone symbolizes the social and professional pressures that can produce a migraine attack. At the same time as it causes the woman's life to telescope in on itself, it also is the medium through which to communicate apologies for missing work and meetings, cancelled outings, and social absences.[55] The noise of the telephone is central to other images too, such as a phone that rings incessantly while a woman pleads "go away, go away, go away." In another piece by the same artist, the phone is off the hook, a denial or refusal of contact with the world outside. Cancelled appointments are a prominent theme, particularly in terms of the isolation and loneliness that come with missing parties and days at the seaside.

"How can you drive when the road looks like this?," one artist asked, depicting a uniform stretch of grey obscuring the lower three-quarters of a circular field of vision.[56] Several of the images hint at the frightening experience of driving as an aura develops. In *The Onset of Migraine* (fig. 9.9), a storyboard takes the viewer through six stages of the aura, beginning with a small white star in the middle of the visual field that gives the first warning of an attack's approach. Within six minutes, the flashing, spiky, C-shaped scotoma dominates the left-hand side, as blurred vision creeps in from the right. Once sight is entirely blurred, there is a brief sense of relief—"normal in three minutes"—until a violent headache follows. One artist simply drew a large cross next to her car, indicating one of the many aspects of her life, including wine, computers, and cheese, that migraine placed off limits. The judges for the third art competition were particularly impressed by one driving-themed entry. Stuck in a traffic jam, hands clenching the wheel, the artist looks out through the windshield, with a jagged aura cleaving across the traffic ahead and the cars

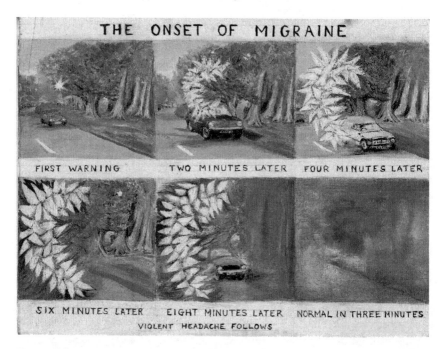

Fig 9.9. The Onset of Migraine, submitted to the Third Migraine Art Competition, 1985, image 337. Courtesy of Migraine Action via the Wellcome Collection, licensed under CC-BY

on the other side of the road disorientatingly stacked on top each of each other.[57]

A number of the images from the Migraine Art Collection make contemporary cultural and social analogies to describe the migraine experience. I began this book by discussing *Programmed In!*, a self-portrait depicting Hubert Airy's drawing of a C-shaped scotoma as the Pac-Man character in a video arcade game. Neurologist Nat Blau was particularly struck by one child who had drawn herself lying in bed, unable to go to school, and who had described migraine as being "like Star Wars."[58] One of the most striking cultural references is in a piece submitted to the third competition, in 1985, in which a woman's hand reaches out against a black background. From her forefinger, a glass bauble labeled "migraine" dangles over the outstretched hand of a young child (fig. 9.10). While it is not clear whether the artist is the recipient or the giver of the bauble (quite possibly she is both), the painting is a simple but moving meditation on the hereditary nature of migraine. The two hands reaching toward each other clearly reference *The Creation of Adam*,

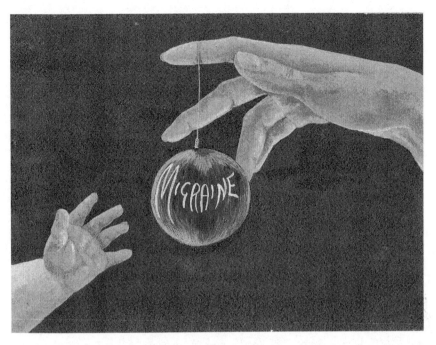

Fig. 9.10. Untitled artwork, submitted to the Third Migraine Art Competition, 1985, image 313. Courtesy of Migraine Action via the Wellcome Collection, licensed under CC-BY

part of Michelangelo's extensive sixteenth-century masterpiece (1508–1512) painted on the ceiling of the Sistine Chapel in the Vatican. This element of the famous fresco has also inspired some of the most resonant cultural images of the late 1970s and early 1980s. On 31 July 1978, *Time* magazine marked the arrival of the world's first test tube baby, a pivotal moment in the history of reproductive medicine, with a cover design showing a test tube containing a glowing fertilized egg between the two reaching hands. If the *Time* cover was a suggestive link to the genetic theme conveyed in the migraine picture, the immediate inspiration for this particular competition entry seems to have been even more recent. In 1982, cinema audiences around the world had been captivated by the story of the extraterrestrial who simply wanted to go home. The poster for *E.T.* had the same blue light against a black background, and a child's hand reaching out. The artist who painted migraine as a bauble to be passed down between generations tapped into a tradition where a very simple motif—two hands reaching toward each other—encapsulated a range of ideas about life, hope, family, and belonging.[59]

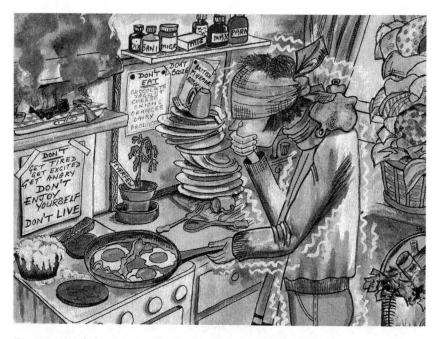

Fig. 9.11. Untitled artwork, submitted to the Third Migraine Art Competition, 1985, image 316. Courtesy of Migraine Action via the Wellcome Collection, licensed under CC-BY

Writer Joan Didion knew her migraine never occurred when she was "in real trouble," but instead when she was fighting "a guerrilla war" with her own life, "during weeks of small household confusions, lost laundry, unhappy help, canceled appointments, on days when the telephone rings too much and I get no work done and the wind is coming up." It was at times like these when Didion's "friend" came "uninvited."[60] Her description of the daily battle with migraine is vividly portrayed by pieces from the art collection depicting the overwhelming minutiae of domestic responsibilities. With bound eyes and forehead, and a hot water bottle on her neck, a shaking, nauseous woman holds her mouth as she cooks breakfast (fig. 9.11). Smoke billows from burning tomatoes and sausages, a saucepan boils over, the trashcan and laundry basket overflow, and the dishes pile up. Surrounded by the chaos of things she *needs* to do, pieces of paper taped to the walls also remind her of all the things she must *not* do. Don't get tired, excited, or angry. "Don't enjoy yourself, don't live," the note above the stove orders, while other notes ban chocolate, yogurt, cheese, onions, oranges, dairy produce, and booze. The shelf above her is crowded by a multitude of pill boxes and medicine bottles, while a potted feverfew plant wilts on the countertop. The artist described how her migraine attacks resulted in a "sense of failure as a wife and mother."[61]

One artist in his seventies entitled his piece *To Fit Again* and reflected on a life avoiding, among others, town centers, shopping trips, sports events, theatres and cinemas, dances, dinners, and receptions.[62] Two images stand out for the detail with which they depict the effects of migraine over the course of an entire life. In *The Five Ages of My Migraine*, the annotated scenes depict important periods in a woman's life (fig. 9.12), from her earliest childhood memories of having vinegar-soaked rags wrapped around her head at the age of three in 1916 through charity work during widowhood in the 1970s. Each small tableau contains a self-portrait of the artist, with arrows running down one side of her face to signify the pain. In each image, apart from the one of her as a child, a zigzag aura partially obscures some of the most important moments in life, affecting her ability to write in school and intruding on her daughter's wedding in 1967. During the "caravan rallies" she and her husband attended between 1956 and 1972, she lies on her bed while, through the window, the fun can be seen continuing outside. Her *Five Ages of My Migraine*

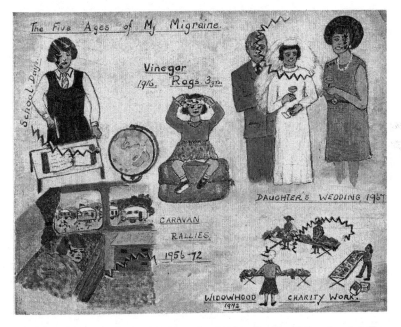

Fig. 9.12. *The Five Ages of My Migraine*, submitted to the First Migraine Art Competition, 1981, image 319. Courtesy of Migraine Action via the Wellcome Collection, licensed under CC-BY

was the first of four drawings this artist submitted, one for each competition. Together, they produce a powerful commentary about the effects of migraine on life and work. *Migraine at the Gala Concert,* submitted to the second competition in 1983, shows a vaporous grey visual aura obscuring the choir, almost as if it was the music wafting its way through the concert hall.[63] In *The Migraine Life,* submitted to the third competition in 1985, the aura appears as if it is lightning striking from a cloud that darkens the sky over St. Paul's Cathedral in central London. As the caption running down the left-hand side of the picture explains, "On the Brightest Day: the Happiest shopping spree, the dreaded MIG may strike, like a thunder storm and ruin everything."[64] In *Sorry Closed for Migraine,* the artist looks out from her shop door as she places a "closed" sign in the window with one hand while covering her left eye and temple with the other. The shop's sign, above the glass, reads "Focal Display," a reference to the visual effects that have forced the lone shopkeeper to close her business.[65] *The Five Ages of My Migraine* made no suggestion that the artist had found any medical relief during a lifetime in which migraine appears as a constant threat, disrupting school, work, important days, significant evenings, and holidays.

A photograph of a young woman in underwear, cut from a magazine, forms the centerpiece of a collage. With ballpoint pen scribbles, the artist identified the areas of her body most affected by migraine: the head that feels "like lead," the sinking feeling in the stomach, the shaky legs, a speech bubble explaining "I love Mars Bars," denoting either a craving or a forbidden luxury. A pair of sunglasses is "a very useful essential." At the bottom of the image, an outline figure of a person, drawn in red ballpoint pen, lies on a cutout photo of a sofa, with the underlined request "PLEASE DO NOT DISTURB." Written notes about the artist's migraine experience fill the margins on the rest of the page, describing in detail its effects on her life. Unusually, the image describes the benefits that pharmaceutical advances had brought to her life. Her migraines began in 1911, "with so-called sick headache," which she battled weekly until 1942. When her doctor prescribed Migril, it "opened out a new world, I could get [up] from my bed and prepare some sort of a meal for my family." In 1976, when she again "was not doing very well," a hospital consultant prescribed the antidepressant drug Nardil, which proved to be another transformation. She would take two Nardil and two Dixarit a day. Now, at age 78, "I have lots of energy. Ride a bicycle[,] garden etc." But this freedom from pain also required discipline: "[I] know when to stop. All this is accomplished by observing a diet." The right-hand side of the page emphasized further the sacrifices required to avoid attacks: "NO TO cheese chocolate jelly ice-cream milk bananas . . . NO TO TV sessions of more than thirty mins no knitting as I pass out, like the final stages of coming out of a fit."[66]

The discipline required to manage migraine is a recurring theme. "I take tablets as prescribed by my doctor. Eat at regular times," one artist wrote.[67] Other therapeutic strategies are more subtle: closed curtains in darkened rooms, quiet isolation, bed rest, sunglasses, ice packs. But the majority of artists who commented on their relationship with medication did so negatively. In *Absolutely Fed-Up with Pills*, the person was transformed into a vessel to be filled with tablets, one of a number of artworks giving a sense of how dependent on medication some entrants felt themselves to be. One artist found solace in her family and Christianity, and she included drugs among the list of other things—despair, loneliness, depression, fear, pain, and vomiting—that threatened a fragile sense of hope. In another image, a monstrous, scaly hand holds out a bottle of pills "to be taken twice a day" to a young woman surrounded by stars and flames.[68] One self-portrait depicts a woman sitting at a table, staring into a small freestanding mirror on the checkered tablecloth, an open bottle of pills on the flat surface in front of her, as if debating whether the benefits of the two tablets that awaited her outweighed their side effects.

When an entrant who had sent her artwork to the migraine art competition as a child was interviewed some years later by Klaus Podoll and Derek Robinson, she recalled:

> I remember never taking the name of "migraine" in vain. When trying perhaps to get a day off school because I didn't feel well, I never once tried to con my mother that I was having an attack. You wouldn't dare treat them with disrespect, mainly as you felt you might be punished with the worst attack of your life; besides it would have been impossible to fake the effects—no one could act that convincingly unless they were truly in pain. . . . There is that feeling that it is taking over your body from within, slowly engulfing you and making you very small, frightened, and powerless.

Her drawing was dominated by an eye, within which a girl sat on the floor.[69] Looking back, from the perspective of someone who no longer considered herself a migraine sufferer, she remembered the profound sense of loneliness she felt during her childhood attacks: "There was never anything anyone could do to make me feel better. . . . You would have to ride out the experience on your own inside your head." Tellingly, this artist was one of many who responded in the past tense to Podoll and Robinson's questions about how migraine had inspired their art. The artist who had drawn herself cooking breakfast stated: "I had no pleasure and seemed to be punished if I veered from the narrow control I had to impose on myself." Another commented on how even the 1980s seemed to represent different expectations, particularly for women: "It seems a bit outdated now. She would be expected to manage a career, job, or study as well as the children and the housework, plus the migraine, nowadays." For her, the more positive viewpoint she could take in hindsight was as much a reflection on the quieter lifestyle, and the knowledge of personal limits, that came with maturity.

In 1991, just three years after the last of the four Migraine Art competitions, Glaxo released sumatriptan, a drug that revolutionized migraine treatment for millions of people around the world affected by this condition.[70] For the first time, many found that a migraine could be aborted at the first sign of an attack. The significance of this change is hinted at by the responses to another series of migraine art competitions, this time in the United States. Between 1989 and 2003, the National Headache Foundation sponsored four of them. Entrants to the first American contest were expressly instructed to create a "vivid interpretation" of pain, a theme that attracted four hundred entries. The second contest, held in 1998, was the first to be held in the posttriptan era, and only 150 submissions were received. There are two explanations for this precipitous drop in the number of entries. The first is that the success of triptans had radically reduced the number of people experiencing severe migraine, and thus cut down on the pool of possible entrants. In addition, the call for submissions to the next contest asked for artworks that would "educate others about the benefits of migraine prevention." Thus a second explanation for why this competition received much less interest is that people with migraine still simply did not feel able to produce creative responses on such a positive theme. By the fourth competition, entitled My Life with Migraine, entries again reached four hundred—suggesting that a theme acknowledging the realities of migraine pain, and the often fraught relationship with medication, even after triptans were available, was a crucial factor in attracting interest.[71]

In recent years, professional artists have also drawn directly on experiences of migraine to inspire their art. Visual artist Blythe Smith describes making art while coping with chronic migraine as "my way of breathing."[72] In 2016, Welsh artist Fran Kelly, a sufferer from hemiplegic migraines, created "Maison Migraine," an installation that invited visitors to immerse themselves in the experience of migraine, with distorted everyday objects, uncomfortable audio effects, a disorientatingly uneven floor, and rotten-tasting candies.[73] Kelly uses her art to try and raise awareness about migraine, as well as to communicate its effects. Another British artist, Debbie Ayles, produces bold paintings in acrylic to reflect not only her experiences of aura, but also as an experiment to see how the process of creating the works might provoke migraine. *View of a Lounge during a Migraine* is deliberately intended to express a feeling of claustrophobia, while the psychedelic *Interior with Clock—Inducing a Migraine* was painted "to see if the bright colours would induce a migraine." Although Ayles comments that the early stages of planning the piece were enjoyable, she suffered migraine attacks as the colors covered the canvas. Her attempts to ease the discomfort with white paper placed over certain areas failed, and "it got too painful and someone else was directed to complete the painting." Working on another piece, *Greenacres Barn*, Ayles discovered that it was not necessarily bright colors that caused visual disturbance, but the way that the tones and colors were distributed.[74]

Conclusion

Since the turn of the new century, online communities for knowledge exchange, support, validation, and censure have emerged. The advent of the internet has radically expanded opportunities for people to share their experiences and creative interpretations of illnesses such as migraine. These include galleries of artwork on Flickr; animations of migraine aura on YouTube; and Facebook, Twitter, and Instagram accounts. YouTube, which hosts a number of video animations of migraine aura, the most popular of which have been viewed hundreds of thousands of times, appears to be a particularly important online space in which men feel comfortable narrating their experiences of migraine in public.[75]

Since 2016, the original Migraine Art Collection has reached a new audience after being digitized and put online in a gallery allowing anyone to download and share any piece from the collection. For the charity Migraine Action, putting the artwork online was a way to raise awareness of migraine generally, as well as start conversations about particular themes or issues facing people with migraine, such as common triggers or the fear of another attack. The aspects of life with migraine portrayed by artists in the 1980s continue to resonate. Migraine has by no means gone away.

The Migraine Art competitions in the 1980s were an important opportunity for ordinary people to depict their experiences with this extremely common disorder. The body of work that was submitted to the contests over nearly a decade is a unique witness to the sensations of migraine in the body and its devastating effects on lives, even at a very early age. While some of the metaphors and experiences seem to reflect ongoing themes that echo across the centuries, there is also much that is very modern in these pieces. The collection is a vivid visual confirmation of how inadequate our treatments of migraine have been, culturally, socially, phenomenologically, and medically.

CHAPTER TEN

Conclusion

At the annual scientific meeting of the American Headache Society (AHS) in June 2017, researchers were excited. Four different companies were announcing positive results from large-scale phase 3 trials for monoclonal antibody therapies to prevent migraine. The data were good: overall, the antibodies halved the number of days with migraine for almost 50 percent of the patients in the trials—a gold standard for preventive treatment.[1] All of the drugs (known as mAbs) target the neurotransmitter calcitonin gene-related peptide (CGRP) or its receptors.[2] CGRP is a molecule produced by nerve cells in the peripheral and central nervous systems. It is the most potent vasodilator we yet know of in the human body, plays a role in the transmission of pain, and is essential for the maintenance of normal brain circulation. CGRP is most concentrated in the nerves of the trigeminovascular system— the part of the brain responsible for head and face pain—where neuroscientists now think a migraine attack is initiated when the nerves are irritated or stimulated in some way. CGRP was first identified as playing a potentially important causative role in migraine attacks in the 1980s, when researchers observed that increased levels of CGRP (and only CGRP) were present in the cranial blood circulation and in saliva during acute migraine attacks.[3] Intravenously infused CGRP was found to induce a migraine-like attack both in patients having migraine with aura and those without aura, supporting the theory that the mechanism of headache induction in both types of migraine could be similar. In chronic migraine, CGRP levels remain elevated.[4]

MAbs are not the first migraine drugs to target CGRP. At the turn of the current millennium, migraine researchers hoped to develop a new class of drugs—gepants—that would act as CGRP receptor blockers without the vascular complications of triptans. Enthusiasm for them was unexpectedly short lived, as these drugs were proven to have potentially serious side effects on the liver with prolonged use.[5] It was then that scientists began to wonder whether monoclonal antibodies might provide an answer. This was a fast-growing sector of the pharmaceutical industry, promising treatments for diseases including cancer, multiple sclerosis, asthma, and rheumatoid arthritis.[6] Could antibodies work for a disorder characterized by pain? It seemed unlikely if the molecules were too big to pass through the blood-brain barrier and into the brain, which is where most researchers thought any effective drug for migraine would need to act.[7] Given these doubts, the announcement at the 2017 AHS meeting that a class of migraine-specific prophylactic mAbs had been successfully created—drugs that were able to prevent attacks over a period of several months—was "a genuine watershed moment," Peter Goadsby declared.[8] While further research was needed to understand their long-term effects and safety, in the short to medium term, all of the monoclonal antibody drugs, which are injected either under the skin or into a vein, appeared to be safe, effective, and more tolerable than triptans.

In May 2018, the FDA approved the first of these drugs (erenumab, marketed by Amgen and Novartis as Aimovig, a self-administered monthly injectable medication) for the preventive treatment of adult migraine. The drug was approved in Europe a few months later. In September 2018, a second FDA approval for Teva's drug Ajovy (fremanezumab) followed. Drugs that target CGRP are not a panacea, however. They do not reduce pain in all cases, and—although at around $7,000 per year the initial cost to consumers is lower than expected—such a price tag still raises pressing questions of access.[9] Among those patients for whom the mAbs work, who will get treatment? Moreover, who will pay for it? In the United States, headache specialists are concerned that insurance companies are restricting access to new therapies that will need to be taken on a chronic basis, when cheaper existing drugs appear to offer similar effects.[10] For anyone without insurance, the cost could be prohibitive. This question of access to pain relief is not a new one, nor is it likely to be resolved in the near future. Even triptans, now available in generic and over-the-counter form in some countries, can still be prohibitively expensive for people with a limited income, as well as in low- and middle-income countries. In 2010, a study published in *Neurology* concluded that uninsured American patients with migraine and those reliant on Medicaid were less likely to receive standard abortive or prophylactic migraine treatment, partly because they were more often treated in emergency rooms than in a physician's office. The result of the study, the authors comment, is "a reminder that access to some forms of insurance is not the same as access to adequate care." Moreover, they acknowledge that "inadequate insurance magnifies the already high burden of migraine on low-income families."[11] In England, the National Institute for Health and Clinical Excellence (NICE, the licensing body for NHS treatments) has agreed to include prescriptions for Botox injections for chronic migraine since 2012, and in Scotland, approval was granted in 2017. The NHS has also funded occipital nerve stimulation for adult patients with intractable chronic migraine since 2015. But this new generation of monoclonal antibodies will have to prove their cost effectiveness to be accepted by insurance companies, the NHS, and other medical systems under a great deal of political, social, and fiscal pressure.[12] Financial and ethical decisions will need to be made about whose migraine is treated. If these discussions are difficult in wealthy countries that experience socioeconomic, racial, and gender disparities in population health and medical care, they will be even harder in resource-poor countries facing other pressing public health crises, such as HIV, tuberculosis, or malaria. Migraine-specific drugs are not included in the WHO lists of essential medicines, and, as Paulo Martelletti argues, unless we are to treat a billion such sufferers worldwide, the priority will be in preventing and reducing chronic migraine.[13]

Our understanding of migraine, and its global burden, has changed rapidly in recent decades. During the 1970s, neurologists undertaking hospital-based studies had assumed that migraine was rare in Africa. Later research presented a more complicated picture but nevertheless suggested that a lower prevalence among Africans might be attributable to a variety of reasons, including underdiagnosis, greater pain tolerance in rural communities, and genetic factors. In the 1990s, studies conducted in the United States indicated that migraine prevalence was lower among African Americans and Asian Americans than populations with a Caucasian background—a finding for which the authors suggested race-related differences in genetic vulnerability were a likely explanatory factor.[14] More recently, surveys carried out in the United States using the *ICHD* criteria have indicated that inequalities in migraine diagnoses, medical care, and treatments are likely to account for disparate burdens across different racial and ethnic groups. While confirmed migraine is more prevalent in non-Hispanic whites, researchers have found the incidence of *probable* migraine to be higher among African Americans. Moreover, African Americans experience a greater burden from migraine, with it being "more frequent, more severe, more likely to become chronic and associated with more depression and lower quality of life."[15] Other research has indicated that the occurrence of migraine might be greatest among Native Americans, a highly disadvantaged group.[16] These results should not be surprising. Minorities have been systematically underrepresented in clinical trials for migraine, while women (unusually) are overrepresented. As a result, the clinical trial population does not adequately characterize either the general population with migraine or the multiple varieties of the disease.[17] We also know that persistent racial and ethnic disparities and biases lead to the systematic undertreatment of minorities for all kinds of pain, whether that pain is acute, chronic, caused by cancer, or amenable to palliative care.[18]

In 2003, in *World Health Report 2001*, the World Health Organization published the results of its first Global Burden of Disease (GBD) survey, conducted in 2000, and ranked migraine nineteenth in global causes of disability, responsible for 1.4 percent of all years lived with disability (YLD).[19] For the headache research community, the report's recognition of migraine's public health burden gave credibility to their repeated calls for greater research investment, funding, and political action. Nevertheless, leading experts in the field of headache disorders argued that disability from migraine (with and without aura) remained underreported. In an editorial published simultaneously in the journals *Cephalalgia*, *Headache*, and the *Journal of Headache and Pain* in 2010, three leading experts criticized the 2000 Global Burden report for considerably underreporting migraine disability and for generally giving a "very poor account" of headache disorders. Primarily, this had been because of a lack of evidence, particularly for China, India, Southeast Asia, Africa, the Eastern Mediterranean and Eastern Europe.[20] In the years since the first GBD survey, Lifting the Burden's Global Campaign Against Headache, a worldwide collaboration between the World Health Organization, nongovernmental organizations, academic institutions, and individuals, has collected a great deal of new evidence.[21] As a result of this effort, as well as the increasing international acceptance of standardized criteria for migraine, the 2010 Global Burden of Disease report radically updated earlier findings related to the burden of headache disorders. Steiner and colleagues cited the 2010 survey's estimated worldwide prevalence of migraine to be 14.7 percent—making it the third most common disease in the world, behind dental caries and tension-type headaches, and the seventh highest specific cause of disability globally. Migraine had become, "by a large margin, the leading cause of disability among neurological disorders."[22] While this recognition was a breakthrough for the field, the implications of this new status for headache disorders were unwelcome. Experts were "appalled" to find largely treatable headache disorders "among these ignominious top ten."[23]

By the 2013 Global Burden of Disease report, migraine, by itself, was up to sixth in the leading causes of disability worldwide. When combined with "medication overuse headache" (at eighteenth), headache disorders ranked third among all causes of disability worldwide. While data on migraine in earlier reports had predominantly come from Europe and the Americas, the 2015 Global Burden of Disease report confirmed that migraine ranked between fifth and eighth among causes of disability in *all* regions of the world, an important rebuttal to racialized assumptions about lower migraine prevalence among Africans, in particular. As new studies provide more accurate data, researchers predict that the proportion of global disability correctly attributed to headache disorders will continue to rise.[24] Nonetheless, much more research is needed to understand how migraine burdens around the world relate to gender, socioeconomic status, race and ethnicity, and access to effective treatments.

Having easy access to modern drugs is not the only answer, however. Increasingly, physicians and researchers interested in migraine are concerned that the frequent use of acute medication can lead to medication overuse headache, which can be a major factor in the transformation from episodic to chronic migraine. Perhaps the most significant change in the second edition of the *International Classification of Headache Disorders* in 2004 was the introduction of chronic migraine as a diagnosis for patients who fulfilled diagnostic criteria for migraine (without medication overuse) on more than fifteen days per month for three months or more.[25] Most recently, *ICHD-3* has incorporated chronic migraine into the main body of its classification, identifying it as a major type of migraine, alongside migraine without and with aura.[26] As recent research has shown, however, what the distinction between episodic and chronic migraine actually means in practice is not clear. One study argues that patients with ten days of migraine a month (high frequency episodic migraine) experience as great a level of emotional and functional impact through disability, loss of quality of life, and direct and indirect costs as patients who reach fifteen days and come into the official chronic category.[27]

Moreover, we are still by no means certain what migraine actually is. While some researchers hope to discover a common biochemical pathway in the brain that will eventually unify all of migraine's diverse symptoms into a single mechanism, genetic research suggests an alternative picture. Early on, this research into migraine identified three ion channel genes that could cause rare and severe forms of migraine disorder, such as familial hemiplegic migraine. These "simple" gene mutations for specific subtypes, however, did not appear to be linked to common migraine. Following the completion of the human genome project in 2003, researchers have been able to undertake much larger genome-wide association studies that identify genetic contributions to a whole range of diseases. At the time of this writing, in 2018, more than forty genetic variations have been found to affect susceptibility to common migraine. Significantly, these genes appear to be involved with vascular and neuronal processes in the two main types of migraine (with and without aura), a finding that opens the door to yet another potential reassessment of the role of vascular processes in migraine.[28] Advances in genetics promise greater insight into the molecular mechanisms of migraine attacks, which, in turn, may help improve patient care and individualized treatment. But, yet again, a great deal remains unknown, including how genetic variations might interact with environmental or socioeconomic factors.[29] Determining the extent to which global regional differences in migraine prevalence might be genetic—rather than the result of underreporting, disparities in the provision of healthcare, political decisions about funding and drug approval, and the inherent weaknesses and biases of diagnostic models that rely on self-reported pain—will require very carefully considered research, robust data, and sensitive interpretation.[30] As the authors of one recent paper point out, undertaking population studies large enough to enable convincing genetic conclusions will require a huge amount of resources, as well as international collaborations across a range of academic, clinical, and commercial partners.[31]

Standardized, globally accepted classifications have allowed more robust, comparable analyses, and new neurobiological frameworks for migraine have afforded better recognition and increased funding, improving the professional status of an unfashionable field. Neuroimaging of patients both during and between attacks offers the possibility for much greater understandings of how drugs act in the brain; how episodic and chronic migraine affect brain structure, function, and neurochemistry; and why patients respond differently to therapies.[32] Yet, as Joanna Kempner argues, greater understanding of migraine's biological reality does not necessarily endow legitimacy or reduce stigma. People with migraine continue to be seen in terms of moral and social failure—weak, excitable, sensitive, neurotic hypochondriacs who are unable to cope with everyday life.[33] As our knowledge continues to evolve, and in whatever biological leads we choose to follow in the hunt for migraine's causes and mechanisms, we must take care that we don't ignore the varied experiences of people who are in pain, as well as the conditions in which they live their lives and access medical care. In particular, we should not sideline people whose pain (especially chronic pain) is *not* reduced by pharmaceutical advances, or whose symptoms do not conveniently fit the classificatory boundaries we select in order to define what does, or does not, constitute migraine at any given moment.

At various times and places, migraine has meant a number of things, and changing definitions have emphasized different symptoms to fit explanatory models. Yet the constancy and severity of pain at the heart of migraine, and people's attempts to manage that pain, have woven their way through the entire history this book has recounted. From the classical period, throughout the Middle Ages, and into the early modern period, pain was the central component of a disease understood in terms of humors. Descriptions of it are visceral, and sometimes violent, and they provide a compelling logic for its severity. In the seventeenth century, concepts of migraine began to broaden. First, we can see a shift in the vernacular meaning of megrim to incorporate sensations of dizziness, turning, or nausea. Then, by the late eighteenth century, European medical writers began to emphasize visual symptoms, while, in the wider culture, migraine came to imply nervous weakness, effeminacy, and even an association with quackery. As lay and professional medical understandings of sick headache and bilious headache diverged in the nineteenth century, the records of how working-class patients talked about their own chronic pain (and the way that pain was used in the service of pharmacological development) is in marked contrast to accounts of a painless visual aura that captivated an intellectual elite. The assumption that migraine was a hereditary disorder of educated, scientific men was only one aspect of wider discussions about the disease, but it suited physicians to emphasize migraine's class-related credentials in an age of concern about the role of nervous disorders in social and moral degeneration. Even as more-standardized pharmaceutical sedative treatments for pain became available in the late nineteenth century, physicians were elevating visual aura as the key diagnostic characteristic of migraine. The conceptual primacy that has since been accorded to the visual manifestations of aura can be seen in the diagnosis of Hildegard of Bingen, the persistent celebration of Hubert Airy, and in the Migraine Art competitions, when organizers simply did not anticipate the extent to which entrants (the vast majority of whom were women) would be motivated to represent pain with such visceral clarity. Tellingly, the winning image in the first competition conformed to a very particular neurological aesthetic of representing migraine "objectively": one detached from the body, in which pain was absent. On the one hand, emphasizing the visual element of migraine adds important weight to the claim that it is much more than "just a headache." On the other hand, it paradoxically deflects attention from the aspect of the migraine experience that most requires our attention—severe, debilitating, and radically undertreated pain.

One of the key contributions of this book has been to show how the widely accepted statistic that women account for two-thirds of the people with migraine has been formalized only in the past few decades, despite a long history of discussion about the kinds of people migraine affects. Such an apparently straightforward figure hides a great deal of complexity. Overall, migraine seems not only to be more common, but also be fundamentally more painful and less visual for women, a finding that has real significance when we consider the way migraine has been represented and researched as a highly gendered neurological disorder since the nineteenth century.

If people with migraine are to receive consistent, appropriate, and, most importantly, effective treatment, those driving health research and policy, whether in individual clinics or at the level of long-term global initiatives to address health inequalities, need to be interested in and well informed about how our current understanding of migraine's neurobiology is founded on a centuries-long social, cultural, and medical history, of which neurology is only a part. That history has shaped our knowledge about the disease, our attitudes towards the people who become patients, and the measures we take to address pain. Even more to the point, when we attempt to comprehend historical ideas and practices on their own terms—particularly when those ideas seem alien to our own concepts, or when the implications of past practices might still resonate uncomfortably—such a history reminds us that our own ideas (not to mention our medicines), however confident we may be now of their value, are also contingent, temporary, and—above all—can be bettered.

Note on Terminology and Names

1. Kempner, *Not Tonight*, 102; Young, "De-stigmatizing Migraine."

Chapter 1 · Introduction

1. Pac-Man gained the status of a cultural icon of the video game era in the early 1980s, particularly as Namco's designers deliberately designed the game to appeal to women, as well as men, by avoiding the standard shooting format of other popular games, such as Space Invaders.

2. Ludmilla Jordanova has noted that artists who paint self-portraits often show a vivid historical awareness at the same time as they reflect preoccupations in the here and now. See Jordanova, "Body of the Artist," 45.

3. Rose, "History of Migraine," 1–3.

4. Other words from the early modern period include the following: migram, migrime, meagrim, mygrame, meigrame, megryme, meagrom, meegreeme, mygryme, migrin, migrine, mygrime, and mygrim.

5. Allbutt, "Clinical Lecture," 203.

6. For the current internationally accepted, research-driven definitions of migraine and other headache disorders, see Headache Classification Subcommittee, *International Classification of Headache Disorders*, 3rd ed. [hereafter cited as *ICHD-3*]. For a useful overview of current understandings and issues relating to headache disorders, including migraine, see World Health Organization, "Headache Disorders."

7. *AL Kennedy's Migraine*, radio program.

8. Carrington, *Rudyard Kipling*, 75.

9. Headache Classification Subcommittee, *ICHD-3*, 8–9; Puledda and Goadsby, "An Update," 2031–2039; Steiner et al., "GBD 2015," 104–107.

10. Buse et al., "Sex Differences," 1279–1280.

11. National Migraine Centre website, "Migraine and Headaches."

12. Maniyar and Goadsby, "Migraine—Some Theories and Controversies," 19–21, 25.

13. Lipton et al., "Headache," 49–50.

14. Headache Classification Subcommittee, *ICHD-3*, 18–22. Other, less common forms of migraine with aura include migraine with brainstem aura and hemiplegic migraine, which includes motor weakness as well as headache and aura symptoms.

15. Moisse et al., "Grammy Reporter."

16. Buse et al., "Sex Differences," 1279–1280; Woldeamanuel and Cowan, "Migraine Affects 1 in 10," 307.

17. MacGregor, "Menstrual Migraine," 17–23; MacGregor et al., "Sex-Related Differences," 852.

18. Abu-Arafeh et al., "Prevalence," 1088–1097.

19. Burch et al., "Prevalence and Burden," 21–34.

20. Kempner, *Not Tonight*, 103–104.

21. Kempner, "Invisible People."

22. Bendelow, *Pain and Gender*; Canning, "Body as Method?"; L. Smith, "An Account."

23. There is a diverse body of literature on pain from a range of disciplinary approaches. A classic study is Scarry, *Body in Pain*. Significant historical studies include Bending, *Representation of Bodily Pain*; Bourke, *Story of Pain*; E. Cohen et al., *Knowledge and Pain*; Moscoso, *Pain*. I have found Drew Leder's phenomenological approach particularly thought provoking in Leder, *Absent Body*.

24. Kamen, *All in My Head*, 86–89.

25. Kempner, *Not Tonight*, xii; Migraine Trust, "Diagnosis and Management."

26. Olesen et al., "Funding," 995.

27. National Institutes of Health, "Estimates of Funding."

28. Kempner, *Not Tonight*, 6, 10–14.

29. Kempner, *Not Tonight*, 12.

30. Pressman, *Last Resort*, 415.

31. For an example of the combative language used in this rejection, see Goadsby, "Vascular Theory." On the segregation of blood from modern neurological representations of the brain, see Martin, "Blood and the Brain."

32. Edvinsson, "Trigeminovascular Pathway," 48, 50; Moskowitz, "Holes."

33. Duden, *Woman beneath the Skin*; Kassell, "Casebooks"; Pilloud and Louis-Courvoisier, "Intimate Experience"; Risse and Warner, "Reconstructing Clinical Activities." A number of projects have placed digitized casebooks and correspondence online. See The Casebooks Project; The Cullen Project; The Sloane Letters Project.

34. Jacyna and Casper, *Neurological Patient*, vii; Porter, "Patient's View," 182–183.

35. On the use of historical visual material, see Jordanova, *Look of the Past*. On medical imagery, see P. Hansen, *Picturing Medical Progress*; Latour, "How to Be Iconophilic."

36. Levy, *A Brain Wider*, 99.

37. In this approach, I am indebted to the social and cultural historians of medicine who, since the 1960s and 1970s, have shied away from a focus on medicine's "great men" and instead attempted to reconstruct how communities and individuals in the past have responded socially, politically, and culturally to illnesses and epidemics. For discussions of this field, see, for example, Jordanova, "Social Construction"; Rosenberg, "What Is Disease?"; Rosenberg and Golden, *Framing Disease*.

38. I discussed my approach to migraine in the "Note on Terminology and Names" at the beginning of this book. On terminology more generally, see Boyd, "Disease, Illness," 9–17; Carel, *Illness*; Cooper, "Disease."

39. Methodological discussions of retrospective diagnosis include C. Bynum, *Holy Feast*; Latour, "On the Partial Existence"; McGough, "Syphilis."

40. There is a large body of literature on the history of disease. For good introductions to some of the methodological issues, see Cunningham, "Identifying Disease"; M. Jackson, "Perspectives."

41. Coleborne, *Madness*, 125. Studies of such disorders include Anderson and Mackay, *Intolerant Bodies*; M. Jackson, *Allergy*; Murray, *Multiple Sclerosis*; M. Smith, *Another Person's Poison*.

42. Fee and Fox, *AIDS*; Moore, "Reorganising Chronic Disease Management"; Peitzman, *Dropsy, Dialysis, Transplant*; Talley, *History of Multiple Sclerosis*; Weisz, *Chronic Disease*.

43. Cunningham, "Identifying Disease,"13.

44. Lawlor, *From Melancholia*, 2–5.

45. Mukherjee, *Emperor*, xvii.

46. M. Jackson, *Asthma*, 10–12, 200–201.

47. A. Wilson, "On the History," 273, 283.

48. On diagnosis, see Cunningham, "Identifying Disease"; Stein, "'Getting' the Pox," 53–60.

49. On the fraught relationship between social construction and biological reality, see Arrizabalaga, "Problematising."

50. Studies of headache and migraine from a neurological viewpoint include Diamond and Franklin, *Headache*; Eadie, *Headache*; Pearce, "Historical Aspects"; Rose, "History of Migraine." In addition, Levy, *A Brain Wider*, contains considerable historical material; Kempner, *Not Tonight*, covers nineteenth- and twentieth-century material, particularly relating to gender.

51. Eadie, *Headache*, 73.
52. Eadie, *Headache*, 268.
53. Puledda and Goadsby, "An Update."
54. Gorsky, "Sources and Resources"; Hampshire and Johnson, "Digital World."
55. Kassell, "Paper Technologies."
56. Literature on history writing and digitization is a rapidly emerging field. Some good introductions to the ethical, practical, and methodological questions historians need to consider include Jordanova, "Historical Vision"; Weller, *History in the Digital Age.*
57. Hitchcock, "Confronting the Digital."
58. I discuss some of these issues further in Foxhall, "Digital Narratives."

Chapter 2 · The "Beating of Hammers"

1. "*Leechbook.* Book 1," in Cockayne, *Leechdoms*, 21–23 [hereafter cited as Bald's *Leechbook*]. The original Middle English text reads: "Wiþ healfes heafdes ece: genim þa readan netlan anstelede, getrifula, meng wið eced 7 æges þæt white, do eall togædere, smire mid. / Wiþ healfes heafdes ece: laures croppan getrifula on eced mid ele, smyre mid þy þæt wenge. Wið þon ilcan genim rudan seaw, wring on þæt næpyrel þe on þa [s]aran healfe bið. Wiþ healfes heafdes ece: genim laures croppan dust 7 senap, meng togædere. Goet eced on, smire mid þa saran healfe mid þy."
2. Bald's *Leechbook*, 21–23.
3. Cameron, "Bald's *Leechbook*," 153; C. Wright, *Bald's Leechbook*, ff. 7v, 8r.
4. Banham, "Dun, Oxa, and Pliny," 57–73; Crawford, "Nadir," 46.
5. Deegan, "Critical Edition," vol. 1, xxxvii–xxxix.
6. Cameron, *Anglo-Saxon Medicine*, 5–18; Crawford, "Nadir," 43.
7. For more on this organizing principle, see Demaitre, *Medieval Medicine*, xi–xii.
8. Cameron, *Anglo-Saxon Medicine*, 82–83. See also Adams and Deegan, "Bald's *Leechbook*," 88.
9. Bald's *Leechbook*, 83.
10. Deegan, "Critical Edition," vol. 1, xxv.
11. Other influences include the fifth-century *Herbarium of Pseudo-Apuleius*, a text that was widely disseminated across Europe; sixth-century Greek physician Alexander of Tralles; and Oribasius, the fourth-century author of seventy books and physician to the Roman emperor. See Deegan, "Critical Edition," vol. 1, vxiii–xxvii; Van Arsdall, *Medieval Herbal Remedies*, 35.
12. Pearce, "Historical Aspects," 1098.
13. On humors, see Arikha, *Passions and Tempers*, 6–10; Rawcliffe, *Medicine and Society*, 32–34.
14. Rawcliffe, *Medicine and Society*, 54; Wear, *Knowledge and Practice*, 65, 78, 88–92.
15. Crawford, "Nadir," 46.
16. Ghalioungui, *Ebers Papyrus*, entry no. 250, 83.
17. Rose, "History of Migraine," 1.
18. W. Smith, *Hippocrates*, 207.
19. Koehler and van de Wiel, "Aretaeus," 256.
20. Lu and Needham, *Celestial Lancets*, 118. The authors identify the point as modern day R1, indicated for similar disorders.
21. Lu and Needham, *Celestial Lancets*, 129. *Pai-hui* corresponds to modern day GV20, or "hundred meeting point" on the top of the skull. More recently, the authors explain, there has been an increase in the number of acupuncture points that are not indicated on any of the traditional tracts, and these have been found to be valuable in treating a number of disorders, including migraine. In addition, the known power of acupuncture in treating afflictions such as migraine and arthritis has led to its use for pain relief during surgical operations since the 1950s. See Lu and Needham, *Celestial Lancets*, 163–164, 200.

22. E. Wallis, *Medieval Medicine*, 17.

23. Horden, "What's Wrong," 11.

24. E. Wallis, *Medieval Medicine*, 18–19.

25. On Hildegard's authorship of *Causae et Curae*, see Sweet, *Rooted in the Earth*, 35–49.

26. Throop, *Causes and Cures*, 74–75, 135.

27. "Recette contre la migraine," in Wickersheimer, "Textes médicaux chartrains," 166. I am grateful to Prof. Anne Duggan for translation from the Latin.

28. Pughe, *Physicians of Myddvai*, 339.

29. Fabbri, "Treating Medieval Plague," 176–177.

30. Van Arsdall, *Medieval Herbal Remedies*, 47–48.

31. Original text: "The heed is greued wiþinne wiþ an ache and an yuel þat phisicians clepiþ emigranea. So seiþ Constantinus. And as he seiþ, þis ache and iuel is most greuous, for who þat haþ [þ]at yuel feliþ in his heed as it were betynge of hamoures and may not suffre noyse, noþir voys, noþir voys, noþir liȝt, noþir schinynge. And yis yuel comeþ of colerik smoke wiþ hoot winde and ventosite. þerfore he feliþ in his heed picchinge and prickenge, brennynge and ringing." Seymour, *On the Properties*, vol. 1, 344.

32. Seymour, *Bartholomaeus*, 19.

33. M. Green, "Constantine the African," 145–146; Green, "Medical Books," 282–283.

34. Getz, *Medicine*, 38, 49; Long, "An Eleventh-Century WebMD"; Rawcliffe, *Medicine and Society*, 37.

35. The books were on themes as diverse as theology, geography, the nature of human life, and the natural world, while medical topics included the humors, anatomy, the life cycle, and treatments.

36. E. Wallis, *Medieval Medicine*, 249–250.

37. Woman's milk was, if not a common component, certainly a recognized ingredient in medical remedies. Bald's *Leechbook* used woman's milk in treatments for eyes and ears, and, for palsy, specified milk from a woman who had given birth to a male child. This seems to be a tradition that can be traced in Egyptian texts. See Buck, "Woman's Milk," 470–472.

38. E. Wallis, *Medieval Medicine*, 251.

39. Keen, *Journey of a Book*, 5; Seymour, *Bartholomaeus*, 12–15; E. Wallis, *Medieval Medicine*, 248.

40. "A Collection of Remedies," ff. 52v, 94r. For a transcription and translation, see Dawson, *Leechbook*, entries 605–607, 1042, 1063–1066.

41. Lev and Amar, *Practical Materia Medica*, 289–292.

42. Dawson, *Leechbook*, entry 607.

43. Original text: "My heid did yak yester nicht / This day to mak that I na micht. / So sair the magryme dois me menyie / Perseing my brow as ony ganyie, / That scant I luik may on the licht." I am grateful to Dr. Jenni Nuttall for her permission to reproduce her translation of the text. For the full poem, see Nuttall, " 'On His Heid-Ake'." See also Dunbar's "The Headache," in Conlee, *William Dunbar*.

44. Dunbar was from southeastern Scotland and attended St. Andrews University, where he trained as a cleric. From 1501 to 1513, he served at the court of King James IV of Scotland. He received an annual pension, and, while his precise role is not clear, historians have suggested that he may have served as a secretary or a chaplain, as well as a "makar," or court poet. See Conlee, *William Dunbar*.

45. Original text: "A maladyȝe yat takyth half a man is hed & doth him lesyn is syȝthe of his yie." See Voigts, "Fifteenth-Century English Banns."

46. Voigts, "Fifteenth-Century English Banns," 264–265.

47. Bildhauer, "Medieval European Conceptions," S60–S64.

48. E. Wallis, *Medieval Medicine*, 281–282.

49. Original text: "Þpe vayne betwyx þe fyngers & þe thombs es gud to be opyd for het of warke in þe swldyrs & migram in þe heue [hede]." See Furnivall and Furnivall, *Anatomie of the Bodie*, 229–230.

50. Kamen, *All in My Head*, 73.

51. Voigts and McVaugh, *Latin Technical Phlebotomy*, 4–8.

52. Taavitsainen, "Transferring Classical Discourse," 62.

53. Bildhauer, "Medieval European Conceptions," S66.

54. E. Wallis, *Medieval Medicine*, 96.

55. Yearl, "Time of Bloodletting," 55.

56. Bald's *Leechbook*, 72, 149.

57. Clowes, *A Prooued Practise*, 176–179.

58. Paré, *Workes*, 692–693.

59. Gil-Sotres, "Derivation and Revulsion," 122–132; Voigts and McVaugh, *Latin Technical Phlebotomy*, 8; Yearl, "Time of Bloodletting," 26.

60. E. Wallis, *Medieval Medicine*, 285.

61. Mediolano, *Regimen Sanitatis Salerni*.

62. Gyer, *English Phlebotomy*, 218–219.

63. Bullein, *Neewe Booke*, f. xxii.

64. Guillemeau, *Frenche Chirurgerye*, f. 30.

65. E. Wallis, *Medieval Medicine*, 325.

66. Yearl, "Time of Bloodletting," 53–64.

67. Curth, *English Almanacs*, 110.

68. Carlebach, *Palaces of Time*, 33.

69. See, for example, Anonymous [hereafter cited as Anon.], *Shepheards Kalendar*, unpaginated, images 63–65.

70. E. Wallis, *Medieval Medicine*, 287.

71. *Almanac in Latin and English*, f. 15r.

72. Monica Green makes this important point about the scarring, often deliberate, of medieval bodies. See M. Green, "Introduction," 3, in *Cultural History*.

Chapter 3 · *"Take Housleeke, and Garden Wormes"*

1. Corlyon, *Booke*, 11.

2. Corlyon, *Booke*, 12–13, 19–20.

3. Corlyon, *Booke*, 4–10, 11–16.

4. The recipes have been gathered by systematically researching the Wellcome Library's collection of recipe books, both archival and digitized, and searching EEBO for remedies with keywords such as megrim, meagrim, meagrom, mygryme, and hemicrania.

5. See "For Pluerese When a Man Is Past Blud Leting," Anne Brumwich and others, collection of receipts, 73; "An Aproved Medecine for a Pluresie, if They Cannot Have ye Helpe of Letinge Blood," Sir Thomas Osborne, recipe book; "An Approved Medicine for a Pleurisy if They Cant Have ye Help of Letting Blood," Bridget Hyde, recipe book; "How to Let on Blood yt Hath a Plague Sore," Jane Parker, recipe book. On the overlap between surgical and domestic medical remits, see LeJacq, "Medical Recipes."

6. Comparing the handwriting in this book with a letter Alathea wrote to her mother in 1607—about the "strange operation" of the "physicke" she had taken that "distempered me exceedingly for some dayes after"—shows without doubt that the book was written in Alathea's hand. Alathea Talbot letter to the Countess of Shrewsbury, f. 135.

7. Field, "'Many Hands Hands,'" 53.

8. Mrs. Corlyon's *Booke* has gained the attention of historians, whose interests range from her remedies for pimples to those for curdled milk in the breast. See various contributions to The Recipes Project.

9. The Wellcome Library in London contains more than 270 volumes of manuscript recipe books dating from the sixteenth to the nineteenth centuries, many of which can be searched for online and viewed in high-quality reproductions. The Folger Shakespeare Library in Washington, DC, contains around a hundred, and there are many others in local archives and medical libraries.

10. Leong, "Making Medicines."

11. Studies of recipe books include DiMeo and Pennell, *Reading and Writing*; Osborn, "Role of Domestic Knowledge"; L. Smith, "Women's Health Care."

12. Leong, "Collecting Knowledge," 83–84; Rankin, *Panaceia's Daughters*, 8–17.

13. Eamon, "How to Read," 41; Evans, "'Gentle Purges,'" 2–19; L. Smith, "Imagining Women's Fertility," 69–79.

14. Elyot, *Castel of Helth*, 52.

15. Corlyon's *Booke*, 37, 99.

16. Fissell, "Marketplace of Print," 114; Leong, "'Herbals She Peruseth,'" 559–562; Slack, "Mirrors of Health," 246–247.

17. Boorde, *Breuiary of Helthe*. Andrew Boorde began his career as a monk before leaving the church to study medicine on the continent. He compiled the *Breuiary* after many years of traveling around Europe, and it became very successful, being reprinted in at least five more editions between 1552 and 1598. See Furdell, "Boorde, Andrew."

18. Boorde, *Breuiary*, ff. ii–iii; Slack, "Mirrors of Health," 256–260.

19. Boorde, *Breuiary*, f. lxxiii.

20. Boorde, *Breuiary*, f. lxxiii.

21. Barrough, *Methode of Phisicke*, 1.

22. Barrough, *Methode of Phisicke*, 2.

23. Barrough, *Methode of Phisicke*, 13–14.

24. Paré, *Workes*, 640.

25. Crooke, *Mikrokosmographia*, 122.

26. Boorde, *Breuiary*, f. lxxiii.

27. Barrough, *Methode of Phisicke*, 2–3.

28. Collins, *Choice and Rare Experiments*, 5, 7; Partridge, *Widowes Treasure*, unpaginated [image 10].

29. "For ye megrom." Miss Shaw, Collection, 248.

30. Slack, "Mirrors of Health," 327.

31. Moulton, *This Is the Myrour*, lxxxxviii.

32. Cartwright, *Hospitall*, 56.

33. Anon., *Admirable Vertue*.

34. Copland, *A Boke*, unpaginated.

35. Cogan, *Hauen of Health*, 81.

36. Gerard, *Herball*, 758–759.

37. Anon., *Here Begynneth*, f. xi.

38. "A Collection of Remedies," f. 52v.

39. Vicary, *English Man's Treasure*, 175.

40. "Ye Toothach Megrim and Head Ach," Townshend Family collection, 19.

41. Migraine Trust, "Feverfew." In the 1980s, in a study of seventeen patients, some researchers found evidence that eating fresh feverfew leaves daily had a preventive effect. See E. Johnson et al., "Efficacy of Feverfew," 569–573; Volger et al., "Feverfew."

42. Culpeper, *English Physitian Enlarged*, 98; Pechey, *Compleat Herbal*, 91. My thanks to Sally Foxhall for finding this example.

43. Anon., *Here Begynneth*, f. xi; Langham, *Garden of Health*, 39–42.

44. Leong, "Just Who"; St. John, *Her Booke*, 32, 54.

45. Corlyon, *Booke*, 32.

46. "For the Migrime in the Forehead," J. Jackson, recipe book, f. 37; "For the Megrim Convulsions Fitts or Falling Sickness," St. John, recipe book, f. 78; "For ye Megrim or Giddiness of ye Head," Lady Ayscough recipe book, f. 125.

47. Pughe, *Physicians of Myddvai*, 339.

48. Dawson, *Leechbook*, recipe nos. 41, 263, 496, 498, 502, 761, 852, 1021, 1024. For the migraine recipe, see no. 606. The transcription cites "stonescar," which is an error.

49. Corlyon, *Booke*, 115.

50. Corlyon, *Booke*, 9, 47, 76.

51. Culpeper, *Pharmacopeia Londinensis*, 31–32. Brockbank, "Sovereign Remedies," 4, 6.

52. Pope John XXI, *Treasury of Healthe*, unpaginated [image 54].

53. Collins, *Choice and Rare Experiments*, 6.

54. Sleigh and Whitfeld, collection of medical receipts, 77.

55. Anon., *Closet*, 160.

56. Some historians have suggested that Alathea Talbot, the owner of Mrs. Corlyon's *Booke*, was the probable author of this anonymously (and posthumously) published book, with a preface to the reader signed "Philiatros," the frontispiece of which bears a portrait of the countess. This association is by no means certain, however, and certainly *Natura Exenterata* bears little direct resemblance to the recipes in Mrs. Corlyon's *Booke*. See Philiatros, *Natura Exenterata*, 28; Travitsky and Prescott, *Seventeenth-Century English Recipe Books*, xxxv.

57. Slack, "Mirrors of Health," 261.

58. Corlyon, *Booke*, 5.

59. Gerard, *Herball*, 637.

60. Demaitre, *Medieval Medicine*, 123.

61. Boorde, *Breuiary*, f. 29r.

62. Barrough, *Methode of Phisicke*, 14.

63. J. Jackson, recipe book, ff. 4 and 17, 16, 27.

64. J. Jackson, recipe book, f. 41v, 52.

65. J. Jackson, recipe book, f. 95, 101.

Chapter 4 · A "Deadly Tormenting Megrym"

1. A. Smith, *Servant of the Cecils*, 54–67.

2. Francis Thomson to Mr. Hicks.

3. Blount, *Glossographia*, unpaginated.

4. Walsham, "Holywell," 212; Walsham, *Reformation of the Landscape*, 395.

5. W. Thomson, *Spas That Heal*, 81–82.

6. M. Langham and Wells, *History of the Baths*, 9–13, 15.

7. William Bassett letter to Cromwell, 1538, in T. Wright, *Three Chapters*, 143–144.

8. Hembry, *English Spa*, 22.

9. Jones, *Benefit*, f. 2v.

10. Speed, *Theatre of the Empire*, 67.

11. W. Thomson, *Spas That Heal*, 82.

12. Langham and Wells, *History of the Baths*, 22.

13. Jones, *Benefit*, f. 2r.

14. Langham and Wells, *History of the Baths*, 20.

15. Hembry, *English Spa*, 24.

16. Walsham, *Reformation of the Landscape*, 413.

17. By the 1580s, recusants could be tried at Quarter Sessions and fined up to £20 per month for missing an Anglican service. See Richardson, "Topcliffe, Richard."

18. Jones, *Benefit*, ff. 4–6, 21.

19. Hembry, *English Spa*, 14.

20. W. Thomson, *Spas That Heal*, 16; Walsham, *Reformation of the Landscape*, 406, 408.

21. Deane, *Spadacrene Anglica*, 17.

22. Deane, *Spadacrene Anglica*, 13–15.

23. Kassell, *Medicine and Magic*, 6–8.

24. The Casebooks Project is an ongoing effort to provide an online digital edition of the entire collection of Foreman's and Napier's medical records. At the time of this writing, searching the project's website for the keyword migraine reveals eighteen cases of megrym or megrim, all from Napier's practice, one of whom was seen by his assistant, Gerence James.

25. Kassell, "Casebooks," 609; MacDonald, *Mystical Bedlam*, 26, 30.

26. MacDonald, *Mystical Bedlam*, 28.

27. Kassell, "Casebooks," 606; MacDonald, *Mystical Bedlam*, 26.

28. Casebooks Project, case 39010, accessed 28 January 2018 [as were all other cases from this website mentioned in the notes]; Casebooks Project, case 17104.

29. Casebooks Project, case 13499.

30. Casebooks Project, case 14625.

31. Casebooks Project, case 22924; email correspondence with Lauren Kassell, 29 January 2018.

32. Casebooks Project, case 15476.

33. My thanks to Lauren Kassell for her assistance with transcribing and interpreting these cases and for explaining jeralog.

34. "A Collection of Remedies," f. 94r, 136.

35. Casebooks Project, case 11809.

36. Casebooks Project, case 10738.

37. Casebooks Project, case 11613.

38. Anon., *Great and Wonderful Prophecies*, 3.

39. Fissell, "Marketplace of Print," 110.

40. Withey, "'Persons That Live Remote,'" 242.

41. Barrough, *Methode of Phisicke*, 1.

42. Apothecary's cash-book, ff. 13r, 27r, 33v, 36v.

43. Williams, *Read All about It!*, 5.

44. Salmon, *Phylaxa Medicina*, 88–89.

45. See, for example, "Advertisements," *Post Boy* (London), 20–23 December 1701, BCN.

46. "The True Cephalick or Head Snuff," *Daily Courant* (London), 29 January 1705, BCN.

47. "The Most Noble Volatile Smelling Bottle," *Daily Courant* (London), 20 February 1708, BCN.

48. P. Wallis, "Consumption, Retailing, and Medicine," 30–31.

49. Addison, "Royal Exchange."

50. "The True Royal Snuff for Purging the Head," *The Spectator* (London), Friday, 23 May 1712, BCN.

51. "Advertisements," *Post Boy* (London), 30 June–2 July 1713, BCN.

52. Cave, "The Head-Ache," 249. I'm grateful to Ludmilla Jordanova for introducing me to this poem.

53. Cody, "'No Cure, No Money,'" 103.

54. Porter, *Health for Sale*, 25.

55. Kamen, *All in My Head*, 114–115.

56. Kamen, *All in My Head*, 178.

57. Berkeley, *Siris*, 4–35; Breuninger, "Panacea for the Nation."

58. Prior, *Authentic Narrative*. On the opposition to Berkeley, see Benjamin "Medicine, Morality," 180.

59. Prior, *Authentic Narrative*, case 96: 26–27, case 142: 39, case 273: 64–65.

60. J. Kelly, "'Drinking the Waters,'" 133–135.

61. Barrington, *Personal Sketches*, 125–132.

62. Anon., *Report of the Cases*, 14.

63. Anon., *Report of the Cases*, case 68: 38.

64. Anon., *Report of the Cases*, case 120: 61.

65. Anon., *Report of the Cases*, case 77: 42, case 82: 44–45.

66. Barker, "Medical Advertising and Trust," 391; Shaw, *Miracles in Enlightenment England*, 75.

67. Cody, "'No Cure, No Money,'" 109; Porter, *Health for Sale*, 52.

68. Dr. William Cullen to Dr. John Alves, regarding Mrs. Baillie, 21 April 1777, letter ID 4045, The Cullen Project.

69. Dr. John Alves to Dr. William Cullen, regarding Mrs. Baillie, 16 April 1777, letter ID 1396, The Cullen Project; Dr. John Alves to Dr. William Cullen, regarding Mrs. Baillie, 3 May 1777, letter ID 1400, The Cullen Project.

70. Bacon, *Sylva Sylvarum*, 187–188.

71. Lardreau, "A Curiosity," 33.

72. Adams, *Diseases of the Soule*, 3–5; Mornay, *Discourse*, C4.

73. Original French text: "Migraine est proprement quand la douleur ne tient que la moitie de la teste [tête], dextre ou senestre." See Paré, *The Workes*, 410.

74. Brooke, "The Imposter," 81.

75. Lardreau, "A Curiosity," 35.

76. Lardreau, *La migraine*, 36–37.

77. Thomas Curtis, letter to Charles Blagden.

78. One contemporary travel guide described "a well that ebbs and flows as the sea does" at Newton. A later guidebook was not complimentary: "There is no inn at this place . . . but at a distance below the village one solitary building of public resort, Newton bathing house, rears its diminutive form to view in the midst of an arid desert." See Donovan, *Descriptive Excursions*, vol. 2, 372–373; Paterson, *Paterson's British Itinerary*, 207.

79. Charles Blagden, letter to Thomas Curtis.

80. Mead, *Treatise*, 84–86.

81. Liveing, *On Megrim*, 447.

82. Mead, *Treatise*, 84–86, 88.

83. Harrison, "From Medical Astrology," 31–32.

84. Tissot, *Traité des nerfs*, 90–92.

85. Liveing, *On Megrim*, 256.

86. Cheyne, *English Malady*, 52–55.

87. Cullen grouped diseases, according to their characteristic symptoms, into classes, orders, genera, and species, in the same way as botanical natural history. Cullen's relatively simple system identified just four classes in his symptom-based nosology: pyrexiae were characterized by fever; second came neuroses; then cachexia, or wasting diseases; and, finally, locales, an "unsatisfactory rag-bag of disorders." See W. Bynum, "Cullen and the Study," 137–188; Cullen, *Nosology*, 97–135.

88. Fothergill, "Remarks," 103–104, 108, 112–114.

89. "King's Theatre Masquerade," *Gazette and New Daily Advertiser* (London), 6 May 1782, 3, BCN.

90. Andrews, *Comparative View of the French and English Nations*, 72, cited in M. Cohen, *Fashioning Masculinity*, 9.

91. Castle, "Eros and Liberty," 156–176.

92. Lardreau-Cotelle, "Migraine."

93. "Parisian Intelligence," *General Evening Post* (London), issue 8383, 16–18 August 1787, 4, BCN.

94. Frederica, Duchess of York, letter to Sir Henry Halford.

Chapter 5 · *"The Pain Was Very Much Relieved and She Slept"*

1. J. H. Jackson, "Case of Elizabeth B.," April 1895, 18. In accordance with the Queen Square Archives' policy to ensure patient anonymity, and following advice from the archivist, I refer to patients of the National Hospital only by their first name in the text, with a first name and initial of the surname in the endnotes.

2. Contemporaneous advice for employers and servants includes Anon., *Servants' Guide*; B. Smith, *Sunshine in the Kitchen*. My thanks to Lauren Butler, Mary-Anne Boermans, Carly Silver, and Judith Flanders for a discussion of this point via Twitter.

3. J. H. Jackson, "Case of Elizabeth B.," April 1895.

4. Liveing, *On Megrim*, 44–45, 226.

5. Trotter, *View of the Nervous Temperament*, xi, xvii, 72, 169, 186–191.

6. Mease, *Treatise on the Causes*, 5.

7. Anon. "Medical Society of London," 57–58.

8. C. Parry, *Elements*, 244–245.

9. Labarraque, "Essai," 39, 65–66. On the influence of Labarraque, see Eadie, *Headache*, 183; Liveing, *On Megrim*, 256.

10. Hall, "On the Threatenings of Apoplexy," cited in Liveing, *On Megrim*, 117.

11. Murphy, "On Headache" (18 February), 182. During the early 1830s, "Dr. G." had been widely quoted in British and American medical journals for enthusiastically recommending the use of leeches to let blood from "robust and plethoric young women" with headaches, while recommending cold compresses to the forehead, dry cupping, spirits of turpentine, and nitrate of silver for "hysterical" women with a more delicate constitution. See, for example, Anon., "Dr. Graves," 145–148.

12. Murphy, "On Headache" (18 February), 183.

13. Buchan, *Domestic Medicine*, 352–354; Murphy, "On Headache" (25 February), 209.

14. Murphy, "On Headache" (20 May): 540–541.

15. In the late seventeenth century, Thomas Willis and Thomas Sydenham (in a letter addressed to Dr. William Cole, published in *Dissertatio epistolaris* [Epistolary Dissertation], in 1682) had rejected the idea that a woman's womb could actually "wander" around her body and, between them, located hysteria's causes in the brain and nervous system. Sydenham saw this as a disorder of the "animal spirits," and he came to believe that both men and women could equally suffer from hysteria, or hypochondriasis. On this history, see Micale, *Hysterical Men*, 19–21, 49, 59–61.

16. Turner, "Disability and Crime," 55.

17. George Phillips, "Breaking Peace: Wounding," 11 January 1865, reference t18650111-186, POB.

18. Jane Milburn, "Theft: Stealing from Master," 12 May 1845, reference t18450512-1153, POB.

19. Turner, "Disability and Crime," 56.

20. Ann Noakes, "Killing: Murder," 26 April 1880, reference t18800426-428, POB.

21. Lees, "Tetrachloride," 810; Bristowe, "Cavendish Lecture on Hysteria."

22. Ross, *Treatise*, 689–690, cited in Kempner, *Not Tonight*, 33.

23. Ross, *Treatise*, 694.

24. Kempner, *Not Tonight*, 33.

25. Although Thomas Willis had coined the English term "neurologie" in the later translation of his 1664 work in Latin, *Cerebri Anatome*, it was only in the 1830s that the modern term "neurologist" emerged to denote a nerve specialist. See Willis, *An Essay*, 5. On the history of the terminology, see Casper, *The Neurologists*, 11; Oppenheim, *Shattered Nerves*, 16.

26. W. Bynum, "The Nervous Patient," 90.

27. Oppenheim, *Shattered Nerves*, 27.

28. W. Bynum, "The Nervous Patient," 96.

29. Booth, *Cannabis*, 38, 57; Clendinning, "Observations."

30. Clouston, "Observations and Experiments."

31. Anstie, *Neuralgia*, 190–191.

32. Sussex County Lunatic Asylum, *Thirteenth Annual Report*, appendix B.

33. By 1873, these appendices came to fifty-seven pages, double the length of the annual reports themselves. At this point, the Medico-Psychological Association agreed that a section of the *Journal of Mental Science*, a "much more appropriate and convenient vehicle," could be set aside for such reports. See Sussex County Lunatic Asylum, *Fifteenth Annual Report*, 25–26.

34. Greene, "Treatment of Migraine," 35–38.

35. See, for example, Anon., "Report on the Treatment" (21 December), 683; Leconte, "Guarana," 313; Samelson, "Guarana against Sick-Headache," 498.

36. Aminoff, *Brown-Sequard*, 103.

37. Scott et al., *William Richard Gowers*, 84–87.

38. J. H. Jackson, "Case of Elizabeth B.," April 1895.

39. J. H. Jackson, "Case Illustrating the Relation," 244–245.

40. J. H. Jackson, "Case Notes, Female," 1895.

41. Gowers and Jackson, "George F.," July 1877, 67.

42. Gowers and Jackson, "Susan T.," April 1873, 243–244.

43. J. H. Jackson, "Case of Hemiopia," 306–307.

44. Bury, "Chronic Illness," 173–174.

45. Ferrier, "Mary Ann W.," October 1896.

46. Beevor, "Janet W.," February 1899.

47. J. H. Jackson, "Emma Jane C.," July 1892.

48. Gowers, "Augustus A.," September 1898.

49. Cornwell, *Hard-Earned Lives*, 130–131.

50. Bastian, "George R.," October 1891.

51. Buzzard, "Jane H.," May 1881.

52. Entract, "'Chlorodyne' Browne."

53. Earles, "Introduction of Hydrocyanic Acid," 305–312.

54. Anon., "Report on the Treatment" (21 December), 683.

55. Gowers, "Annie W.," March 1899.

56. This would be included in the first seven editions of Lord Russell Brain's *Diseases of the Nervous System*, from 1933 until 1969. As late as the 1970s, a recipe for Gowers' Mixture was being published in migraine texts. See Clarke, "Gowers' Mixture," 215–216; Foster, "General Aspects of Management," 140; Scott et al., *William Richard Gowers*, 226.

57. Potter, *Handbook of Materia Medica*, 684–685.

58. Chemist and Druggist, *Pharmaceutical Formulas*, 125.

Chapter 6 · "As Sharp as If Drawn with Compasses"

1. Gowers, "Subjective Visual Sensations," 21–22, 33–35.

2. Gowers, "Subjective Visual Sensations," 25, 37–38.

3. Anon., "Subjective Visual Sensations," 563.

4. Daston and Galison, *Objectivity*, 17–27.

5. This modern idea of scientific objectivity, the virtue of "seeing" or "knowing" scientifically without prejudice, interference, interpretation, or intelligence, in order to prevent the scientist's subjectivity from intruding, is why, although many modern headache specialists enter the field because they have migraine themselves, they rarely write about their personal experiences. See Kempner, *Not Tonight*, xiv.

6. Tissot, *Traité des nerfs*, 112–113.

7. Fothergill, "Remarks," 120–121.

8. Heberden, *Commentaries on the History*, 78.

9. C. Parry, *Collections*, vol. 1, 558.

10. Andral, "Lectures on Medical Pathology," 2.

11. Snyder, *Philosophical Breakfast Club*, 301, 335.

12. Herschel, "On Sensorial Vision," 401–406.

13. Herschel, "On Sensorial Vision," 406–409. In 1852, Herschel and Airy had corresponded on the topic of some optical phenomena seen by the sister of Herschel's assayer. It is likely that this is the woman to whom Herschel was referring. See Musselman, *Nervous Conditions*, 129.

14. Herschel, "On Sensorial Vision," 411–413.

15. Herschel, diary, 11 June 1846.

16. Herschel, diary, 19 February 1854 and 18 August 1855.

17. Herschel, diary, 12 February 1865 and 30 July 1866.

18. Wollaston, "On Semi-Decussation," 222–231.

19. Musselman, *Nervous Conditions*, 117.

20. Brewster, "On Hemiopsy," 503–507. In 1790, William Rowley described hemiopsia as "a defect of vision in which the patient sees the half, but not the whole, of an object." See Rowley, *Treatise*, 328.

21. G. Airy, "Astronomer Royal on Hemiopsy," 19–21.

22. Buchan, *Domestic Medicine*, 54–57.

23. Madden, *Infirmities of Genius*, 78–79.

24. Brewster, "On Hemiopsy," 506.

25. G. Airy, "Astronomer Royal on Hemiopsy," 21.

26. W. Airy, *Autobiography*, 12.

27. Herschel, diary, 5 May 1868.

28. H. Airy, "On a Distinct Form," 252–253.

29. H. Airy, "On a Distinct Form," 247.

30. H. Airy, "On a Distinct Form," 247–248.

31. H. Airy, "On a Distinct Form," 256, 258.

32. H. Airy, "On a Distinct Form," 264.

33. Daston and Galison, *Objectivity*, 130–131.

34. Lithography, invented in 1798, did away with the need to etch or grind a plate. Images could be drawn directly onto the polished printing stone with waxy crayons, pencils, or pens, or transferred from paper. Lithography ensured that precise texts and lines could be reproduced and lent itself to the large areas of black that were so characteristic of astronomical images and Airy's diagrams. In 1837, Godefroy Engelmann patented the color technique of chromolithography, the first true method for printing multiple colors (rather than tinting by hand). By the 1860s, chromolithography was widely used for mass-producing posters, advertisements, and book illustrations.

35. Liveing, *On Megrim*, 81.

36. Liveing, *On Megrim*, 1–2.

37. Symonds, "On Headache," 419–420.

38. Liveing, *On Megrim*, 4.

39. Liveing, *On Megrim*, 336.

40. Liveing, *On Megrim*, 390–391.

41. Liveing, *On Megrim*, 49.

42. Liveing, *On Megrim*, 107, 113.

43. Liveing, *On Megrim*, 25, 430–436.

44. Levy, *A Brain Wider*, 38–39.

45. Liveing, *On Megrim*, 29.

46. Latham, *On Nervous or Sick-Headache*; Latham, "On Sick-Headache," 7–8.

47. Latham, *On Nervous or Sick-Headache*, 16–23.

48. For a fuller discussion of Liveing and Latham, their influence, and the modern reputation of their work, see Weatherall, "Migraine Theories."

49. Alexander Auld was not convinced, and he proposed that "not a few cases of so-called developmental migraine, supposed to be epileptic manifestations, may with greater truth be referred to hysteria." Auld, *Asthma*, 106–107.

50. J. H. Jackson, "A Case of Hemiopia," 306–307.

51. John Hughlings Jackson's understanding of Thomas R.'s symptoms reflected a belief common among neurologists in Europe and America: the presence of pain must indicate the existence of a lesion, whether or not contemporary techniques could find it. This was an important change in understanding disease, differing from the humoral framework, which had emphasized imbalances and their ability to move around the whole bodily system, rather than identifying precise locations for and agents of disease in tissue. See Goldberg, "Pain without Lesion."

52. Allbutt, "Clinical Lecture," 205–206.

53. Liveing, *On Megrim*, 399, 404.

54. Haig, *Uric Acid*, ix.

55. Haig, *Uric Acid*, 222–226, 231.

56. Haig, *Uric Acid*, 238–239.

57. The term "neurasthenia" came from Scottish physician John Brown's eighteenth-century grouping of diseases into two categories: "sthenic" diseases, which were characterized by too much excitability, and "asthenic," by too little. On Brown's terminology, see Oppenheim, *Shattered Nerves*, 94–95. The most comprehensive study of neurasthenia is Schuster, "Neurasthenic Nation."

58. Sengoopta, "Mob of Incoherent Symptoms," 97–99.

59. Beard, *Practical Treatise*, 13.

60. Beard, *Practical Treatise*, 24–25.

61. Beard, *Practical Treatise*, 148–149.

62. Beard, *Practical Treatise*, 103.

63. Liveing, *On Megrim*, 434.

64. Sengoopta, "Mob of Incoherent Symptoms," 98.

65. Crichton-Browne, "An Oration," 1017.

66. Bolton Tomson, "Vaso-motor Neuroses," 877–879.

67. Wilks, "Epilepsy and Migraine," 263.

68. Stone, "Samuel Wilks," 263–265.

69. Allan, "Inheritance of Migraine," 590.

70. Rachford, *Neurotic Disorders of Childhood*, 192–193.

71. Maudsley, *Pathology of Mind*, 108–111.

72. Crichton-Browne, "Circles of Mental Disorder," 262–267, 265.

73. Liveing, *On Megrim*, 27, 430–431.

74. Beard, *Practical Treatise*, 164.

75. Liveing, *On Megrim*, 22, 86, 252.

76. Wilkinson and Isler, "The Pioneer Woman's"; Anon., "Report on the Treatment" (13 January), 46.

77. Anon., "Report on the Treatment" (21 December), 683; Latham, "Guarana (Paullinia) Powder," 446–447.

78. Rachford, *Neurotic Disorders of Childhood*, 193–194.

79. Eadie, *Headache*, 99–100.

80. Gowers, *Manual of Diseases*, 776–794.

81. Gowers, *Manual of Diseases*, 793–795.

82. Gowers, *Manual of Diseases*, 778–791.

83. Gowers, *Border-Land*, 100–103.

84. Eadie, "Hubert Airy," 263–267.

85. Levene, "Sir G. B. Airy," 15–23.

86. For a good example of how aura has fascinated neurologists, see Oliver Sacks's essay on "Patterns" in *Hallucinations*, 122–132.

87. Weatherall, "Migraine Theories," 8.

88. Gowers, *Manual of Diseases*, 777.

Chapter 7 · *"A Shower of Phosphenes"*

1. Singer, *From Magic to Science*, 8.

2. At the turn of the twentieth century, Hildegard's works, including the Wiesbaden copy of the *Scivias* manuscript (c. 1165), had begun to attract a great deal of attention, particularly from feminist medical historians, who enthusiastically adopted Hildegard as a model of female medical practice, the experimental method, and natural observation. See M. Green, "In Search," 39, 44–45.

3. Singer, *From Magic to Science*, viii.

4. Singer, "Scientific Views," 51–55.

5. Lorch, "Language and Memory Disorder."

6. Cooter, "The Life of a Disease?," 111. See also McGough, "Syphilis in History," 573–574.

7. C. Bynum, *Holy Feast*, 194–218. See also Brumberg, *Fasting Girls*.

8. Shuttleworth, *Mind of the Child*, 22.

9. Rose, "Overview from Neolithic Times," 347–352.

10. Rocca, "Galen," 253–271.

11. Ganidagli et al., "Approach to Painful Disorders," 167.

12. Rapoport and Edmeads, "Migraine," 1221; Willis, *London Practice of Physick*, 380.

13. Rose, "Overview from Neolithic Times," 357; Eadie, *Headache*, 35.

14. Brunton, "Discussion on Headaches," 1241–1243.

15. Brunton, *Hallucinations*, 25–26.

16. Brunton, *Hallucinations*, 27–28.

17. Clower and Finger, "Discovering Trepanation," 1423.

18. Levy, *A Brain Wider*, 25.

19. Osler, *Evolution of Modern Medicine*, 8.

20. T. Parry, "Neolithic Man."

21. For overviews of Hildegard's life and work, see Dronke, "Hildegard of Bingen"; Flanagan, *Hildegard of Bingen*; Newman, *Voice of the Living Light*.

22. Arnold Klebs, letter to Charles Singer, 29 July 1913.

23. Anon., "St. Hildegard," 1–2.

24. Fee and Brown, "Using Medical History," 149.

25. Singer, *From Magic to Science*, ix.

26. Singer quoted extensively from Theodoric's *vita* of the life of Hildegard, which had been reprinted in Migne, *S. Hildegardis Abbatissa*. See Singer, "Scientific Views," 52–53.

27. Singer, "Science," 111.

28. Singer, "Scientific Views," 30–32.

29. Mayer, "When Things Don't Talk," 326–327.

30. Singer, *From Magic to Science*, xii–xiii.

31. Elliott, "Migraine and Mysticism," 449–459.

32. Sacks, *Migraine*, 106–108. Oliver Sacks's book, first published in 1970 and designed for a general readership, quickly became a best seller. Through many editions, as well as being revised and expanded in 1985 and again in 1990, it has attracted millions of readers since its first publication.

33. Sacks, *Migraine* (1985), 55.

34. Sacks, *Migraine* (1985), 192.

35. Sacks, *Migraine* (1992), xv.

36. Silvas, *Jutta and Hildegard*, 226.

37. On Hildegard and medicine, see Glaze, "Medical Writer"; M. Green, "In Search," 51; Sweet, *Rooted in the Earth*.

38. Baird and Ehrman, *Letters of Hildegard*, 80–82; E. Cohen, *Modulated Scream*, 118.

39. Newman, "Hildegard of Bingen," 167.

40. Flanagan, *Hildegard of Bingen*, 200.

41. Newman, "Three-Part Invention," 197–198.

42. Madeline Caviness points to stylistic conventions, such as the depiction of drapery, the privileging of the feminine in several of the illuminations, and the close correlation between text and imagery, as well as the transposition of ideas from Hildegard's other writings, as evidence for the abbess's direct role in creating the images. This argument is explored most fully in Caviness, *Art*, 71–108; Caviness, "Hildegard as Designer."

43. Caviness, "Artist," 110, 113.

44. Charles Singer's own wording on this point changed subtly over time. While, in his original Hildegard article (1917), he claimed there was "strong evidence" that the manuscript was either supervised by Hildegard herself or "under her immediate tradition," in his revised article (1928), this phrase became "little doubt." In the 1928 version, Singer also removed the highly criticized sections from the original article, in which he rejected Hildegard's authorship of the medical manuscript *Causes and Cures*. While not integral to his discussion about migraine, which refers only to *Scivias*, Singer's deletion of the part about *Causae et Curae* further removed any sense of doubt in the piece, allowing historians who have only consulted the 1928 version of his article or the essay on "The Visions of Hildegard of Bingen" in his 1958 book (*From Magic to Science*), to forget that debates about manuscript authenticity were as contested in Singer's time as they are today.

45. "Hildegard of Bingen (Migraine)," Mombu, 6 April 2010, http://www.mombu.com/medicine/medicine/t-hildegard-of-bingen-migraine-4798218.html.

46. Willis, *Two Discourses*, 106, 121–122.

47. Owen, "Famous Case," 571.

48. See, for example, Skwire, "Women, Writers, Sufferers"; Zimmer, *Soul Made Flesh*, 190–199. For an excellent deconstruction of Willis's neurological reputation, see O'Neal, "A Love of 'Words as Words,' " 7–13.

49. Eadie, *Headache*, 6–8, 60–68; Willis, *Two Discourses*, 107. On Willis and heredity, see Liveing, *On Megrim*, 28.

50. Willis, *De Anima Brutorum*, 291; Willis, *Two Discourses*, 106.

51. Eadie, *Headache*, 107–108; Pearce, "Historical Aspects," 1099.

52. Willis, *Two Discourses*, 122.

53. Newman, "Sibyl of the Rhine," 1.

54. Levy, *A Brain Wider*, 122.

55. Ferrari and Haan, "Migraine Aura," 686.

56. Haan and Ferrari, "Picasso's Migraine."

57. Blau, "Somesthetic Aura," 582.

58. Podoll and Robinson, "Lewis Carroll's Migraine Experiences," 1366. William Bowman could not have connected Carroll's visions to migraine, because the link between aura and migraine was not commonly made for another two decades, as chapter 6 discusses.

59. Levy, *A Brain Wider*, 97–106, 115.

60. Sharratt, "Were Hildegard's Visions."

61. Aikin, "Etiology," 485–487.

62. Elliott, "Migraine and Mysticism," 452.

63. Critchley, "Discarded Theories," 241–246.

64. Hurst, "Migraine and Its Treatment," 60–61. Luminal had been discovered in 1912, having been developed first as a sedative for the mentally ill, and then administered for epilepsy at the Leipzig Institute for Brain Research. By the 1920s, it was being widely recommended as a treatment for migraine.

65. Symonds, "Discussion on Migraine," 1097–1106.

66. Symonds, "Discussion on Migraine," 1106–1107.

67. Symonds, "Discussion on Migraine," 1108–1110.

68. This situation echoes historian Mathew Thomson's observations about neurasthenia as a way of dumping together "a vast range of conditions which had no other obvious organic origin." Indeed, William Gowers saw neurasthenia as a "convenient" term "for when the patient suffers from so many slight functional disorders that it is difficult to select any one as sufficiently prominent to afford a designation." Gowers urged physicians to resist the "craving for nomenclature," because giving a firm diagnosis in such situations "would involve more error than truth." See Gowers, *Manual of Diseases*, 960; M. Thomson, "Neurasthenia in Britain," 79–80.

69. Atkinson, "Nasal Headaches," 264–266.

70. Lorch, "Language and Memory," 3136.

71. Historian Sally Shuttleworth has observed that medical writers have often used clinical legends anachronistically and unproblematically, for their own ends. Once transformed into cases by scientific authority, such historical stories take on textual lives of their own as they are repeated over decades. See Shuttleworth, *Mind of the Child*, 22.

72. Rebecca O'Neal has noted the neurological community's "highly selective and teleological" embrace of Willis as a forefather. See O'Neal, "A Love of 'Words as Words,'" 7–8.

Chapter 8 · *"Happy Hunting Ground"*

1. Goltman, "Mechanism of Migraine," 352–353.

2. For more discussion of the intellectual climate that fostered the emergence of neurosurgery, see Pressman, *Last Resort*, 47–58.

3. Bliss, *Harvey Cushing*, 169–173; Gavrus, "Making Bad Boys Good," 73–78.

4. Raz, *Lobotomy Letters*, 1–5. The classic study examining the circumstances in which invasive treatments such as lobotomy can be developed and accepted is Pressman, *Last Resort*.

5. Critchley and Ferguson, "Migraine" (21 January 1933), 123.

6. Brain, *Diseases*, 735.

7. Graham, *Treatment of Migraine*, 5–8.

8. Osler, *Principles and Practice*, 957–958.

9. Aikin, "Etiology and Treatment," 486.

10. Clemens von Pirquet's term initially was dismissed in favor of Charles Richet's word "anaphylaxis" (first coined in 1902 in two papers by Paul Portier and Richet, with Richet's continued research leading to a Nobel Prize in 1913), but by the 1930s, anaphylaxis was increasingly being used to describe extreme reactions, while the concept of allergy brought together a broader host of problems, including asthma triggered by the presence of animals, the seasonal nature of hay fever and the discovery of pollen as a causative agent, and the isolation of histamine. For

the history of this terminology and the early history of allergy, see M. Jackson, *Allergy*, 31–38; M. Smith, *Another Person's Poison*, 43–66.

11. Löwy, "Biotherapies of Chronic Disease," 681; Urbach and Gottlieb, *Allergy*, 795; Vaughan, "Allergic Migraine," 1383–1386.

12. Bray, *Recent Advances in Allergy*, 333–335.

13. Vaughan, *Allergy and Applied Immunology*, 321.

14. M. Smith, *Another Person's Poison*, 91–92.

15. Schwartz, "Is Migraine an Allergic Disease?," 428.

16. Walker, "Place of Allergy," 24.

17. Critchley, "Migraine: General Remarks," 165.

18. For this early history of hormones, see Sengoopta, *Most Secret Quintessence*, 1–2.

19. Pardee, "Pituitary Headaches," 174–184.

20. Bramwell, "Discussion on Migraine," 768; Sengoopta, *Most Secret Quintessence*, 4.

21. Moffat, "Treatment of Menstrual Migraine," 614.

22. Glass et al., "Migraine and Ovarian Deficiency," 333–338.

23. Sengoopta, *Most Secret Quintessence*, 156–163.

24. Critchley and Ferguson, "Migraine" (21 January), 124.

25. Critchley and Ferguson, "Migraine" (28 January), 187.

26. Singh et al., "Progesterone," 745–747.

27. Urbach and Gottlieb, *Allergy*, 795–796.

28. Moffat, "Treatment of Menstrual Migraine," 612–615.

29. Urbach and Gottlieb, *Allergy*, 801.

30. The term "eugenics," coined by Francis Galton in 1883, became the name for a movement based on the idea that if a society could control heredity, it could prevent a whole range of social ills—including mental and physical diseases, crime, poverty, and prostitution—to produce happier, healthier, more intelligent communities. Conditions such as syphilis, tuberculosis, mental illness, alcoholism, and epilepsy gravely concerned eugenicists, who diagnosed them as social ills threatening "national degeneracy." Nations around the world embraced a whole range of "social hygiene" policies in the first decades of the twentieth century. Measures such as the promotion of marriage and the sterilization of people deemed "unfit" were aimed at preventing, controlling, or manipulating reproductive practices. See Galton, *Inquiries*, 24. On the history of eugenics, see Levine and Bashford, *Oxford Handbook*, 3–24.

31. Tredgold, "Feeble-Minded," 99, quoted in M. Jackson, *Borderland of Imbecility*, 99.

32. M. Jackson, *Borderland of Imbecility*, 99.

33. Levine and Bashford, *Oxford Handbook*, 3–4.

34. M. Thomson, *Psychological Subjects*, 86.

35. Crookshank, *Migraine*, 75, 82–88, 89–94.

36. Loughran, "Shell-Shock," 79–95, 82, 89.

37. Schimmel, *Sigmund Freud's Discovery*, 122.

38. Karwautz et al., "Freud and Migraine," 22–26.

39. Loughran, "Shell-Shock," 87.

40. See, for example, Slight, "Migraine."

41. Alvarez, *How to Live with Your Migraine*, 1–2.

42. Alvarez, "Migrainous Personality," 1–8.

43. Wolff, *Headache*, 321–322, 328.

44. Wolff, *Headache*, 344–345.

45. Graham, *Treatment of Migraine*, 8, 26, 38.

46. Graham, *Treatment of Migraine*, 87–88.

47. Graham, *Treatment of Migraine*, 89–93.

48. Foster, "General Aspects of Management," 142.

49. Critchley, "Discarded Theories," 245.

50. Graham and Wolff, "Mechanism of Migraine Headache."

51. Kempner, *Not Tonight*, 35–37.

52. Goodman and Gilman, *Pharmacological Basis of Therapeutics*, 878–880.

53. German physician Albert Eulenberg reported success with ergot by injection, but in its natural state, ergot contains a varying alkaloid content, making any dosage unreliable. In 1918, Arthur Stoll, a biochemist at Sandoz, isolated ergotamine tartrate, a much more reliable substance. See Eadie, "Ergot of Rye," 4–7; Tfelt-Hansen and Koehler, "One Hundred Years," 753.

54. Graham and Wolff, "Mechanism of Migraine Headache," 740. I had hoped to reproduce this graph, but gaining permission for the image rights was prohibitively expensive.

55. Graham and Wolff, "Mechanism of Migraine Headache," 762.

56. At that time, the drug was called E.C. 110, and it would later be named Cafergot. Burroughs Wellcome had long been interested in ergot derivatives. Ergotin had been one of its earliest products developed in the 1880s, and the company had continued to work on obstetric applications for ergot through the first decades of the twentieth century. See Church and Tansey, *Burroughs Wellcome & Co.*, 128, 177, 186–187, 309–312.

57. H. Stewart, "Ergometrine for Migraine," 745.

58. "Suggestions for New Product."

59. "Migril," folder 2 (1961).

60. "Migril," folder 1 (1957–1960).

61. Herzberg, *Happy Pills in America*, 182.

62. In modern websites that market migraine drugs, Kempner has found that the dominant imagery is of attractive, well-presented, white, middle-class women. Images of men are "so deeply buried in internal pages that readers might never find them." See Kempner, *Not Tonight*, 107–108.

63. "Migril," folder 7 (1969).

64. Waters, "Controlled Clinical Trial," 325–327.

65. Foster, "General Aspects of Management," 138–40; Tfelt-Hansen and Koehler, "History of Use," 877–881.

66. Graham, *Treatment of Migraine*, 58–67, 70, 72.

67. Walker, "Place of Allergy," 23.

68. Overy and Tansey, *Migraine*, 30–31.

69. Blau, "Problems and Paradoxes," 6–7.

70. Foster, "General Aspects of Management," 140.

71. Graham, *Treatment of Migraine*, 104.

72. Wilkinson, "Migraine," 754–755.

73. Graham, *Treatment of Migraine*, 107.

74. This migraine clinic was founded by Eileen Lecky, a health worker from the London district of Putney, in response to general practitioners who wanted a clinic along the lines of a hospital outpatient department, where they could refer patients unable to afford specialist consultant fees. See Sutherland, *Migraine Clinic*, 10–11, 24–25.

75. Sutherland, *Migraine Clinic*, 32, 53, 63–64.

76. Sicuteri, "Prophylactic and Therapeutic Properties." See also Kempner, *Not Tonight*, 45.

77. Neil Raskin, cited in Solomon et al., "American Headache," 672.

78. Blau, "Problems and Paradoxes," 6–7; Rawson and Liversedge, "Clinical Pharmacology of Migraine," 145, 150–151.

79. In the 1930s, Italian pharmacologist and chemist Vittorio Erspamer had discovered a substance he named enteramine. Later, enteramine and serotonin were both found to be 5-hydroxytryptamine, but Upjohn, the American drug company, was the first to synthesize it and make it available for researchers, and kept the name serotonin. On this history, see Whitaker-Azmitia, "Discovery of Serotonin," 2S–3S.

80. Sanders-Bush, *Serotonin Receptors*, 3–5.

81. Koehler and Tfelt-Hansen, "History of Methysergide," 1127.

82. Anthony and Lance, "Role of Serotonin," 120.

83. James Lance has recalled this era in an interview for the Australian Academy of Science. See Burke, "Professor James Lance, Neurologist."

84. Hanington and Harper, "Role of Tyramine," 84.

85. Hanington, "Migraine: A Platelet Disorder," 720.

86. Anthony and Lance, "Role of Serotonin," 113–119.

87. Sicuteri et al., "Biochemical Investigations." Swiss neurologist Harwig Heyck proposed that during a migraine attack, arteriovenous shunts opened to divert channels of blood, thereby withdrawing blood from the capillaries (thus explaining the characteristic facial pallor) and directing it into the veins, causing them to dilate with the extra pressure. Heyck theorized that there must be a special "neuronal or biochemical stimuli" that caused the shunts to open. See Heyck, "Pathogenesis of Migraine," 14.

88. Cumings, "Speculation Not the Way," 1, 4.

89. Humphrey, "Discovery and Development," 686; Humphrey, "Discovery of Sumatriptan," 4–5.

90. Humphrey, "5-Hydroxytryptamine," S38–S44; Overy and Tansey, *Migraine*, 47.

91. Cady et al., "Treatment of Acute Migraine," 2831.

92. Regush, "Migrainekiller," 26–31, 70.

93. Overy and Tansey, *Migraine*, 44–45. In 2002, in response to evidence that concerns about cardiovascular safety were limiting the use of triptans, the American Headache Society convened the Triptan Cardiovascular Safety Expert Panel to evaluate the evidence. The panel concluded that while adverse cardiovascular events had occurred after the use of triptans, the incidence and risk appeared to be "extremely low" in patients without known coronary artery disease, and "in patients at low risk of coronary heart disease, triptans can be prescribed confidently without the need for prior cardiac status evaluation." See Triptan Cardiovascular Safety Expert Panel, "Consensus Statement," 422–423.

94. Overy and Tansey, *Migraine*, 13.

95. Kempner, *Not Tonight*, 62.

96. Blau, *Headache and Migraine Handbook*, 87–88.

97. Blau, "Migraine Pathogenesis," 438–439.

98. In 1941, after observing his scotoma for a number of years, American psychologist Karl Spencer Lashley had proposed that a wave of intense excitation across the visual cortex was propagated at a rate of three millimeters per minute. In 1943, Brazilian neurophysiologist Aristides Leão, then a PhD student, electrically stimulated rabbits' brains and discovered a marked reduction of electrical activity, which then spread out from the stimulated region across the cerebral cortex. Leão proposed that this "cortical spreading depression" might be related to migraine aura, but it wasn't until 1958 that Peter Milner linked Leão and Lashley's observations. See Leão, "Spreading Depression"; Lashley, "Patterns"; Milner, "Note"; Tfelt-Hansen and Koehler, "One Hundred Years," 757–758.

99. Olesen et al., "Common Migraine Attack," 438–449.

100. Wilkinson, "Are Classical and Common Migraine Different Entities?," 211–212.

101. Ziegler, "Headache Symptom," 273–274.

102. Allan, "Sex Ratio in Migraine"; Waters and O'Connor, "Prevalence of Migraine," 616.

103. Abramson et al., "Migraine and Non-migrainous Headaches," 188.

104. Lance and Olesen, "Preface," 9.

105. Overy and Tansey, *Migraine*, 33–40.

106. Rasmussen, "Epidemiology of Headache," 1468.

107. Overy and Tansey, *Migraine*, 65.

108. Critchley, "Towards a Definition," 1–2.

109. Overy and Tansey, *Migraine*, 59.

110. Humphrey and Goadsby, "Mode of Action."

111. Goadsby, "Vascular Theory of Migraine," 7.

112. As reported by Anne MacGregor to the Wellcome Witness Seminar in 2013. I am grateful to Professor MacGregor for sharing further thoughts on this point by email. See also Epstein, *Inclusion*, 4–5; Overy and Tansey, *Migraine*, 10–11; Peterlin et al., "Sex Matters," 839–842.

Chapter 9 · *"If I Could Harness Pain"*

1. Untitled artwork, submitted to the Third Migraine Art Competition, unnamed artist, 1981, image 14, MAC. All of the images referred to in this chapter (unless otherwise indicated) are from the Migraine Action Art Collection, which, at the time of writing, was in the process of being transferred to the Wellcome Library. From 2016 to 2018 the full collection had been available online at http://www.migraineart.org.uk. This website was the result of a collaboration with Migraine Action to catalog and digitize the art collection, a project funded by the University of Leicester. I am indebted to Dr. Steve Ling for his work cataloging the collection and assisting the website project.

2. Podoll and Robinson, *Migraine Art*, 71. In their book, Klaus Podoll and Derek Robinson reproduce three hundred of the artworks from the collection.

3. Nearly a third of the entrants to the competition paid £1 to have their artwork returned to them.

4. Migraine Action, "Brief History." In 1965, the British Migraine Association split into two organizations. The Association (later to be renamed Migraine Action) would continue to work with and advocate for patients, and the Migraine Trust would focus on medical research and education. In 2018, Migraine Action closed. Its assets were donated to the Migraine Trust to form a single, larger charity, and the Wellcome Library acquired the Migraine Art Collection.

5. P. Johnson, "Consumer's End," 3–4.

6. "Migraine (Treatment)," House of Commons debate, 4 March 1960, http://hansard.millbanksystems.com/commons/1960/mar/04/migraine-treatment/.

7. Wailoo, *Pain: A Political History*, 29–32, 58.

8. Wailoo, *Pain: A Political History*, 58–59, 64.

9. Ham and Alberti, "Medical Profession," 839.

10. At that time, there were two clinics in London: Critchley's own at King's College London, opened in 1955, and another at the National Hospital in Queen Square. Both clinics were held in the evening, so patients could attend without taking time off from work. See Critchley, "Migraine: General Remarks," 167.

11. Marcia Wilkinson's clinic would become the City Migraine Clinic. She later opened it as an independent medical charity, the City of London Migraine Clinic, in 1980. See Anon., "Editorial: Migraine Clinics," 376; Overy and Tansey, *Migraine*, 67.

12. Elizabeth Garrett Anderson was the first woman in Britain to obtain the title of MD. Garrett Anderson herself explained that she chose to study migraine for quite pragmatic reasons: she needed a topic for her MD studies that could be "well-studied without post-mortem observations, of which I can have but very few in either private or dispensary [clinic] practice." Marcia Wilkinson sent for this thesis from Paris in 1966 and translated it into English. Wilkinson was the first recipient of the International Headache Society's Elizabeth Garrett Anderson Award, established in 2000 to reward work by women in the field of migraine. See Wilkinson and Isler, "Pioneer Woman's View," 3.

13. Overy and Tansey, *Migraine*, 21–22.

14. Zilkha, "Clinics," 3.

15. Hanington, "Preliminary Report on Tyramine," 550–551.

16. Hanington and Harper, "Role of Tyramine."

17. Tfelt-Hansen, "History of Headache Research," 748–752.

18. Mathew et al., "Transformation of Episodic Migraine," 66–68.

19. Studies on patients from specialist clinics include Hay, "Treatment of Pain Trigger Areas"; Henryk-Gutt and Rees, "Psychological Aspects of Medicine"; Rydzewski, "Serotonin (5-HT) in Migraine"; Wainscott et al., "Outcome of Pregnancy"; Wilkinson and Woodrow, "Migraine and Weather."

20. G. Green, *Last Angry Man*, 385.

21. Didion, "In Bed," 168–169.

22. Sacks, *Migraine* (1985), 134–135. By the 1990s, however, use of the term "migraineur" seems to have declined. It is perhaps not an accident that this coincides with the rise of neurological theories and the efficacy of triptans.

23. Margoshes, "Don't Say My Migraines."

24. Hogan, *Healing Arts*, 195–196.

25. Hachinski et al., "Visual Symptoms."

26. Cardinal, "Outsider Art," 1462.

27. It is important to acknowledge that the therapeutic value of art is by no means universal. In one study from 2005, looking at the relationship between artmaking and migraine pain, the authors found that more respondents felt creating artwork was likely to trigger or worsen their headaches than to alleviate or lessen their pain, with factors such as the odor of materials or solvents and lighting conditions being identified as important. Many found themselves physically unable to execute their ideas during a migraine. "My creativity seems to increase while having a headache," one respondent commented, "but my ability to put pen to paper must wait for the pain to subside." As the authors of the report suggest, such evidence challenged "a basic truism of art therapy . . . the implication that *all* art is healing to *all* people under *all* conditions." See Vick and Sexton-Radek, "Art and Migraine," 198–199.

28. Clonidine had vasoactive properties and had been used, among other things, for hypertension and menopausal hot flashes. It was first reported as a migraine prophylactic by Marcia Wilkinson in 1969. See Wilkinson, "Clonidine for Migraine," 430.

29. Jean Butter's picture is reproduced in Hay, "Migraine."

30. Podoll and Robinson, *Migraine Art*, 34–37. Across the four competitions, Jean Butter would contribute at least seven pieces.

31. The forms of aura listed by Peter Wilson were "the shimmering stars of teichopsia; the half vision of hemianopia; the bright-edged castellated lines of fortification spectrum; of scintillating scotoma; and tunnel vision." See P. Wilson, "National Migraine Art Competition."

32. Podoll and Robinson, *Migraine Art*, 161–162.

33. Levy, *A Brain Wider*, 55–58.

34. Nat Blau is referring to image 48 from the Migraine Art Collection. See Blau, *Headache and Migraine Handbook*, 76–77.

35. Lomas and Howell, "Medical Imagery."

36. Kettenmann, *Frida Kahlo*, 67–68.

37. Jordanova, "Beth Fisher."

38. Frank, "Rhetoric of Self-Change," 40.

39. John Joseph Brennan, quoted in Podoll and Robinson, "Migraine Experiences," 264. *Migraine Man* (MAC 440) is a surreal figure made of geometric shapes, with crooks reminiscent of Salvador Dali's paintings replacing the left leg, and arcs and spheres suggestive of migraine aura swirling around the figure's head, with the point of a sharp cone piercing the head where an eye should be.

40. Charmaz, *Good Days, Bad Days*, 108–109.

41. Woolf, "On Being Ill."

42. Biro, *Language of Pain*, 77. Elaine Scarry suggested that physical pain "does not simply resist language but actively destroys it." See Scarry, *Body in Pain*. While Scarry's approach has been influential, it has also been criticized. If we assume there is "no language for pain," Lucy Bending responds, then "authority for representing that pain passes over to another group, with the result that those who suffer lose control over their own suffering." See Bending, *Representation of Bodily Pain*, 115.

43. Bourke, *Story of Pain*, 55, 58–65.

44. Podoll and Robinson, *Migraine Art*, 129.

45. Untitled artwork, submitted to the Migraine Art Competition, unnamed artist, n.d., MAC 484.

46. Untitled artwork, submitted to the Second Migraine Art Competition, unnamed artist, 1983, MAC 476.

47. Untitled artwork, submitted to Second Migraine Art Competition, unnamed artist, 1983, MAC 478.

48. Untitled artwork, submitted to Fourth Migraine Art Competition, unnamed artist, 1987, MAC 233.

49. Sacks, *Migraine* (1992), 281–282.

50. *A Migraine Attack*, submitted to the Second Migraine Art Competition, unnamed artist, 1983, MAC 77; *Go Away, Go Away, Go Away*, submitted to the Fourth Migraine Art Competition, unnamed artist, 1987, MAC 106.

51. An unnamed artist, quoted in Podoll and Robinson, *Migraine Art*, 73.

52. Untitled artwork, submitted to the Migraine Art Competition, unnamed artist (under-16 category), n.d., MAC 291.

53. Untitled artwork, submitted to the Migraine Art Competition, unnamed artist (under-16 category), n.d., MAC 18.

54. *Please Be Quiet. Do Not Disturb*, submitted to the Migraine Art Competition, unnamed artist (under-16 category), n.d., MAC 327.

55. *Migraine! Cause and Effect*, submitted to the First Migraine Art Competition, unnamed artist, 1981, MAC 513.

56. *How Can You Drive When the Road Looks Like This?*, submitted to the First Migraine Art Competition, unnamed artist, 1981, MAC 169.

57. Untitled artwork, submitted to the Second Migraine Art Competition, unnamed artist, 1983, MAC 339.

58. Nat Blau is referring to image 48 from the Migraine Art Collection. See Blau, *Headache and Migraine Handbook*, 76–77.

59. "Test Tube Baby," 31 July 1978, *Time* Magazine Covers; Wigley, "Best 80s Sci-Film Posters."

60. Didion, "In Bed," 172.

61. Podoll and Robinson, *Migraine Art*, 71.

62. *To Fit Again*, submitted to the Third Migraine Art Competition, unnamed artist, 1985, MAC 431. The red lion in the left-hand corner represents the logo of the British Migraine Association, and the "Let Me Help" below it suggests the importance of this charity to people with migraine.

63. *Migraine at the Gala Concert*, submitted to the Second Migraine Art Competition, unnamed artist, 1983, MAC 447.

64. *The Migraine Life*, submitted to the Third Migraine Art Competition, unnamed artist, 1985, MAC 385.

65. *Sorry Closed for Migraine*, submitted to the Fourth Migraine Art Competition, unnamed artist, 1987, MAC 57.

66. *Yr 1911*, submitted to the Second Migraine Art Competition, unnamed artist, 1982, MAC 333.

67. Untitled artwork, submitted to the Second Migraine Art Competition, unnamed artist, 1982, MAC 164.

68. Untitled artwork, submitted to the Second Migraine Art Competition, unnamed artist, 1983, MAC 129.

69. Untitled artwork, submitted to the Second Migraine Art Competition, unnamed Artist (under-16 category), 1983, MAC 448; Podoll and Robinson, *Migraine Art*, 50–51.

70. Humphrey, "Discovery and Development," 685.

71. Podoll, "Further Competitions."

72. Glasier, "Stunning Look at Life."

73. F. Kelly, "Experience 'Maison Migraine.'"

74. Debbie Ayles's paintings, photographs, and comments can be viewed on the Wellcome Collection: Images website.

75. For more on this aspect of YouTube, see Foxhall, "Digital Narratives."

Chapter 10 · Conclusion

1. For erenumab, researchers achieved a 50% or greater reduction in the number of migraine days per month for around half of the patients included in the trial. For fremanezumab, the results were a 50% reduction in migraine days for 38% of the people in the group injected quarterly, and 41% in the group injected monthly. Alder Biopharmaceuticals announced that 61% of patients on the eptinezumab trial had achieved a 50% or greater reduction in migraine days over a three-month period. See Goadsby et al., "Controlled Trial of Erenumab"; Silberstein et al., "Fremanezumab."

2. American Headache Society, "AHS Meeting Release CGRP"; Robinson, "News." The four different drugs were eptinezumab (Alder Biopharmaceuticals), galcanezumab (Eli Lilly & Company), fremanezumab (Teva Pharmaceutical Industries), and erenumab (Amgen and Novartis).

3. Edvinsson, "Trigeminovascular Pathway," 47–55; Lassen et al., "CGRP," 54–61; Wrobel Goldberg and Silberstein, "Targeting CGRP."

4. J. Hansen et al., "Calcitonin Gene-Related Peptide."

5. Edvinsson, "CGRP Receptor Antagonists."

6. Wrobel Goldberg and Silberstein, "Targeting CGRP," 447–448.

7. For useful overviews of CGRP and migraine in accessible language, see Underwood, "FDA Just Approved"; Yeh, "Monoclonal Antibodies."

8. American Headache Society, "AHS Meeting Release CGRP."

9. Staines, "Novartis/Amgen's Migraine Drug."

10. T. Smith, "Some Insurance Companies." There are precedents. Health insurers have limited access to PCKS9, a cholesterol-controlling drug with a similar cost.

11. Wilper et al., "Impact of Insurance," 1180–1182.

12. National Health Service, "Botox Gets Nod"; National Health Service England, "Clinical Commissioning Policy." In January 2019, NICE made an initial decision not to recommend erenumab for routine use in the NHS.

13. Martelletti, "Application of CGRP"; World Health Organization, "WHO Model List."

14. Tekle Haimanot, "Burden of Headache"; W. Stewart et al., "Variation in Migraine Prevalence."

15. Charleston and Burke, "Do Racial/Ethnic Disparities Exist?," 879–881.

16. Loder et al., "Prevalence, Burden, and Treatment," 224.

17. Robbins and Bernat, "Minority Representation."

18. Hoffman et al., "Racial Bias."

19. Leonardi and Mathers, "Global Burden."

20. Steiner et al., "Migraine: The Seventh Disabler."

21. See "The Global Campaign," Lifting the Burden, http://www.l-t-b.org/index.cfm/spKey

/the_global_campaign.html. For a history of the Global Burden of Disease reports and links to various findings, see the Institute for Health Metrics and Evaluation website, http://www.health data.org/gbd/about/history/.

22. Steiner et al., "Migraine: The Seventh Disabler."

23. Steiner et al., "Migraine: The Seventh Disabler."

24. Steiner et al., "GBD 2015."

25. Headache Classification Subcommittee, *ICHD-2*. *ICHD-2* also introduced subcategories for medication overuse headache attributed to ergotamine, triptan, an analgesic, an opioid, or a combination of medications. See Silberstein et al., *"ICHD-II*—Revision of Criteria."

26. Headache Classification Subcommittee, *ICHD-3*, 24. This was released for immediate use in beta form in 2013 and published as a final version in 2018. Following a petition from a number of experts in the headache field, in December 2017, the US Food and Drug Administration confirmed that in the future, they would require sponsors of over-the-counter migraine products to include a specific warning: "Headaches may worsen if this product is used for 10 or more days per month."

27. Torres-Ferrús et al., "When Does Chronic Migraine Strike?," 105, 112.

28. Anttila et al., "Genetics of Migraine."

29. Bigal et al., "Migraine in Adolescents."

30. For instance, in early 2018, researchers published a study proposing that while the ancestral allele of the gene TRPM8 was protective of migraine, an adaptation of the gene (which is, as the authors of the study explain, the "only known receptor to mediate the perception of moderate cold temperature in humans") has lost that characteristic. The adapted gene, which correlates strongly with latitude and temperature, is significantly more frequent in Finland than in Nigeria, a result, the authors suggest, of positive natural selection and a possible explanation for higher rates of migraine prevalence among individuals of European descent. See Key et al., "Human Local Adaptation."

31. Gormley et al., "Migraine Genetics," 1.

32. Borsook et al., "Can Imaging Change," 371.

33. Kempner, *Not Tonight*, 160–162.

All websites were accessed in September 2018, unless otherwise noted.

Manuscript Collections

British Library (BL), London, UK.
Case Notes Collections, Queen Square Archives (QSA), London, UK.
East Sussex Record Office (ESRO), UK.
James Ramsay Hunt Casebooks, Hammer Medical Sciences Center, Columbia University, New York, USA.
Louis P. Hamburger Collections, Alan Mason Chesney Medical Archives, Johns Hopkins University, Baltimore, USA.
Royal Society of London Archives (RSL), UK.
Talbot Papers, Lambeth Palace Library (LPL), London, UK.
Wellcome Library (WL), London, UK.

Manuscript Collections, Digitized

The Casebooks Project: A Digital Edition of Simon Forman's & Richard Napier's *Medical Records 1596–1634*. https://casebooks.lib.cam.ac.uk.
The Cullen Project: The Consultation Letters of Dr. William Cullen (1710–1790) at the Royal College of Physicians of Edinburgh. http://www.cullenproject.ac.uk.
Early English Books Online (EEBO). http://eebo.chadwyck.com.
Eighteenth Century Collections Online (ECCO). https://www.gale.com/primary-sources/eighteenth-century-collections-online/.
Migraine Action Art Collection (MAC). http://www.migraineart.org.uk.
Proceedings of the Old Bailey, 1674–1913 (POB). https://www.oldbaileyonline.org.
17th–18th Century Burney Collection Newspapers (BCN). https://www.gale.com/c/17th-and-18th-century-burney-newspapers-collection/.
The Sloane Letters Project. http://sloaneletters.com.
Wellcome Library Digital Collections (WL). https://wellcomelibrary.org/collections/browse/.

Websites

ABC News. http://abcnews.go.com.
Australian Academy of Science. https://www.science.org.au.
Commons and Lords Hansard. https://hansard.parliament.uk/
Europe PMC. https://europepmc.org.
Google Books. https://books.google.co.uk.
The Guardian. https://www.theguardian.com.
Institute for Health Metrics and Evaluation. http://www.healthdata.org.
Internet Archive. https://archive.org.
JSTOR. https://www.jstor.org.
Lifting the Burden Global Campaign Against Headache. www.l-t-b.org.
National Migraine Centre. http://www.nationalmigrainecentre.org.uk/migraine-and-headaches/.
Oxford Dictionary of National Biography. http://www.oxforddnb.com.
PubMed. https://www.ncbi.nlm.nih.gov/pubmed/.
The Recipes Project. https://recipes.hypotheses.org.
Time Magazine Covers. http://content.time.com/time/coversearch/.
US Department of Health and Human Services. https://www.hhs.gov/.
Wellcome Collection: Images. https://wellcomecollection.org/works/.

Radio

AL Kennedy's Migraine, presented by AL Kennedy, 3 April 2017, BBC Radio 4. http://www.bbc.co.uk/programmes/b08kttk1/.

Manuscripts

Almanac in Latin and English, [1464?]. MS 41, WL.

Apothecary's cash-book, c. 1703–1710. MS 7500, WL.

Ayscough, Lady. Recipe book, 1692. MS 1026/62. WL.

Bald's *Leechbook*, c. 950. Royal 12 D XVII, BL.

Bastian, [Henry] Charlton. "Case Notes, Male," 1891. NHNN/CN/5/8, QSA.

Beevor, Charles Edward. "Case Notes, Male and Female," 1899. NHMM/CN/17/8, QSA.

Blagden, Charles. Draft of letter to Thomas Curtis, 7 September 1781. Blagden Correspondence, CB/1/3/160, RSL.

Brumwich, Anne, et al. Collection of medical receipts, c. 1625–1700[?]. MS 160, WL.

Buzzard, Thomas. "Case Notes, Male and Female," 1881. NHNN/CN/4/5, QSA.

"A Collection of Remedies," mid-fifteenth century. MS MSL 136, WL.

Corlyon, Mrs. *A Booke of Diuers Medecines, Broothes, Salues, Waters, Syroppes, and Oyntementes*, 1606. MS 213. WL.

Curtis, Thomas. Letter, written from Penpont, to Charles Blagden, physician to the Army, Plymouth, 25 August 1781. Blagden Correspondence, CB/1/3/161, RSL.

Ferrier, David. "Case Notes, Male and Female," 1896. NHNN/CN/13/12, QSA.

"For ye megrom." English recipe book, c. 1675–1800. MS 7721/134, WL.

Frederica, Duchess of York. Letter to Sir Henry Halford, 28 May [c. 1819]. DG 24/831/22, LR.

"Guild Book of the Barber Surgeons of York," c. 1486. Egerton 2572, BL.

Gowers, Sir William Richard. "Case Book, Female," 1899, NHNN/CN/9/17, QSA.

Gowers, Sir William Richard. "Case Book, Male," 1898. NHNN/CN/9/14, QSA.

Gowers, Sir William Richard, and John Hughlings Jackson. "Case Notes, Male and Female," 1870–1877. NHNN/CN/2/1, QSA.

Herschel, John. Diary, 1800s. MS 583/2/3/4. RSL.

Hyde, Bridget. Recipe book, c. 1676–1690. MS 2990/98, WL.

Jackson, Jane. Recipe book, 1642. MS 373/47, WL.

Jackson, John Hughlings. "Case Notes, Female," 1895. NHNN/CN/8/18, QSA.

Jackson, John Hughlings. "Case Notes, Male and Female," 1892. NHNN/CN/8/12, QSA.

Klebs, Arnold. Letter to Charles Singer, 29 July 1913. Charles Singer Correspondence: K. PP/CJS.A.10, WL.

"Migril." Wellcome Foundation Product Literature (Migril), Folder 1: 1957–1960. WF/M/PL/199, WL.

"Migril." Wellcome Foundation Product Literature (Migril), Folder 2: 1961. WF/M/PL/199, WL.

"Migril." Wellcome Foundation Product Literature (Migril), Folder 7: 1969. WF/M/PL/199, WL.

Osborne, Sir Thomas. Recipe book, c. 1670–1695. MS 3724/54, WL.

Parker, Jane. Recipe book, 1651. MS 3769/59. WL.

Shaw, Miss. Collection of Medical and Cookery Receipts, c. 1675–1800. MS7721/134, WL.

Sleigh, Elizabeth, and Felicia Whitfeld. Collection of medical receipts, c. 1647–1722. MS 751/5, WL.

St. John, Johanna. Recipe book, 1680. MS 4338, WL.

"Suggestions for New Product—Ergot-Caffeine Combination for Migraine." Developmental Rejects, May 1948. WF/M/P/07/01, WL.

Sussex County Lunatic Asylum. *Thirteenth Annual Report for 1871*. Sussex Asylum, Annual Reports, 1869–1878. HC2/2, ESRO.

Sussex County Lunatic Asylum, *Fifteenth Annual Report for 1873*. Sussex Asylum, Annual Reports, 1869–1878. HC2/2, ESRO.

Talbot, Alathea, Countess of Arundel. Letter to the Countess of Shrewsbury, 1607. MS 3205, LPL.

Thomson, Francis, a persecuted recusant. Letter to Mr. Hicks, undated. Landsdowne MS 108/56, BL.

Townshend Family. Collection of medical and cookery receipts, c. 1636–1647. MS 774, WL.

Publications, Pre-1900

Adams, Thomas. *Diseases of the Soule: A Discourse Diuine, Morall, and Physicall*. London: George Purslowe, 1616. EEBO.

Addison, Joseph. "The Royal Exchange." *The Spectator*, 19 May 1711, 281. http://www2.scc.rutgers.edu/spectator/text/may1711/n069.html.

Airy, George Biddell. "III. The Astronomer Royal on Hemiopsy." *London, Edinburgh, and Dublin Philosophical Magazine and Journal of Science*, ser. 4, 30, no. 200 (July–December 1865): 19–21.

Airy, Hubert. "On a Distinct Form of Transient Hemiopsia." *Philosophical Transactions of the Royal Society of London* 160 (1870): 247–264.

Airy, Wilfred, ed. *Autobiography of Sir George Biddell Airy*. Cambridge: Cambridge University Press, 1896.

Allbutt, Clifford. "Clinical Lecture on Migraine." *Medical Times and Gazette* 1807 (14 February 1885): 203–208.

Andral, Gabriel. "Lectures on Medical Pathology: Lecture XVII. Perversions of Sensibility Continued. Vague Nervous Pain of the Head." *The Lancet* 20, no. 500 (30 March 1833): 1–5.

Andrews, John. *Comparative View of the French and English Nations, in Their Manners, Politics, and Literature*. London: T. Longman & G. G. J. & J. Robinson, 1785. ECCO.

Anon. *The Admirable Vertue, Property, and Operation of the Quintessence of Rosemary Flowers*. London: R. Barker, 1615. EEBO.

Anon. *A Closet for Ladies and Gentlewomen*. London: Arthur Johnson, 1608.

Anon. "Dr. Graves on the Treatment of Various Diseases." *Medico-Chirurgical Review and Journal of Practical Medicine* 19 (1833): 145–148.

Anon. *The Great and Wonderful Prophecies of Mr. Patridge, Mr. Coly, Mr. Tanner, and Mr. Andrews*. London: printed for J. C., 1689. EEBO.

Anon. *Here Begynneth a New Boke of Medecynes*. London: J. Rastall, 1526. EEBO.

Anon. "Medical Society of London." *The Lancet* 44, no. 1101 (5 October 1844): 57–58.

Anon. *A Report of the Cases Relieved and Cured in the Baths Appropriated for the Reception of the Poor*. Dublin: J. Chambers, 1777. ECCO.

Anon. "Report on the Treatment of Sick Headache" *British Medical Journal* (13 January 1872): 46–48.

Anon. "Report on the Treatment of Sick Headache." *British Medical Journal* (21 December 1872): 683–684.

Anon. *The Servants' Guide and Family Manual*, 2nd ed. London: John Limbird, 1831. Google Books.

Anon. *The Shepheards Kalendar*. London: Thomas Adams, 1604. EEBO.

Anon. "Subjective Visual Sensations." *British Medical Journal* (29 February 1896): 563.

Anstie, Francis E. *Neuralgia and the Diseases That Resemble It*. London: Macmillan, 1871.

Bacon, Francis. *Sylva Sylvarum; Or, A Naturall Historie*. London: William Lee, 1627. EEBO.

Barrington, Jonah. *Personal Sketches of His Own Times*. London: H. Colburn & R. Bentley, 1830.

Barrough, Philip. *The Methode of Phisicke Conteyning the Causes, Signes, and Cures of Inward Diseases in Mans Body from the Head to the Foote*. London: Thomas Vautroullier, 1583. EEBO.

Beard, George. *A Practical Treatise on Nervous Exhaustion*. New York: W. Wood, 1880. Internet Archive.

Berkeley, George. *Siris: A Chain of Philosophical Reflexions and Inquiries Concerning the Virtues of Tar Water*. London: C. Hitch & C. Davis, 1744. ECCO.

Blount, Thomas. *Glossographia*. London: George Sawbridge, 1661. EEBO.

Bolton Tomson, W. "Vaso-Motor Neuroses." *The Lancet* 140, no. 3607 (15 October 1892): 877–879. doi:10.1016/S0140-6736(01)88094-6.

Boorde, Andrew. *The Breuiary of Helthe for All Maner of Syckenesses and Diseases*. London: Wylllyam Myddelton, 1547. ECCO.

———. *Hereafter Foloweth a Compendyous Regyment or a Dyetary of Helth*. London: Robert Wyer, 1542.

Brewster, David. "LXIX. On Hemiopsy, or Half-Vision." *London, Edinburgh, and Dublin Philosophical Magazine and Journal of Science*, ser. 4, 29, no. 199 (January–June 1865): 503–507. doi:10.1080/14786446508643912.

Bristowe, J. S. "The Cavendish Lecture on Hysteria and Its Counterfeit Presentments." *The Lancet* 125, no. 3225 (20 June 1885): 1113–1117. doi:10.1016/S0140-6736(02)00748-1.

Brooke, Henry. *The Imposter*. Pp. 4–192 in *The Poetical Works of Henry Brooke*, vol. 3, ed. Henry Brooke. Dublin: Henry Brooke, 1792.

Brunton, T. Lauder. "A Discussion on Headaches and Their Treatment." *British Medical Journal* (4 November 1899): 1241–1243.

Buchan, William. *Domestic Medicine*, 11th ed. London: A. Strahan, 1790. ECCO.

Bullein, William. *A Newe Booke Entituled the Gouernement of Healthe*. London: John Day, 1558. EEBO.

Cartwright, Thomas. *An Hospitall for the Diseased*. London: Edward White, 1579. EEBO.

Cave, Jane. "The Head-Ache, Or An Ode to Health" (1794). P. 249 in *Eighteenth Century Women Poets: An Oxford Anthology*, ed. Roger Lonsdale. Oxford: Oxford University Press, 1989.

Cheyne, George. *The English Malady*. London: G. Strahan & J. Leake, 1733. EEBO.

Clendinning, John. "Observations on the Medicinal Properties of the Cannabis Sativa of India." *Medico-Chirurgical Transactions* 26 (1843): 188–210.

Clouston, T. S. "Observations and Experiments on the Use of Opium, Bromide of Potassium, and Cannabis Indica in Insanity." [London?]: [printed by J. E. Adlard], 1870. Internet Archive.

Clowes, William. *A Prooued Practise for All Young Chirurgians, Concerning Burnings with Gunpowder, and Woundes Made With Gunshot, Sword, Halbard, Pyke, Launce, or Such Other*. London: Thomas Orwyn, 1588. EEBO.

Cockayne, Oswald. *Leechdoms, Wortcunning, & Starcraft of Early England*, vol. 2. London: Longman, Green, Longman, Roberts, & Green, 1863. Internet Archive.

Cogan, Thomas. *The Hauen of Health*. London: Anne Griffin, 1636. EEBO.

Collins, Thomas. *Choice and Rare Experiments in Physick and Chirurgery*. London: Francis Eglesfield, 1658.

Copland, William. *A Boke of the Properties of Herbes Called an Herball*. London: Wyllyam Copland, 1552.

Crichton-Browne, J. "Circles of Mental Disorder—Modern Nervous Diseases." *British Medical Journal* (14 August 1880): 262–267.

———. "An Oration on Sex in Education." *The Lancet* 139, no. 3584 (7 May 1892): 1011–1018. doi:10.1016/S0140-6736(02)14447-3.

Crooke, Helkiah. *Mikrokosmographia*. London: printed by R. C., 1615. EEBO.

Cullen, William. *Nosology: Or, A Systematic Arrangement of Diseases*. Edinburgh: William Creech, 1792. ECCO.

Culpeper, Nicholas. *The English Physitian Enlarged*. London: Peter Cole, 1653. EEBO.

———. *Pharmacopeia Londinensis, or, The London Dispensatory*. 1653. London: Peter Cole, 1653. EEBO.

Deane, Edmund. *Spadacrene Anglica or, The English Spaw Fountaine*. London: M. Flesher, 1626. EEBO.

Dodoens, Rembert. *A New Herball, or Historie of Plantes*, trans. Henry Lyle. London: Edm. Bollifant, 1595. EEBO.

Donovan, Edward. *Descriptive Excursions through South Wales and Monmouth in the Year 1804 and the Four Preceding Summers*, 2 vols. London: Bye & Law, 1805. Internet Archive.

Elyot, Thomas. *The Castel of Helth*. London: Thomas Berthelet, 1539. EEBO.

Fothergill, John. "Remarks on That Complaint Commonly Known as Sick-Headache. Read Dec. 14, 1778." *Medical Observations and Inquiries* 6 (1757–1784): 103–137. ECCO.

Furnivall, Percy, and Frederick J. Furnivall, eds. *The Anatomie of the Bodie of Man, by Thomas Vicary*. Oxford: published for the Early English Text Society by N. Trubner, 1888.

Galton, Francis. *Inquiries into Human Faculty and Its Development*. London: Macmillan, 1883.

Gerard, John. *The Herball, or Generall Historie of Plants*. London: Adam Islip, Ioice Norton, & Richard Whitakers, 1633. EEBO.

Gowers, W. R. *A Manual of Diseases of the Nervous System*, vol. 2. London: J. & A. Churchill, 1888.

———. "Subjective Visual Sensations." *Transactions of the Royal Ophthalmological Society of the United Kingdom* 15 (1895): 1–38.

Greene, Richard. "The Treatment of Migraine with Indian Hemp." *Practitioner* 41 (1888): 35–38.

Guillemeau, Jacques. *The Frenche Chirurgerye, or All the Manualle Operations of Chirurgerye*. Dort [Dordrecht], Netherlands: Isaac Canin, 1598. EEBO.

Gyer, Nicholas. *The English Phlebotomy; or, Method and Way of Healing by Letting of Blood*. London: W. Hoskins & J. Danter for A. Mansell, 1592. EEBO.

Hall, Marshall. "On the Threatenings of Apoplexy and Paralysis." *The Lancet* 52, no. 1299 (22 July 1848): 92–96.

Heberden, William. *Commentaries on the History and Cure of Diseases*, 4th ed. London: Payne & Foss, 1816.

Herschel, John. "On Sensorial Vision." Pp. 400–418 in *Familiar Lectures on Scientific Subjects*. New York: George Routledge & Sons, 1872.

Jackson, John Hughlings. "Hospital for the Epileptic and Paralysed: A Case of Hemiopia, with Hemianaesthesia and Hemiplegia." *The Lancet* 104, no. 2661 (29 August 1874): 306–307. doi:10.1016/S0140-6736(02)56459-X.

———. "Hospital for the Epileptic and Paralysed: Case Illustrating the Relation betwixt Certain Cases of Migraine and Epilepsy." *The Lancet* 106, no. 2711 (14 August 1875), 244–245.

Jones, John. *The Benefit of the Auncient Batthes of Buckstones*. London: Tho. East & Henry Myddleton, 1572. EEBO.

Labarraque, Henri. *Essai sur la céphalalgie et la migraine, soit comme affection symptomatique, soit comme maladie essentielle*. Thèse, médecine. Paris: Rignous, 1837.

Langham, William. *Garden of Health*. London: Christopher Barker, 1597.

Latham, P. W. "Guarana (Paullinia) Powder a Remedy for Sick-Headache." *British Medical Journal* (27 April 1872): 446–447.

———. *On Nervous or Sick-Headache, Its Varieties and Treatment*. Cambridge: Deighton, Bell, 1873.

———. "On Sick-Headache." *British Medical Journal* (4 January 1873): 7–8.

Leconte, M. "Guarana." *The Lancet* 100, no. 2557 (31 August 1872): 313–314.

Lees, F. Arnold. "Tetrachloride and Bisulphide of Carbon in Neuralgia." *British Medical Journal* (8 June 1878): 850. doi:10.1136/bmj.1.910.850.

Liveing, Edward. *On Megrim, Sick Headache, and Some Allied Disorders: A Contribution to the Pathology of Nerve-Storms*. London: J. & A. Churchill, 1873.

Lucas-Championnière, Just. *La trépanation guidée par les localisations cérébrales: Étude historique et clinique sur la trépanation du crane*. Paris: V. A. Delahaye, 1878.

Madden, Richard Robert. *The Infirmities of Genius*. Philadelphia: Carey, Lea, & Blanchard, 1833. Internet Archive.

Maudsley, Henry. *The Pathology of Mind*. New York: D. Appleton, 1880. Internet Archive.

Mead, Richard. *A Treatise Concerning the Influence of the Sun and Moon upon Human Bodies and the Diseases Thereby Produced*, trans. Richard Stack. London: J. Brindley, 1748. ECCO.

Mease, James. *A Treatise on the Causes, Means of Prevention, and Cure of the Sick-Headache*. Philadelphia: M. Casey & Son, 1819. Internet Archive.

Mediolano, Joannes de. *Regimen Sanitatis Salerni*. London: Thomas Berthelet, 1528. EEBO.

Migne, Jacques-Paul. *S. Hildegardis Abbatissa*, vol. 197 of *Patrologia Latina*. Paris: Migne, 1855.

Mornay, Philippe de. *A Discourse of Life and Death: Written in French, Done in English by the Countesse of Pembroke*, 2nd ed. London: Matthew Lownes, 1608. EEBO.

Moulton, Thomas. *This Is the Myrour or Glasse of Health*. London: Rycharde Kele, c. 1540. EEBO.

Murphy, Patrick J. "On Headache and Its Varieties. " *The Lancet* 63, no. 1590 (18 February 1854): 182–183.

———. "On Headache and Its Varieties." *The Lancet* 63, no. 1591 (25 February 1854): 209–210.

———. "On Headache and Its Varieties." *The Lancet* 63, no. 1603 (20 May 1854): 540–541.

Osler, William. *The Principles and Practice of Medicine*. New York: D. Appleton, 1892. Internet Archive.

Paré, Ambroise. *The Workes of that Famous Chirurgion Ambrose Parey Translated out of Latine and Compared with the French by Thomas Johnson*. London: T. Cotes & R. Young, 1634. EEBO.

Parry, Caleb Hiller. *Collections from the Unpublished Medical Writings of the Late Caleb Hillier Parry*, 3 vols. London: Underwoods, 1825.

———. *Elements of Pathology and Therapeutics*, vol. 1, 2nd ed. London: Underwood, 1825.

Partridge, John. *The Widowes Treasure*. London: Edward White, 1588. EEBO.

Paterson, Daniel. *Paterson's British Itinerary, Being a New and Accurate Delineation of the Direct and Principal Crossroads of Great Britain*. London: Carrington Bowles, 1785. ECCO.

Pechey, John. *The Compleat Herbal of Physical Plants*. London: R. & T. Bonwicke, 1707.

Philiatros. *Natura Exenterata*. London: H. Twiford, 1655. EEBO.

Pope John XXI. *The Treasury of Healthe Conteynyng Many Profitable Medycines*. London: Wyllyam Coplande, 1553. EEBO.

Potter, Samuel O. L. *Handbook of Materia Medica, Pharmacy, and Therapeutics*, 5th ed. Philadelphia: P. Blakiston & Son, 1897.

Prior, Thomas. *An Authentic Narrative of the Success of Tar-Water, in Curing a Great Number and Variety of Distempers*. Dublin: W. Innys, C. Hitch, M. Cooper, & C. Davis, 1746. ECCO.

Pughe, John, trans. *The Physicians of Myddvai*, ed. John Williams ab Ithel. Welsh MSS Society. Llandovery, Wales, UK: D. J. Roderic, 1861.

Ross, James. *A Treatise on the Diseases of the Nervous System*, vol. 1, 2nd ed. New York: William Wood, 1883.

Rowley, William. *A Treatise on One Hundred and Eighteen Principal Diseases of the Eyes and Eyelids*. London: printed for J. Wingrave, E. Newbery, & T. Hookham, 1790. Google Books.

Salmon, William. *The London Almanack: For the Year of Our Lord, 1701*. London: W. Horton, 1701. ECCO.

———. *Phylaxa Medicina: A Supplement to the London-Dispensatory, and Doron: Being, a Cabinet of Choice Medicines Collected, and Fitted for Vulgar Use*, 2nd ed. London: Simon Neale, 1688. Google Books.

Samelson, A. "Guarana against Sick-Headache." *British Medical Journal* (11 May 1872): 498. JSTOR.

Smith, Benjamin. *Sunshine in the Kitchen; or, Chapters for Maidservants*. London: Wesleyan Conference Office, 1872. Google Books.

Speed, John. *The Theatre of the Empire of Greate Britaine*. London: J. Sudbury & G. Humble, 1611/12.

Symonds, John Addington. "On Headache: Lecture II, Concluded." *Medical Times and Gazette* (24 April 1858): 419–422.

Tissot, Samuel A. D. *Traité des nerfs et de leurs maladies*. Lausanne: François Grasset, 1789. Internet Archive.

Trotter, Thomas. *A View of the Nervous Temperament*. Boston: Wright, Goodenow, & Stockwell, 1808.

Vicary, Thomas. *The English Man's Treasure*. London: Thomas Creede, 1613. EEBO.

Wilks, Samuel. "Epilepsy and Migraine." *The Lancet* 132, no. 3389 (11 August 1888): 263–264. doi: 10.1016/S0140-6736(02)24647-4.

Willis, Thomas. *An Essay of the Pathology of the Brain and Nervous Stock*. London: T. Dring, 1681.

———. *De Anima Brutorum quae Hominis Vitalis ac Sentitiva Est: Exercitationes Duae*. Oxford: Ric. Davis, 1672. EEBO.

———. *The London Practice of Physick*. London: Thomas Basset & William Crooke, 1685. EEBO.

———. *Two Discourses Concerning the Soul of Brutes, Which Is That of the Vital and Sensitive of Man*, trans. Samuel Pordage. London: Thomas Dring, Ch. Harper, and John Leigh, 1683. http://tei.it.ox.ac.uk/tcp/Texts-HTML/free/A66/A66518.html and EEBO.

Woakes, Edward. "On Ergot of Rye in the Treatment of Neuralgia." *British Medical Journal* 2, no. 491 (3 October 1868): 360–461.

Wollaston, William Hyde. "On Semi-Decussation of the Optic Nerves." *Philosophical Transactions of the Royal Society of London* 114 (1824): 222–231. doi:10.1098/rstl.1824.0013.

Wright, Thomas. *Three Chapters of Letters Relating to the Suppression of Monasteries*. London: Camden Society, 1843.

Publications, Post-1900

Abramson, J. H., C. Hopp, and L. M. Epstein. "Migraine and Non-migrainous Headaches: A Community Survey in Jerusalem." *Journal of Epidemiology and Community Health* 34, no. 3 (1980): 188–193. doi:10.1136/jech.34.3.188.

Abu-Arafeh, Ishak, Sheik Razak, Baskaran Sivaraman, and Catriona Graham. "Prevalence of Headache and Migraine in Children and Adolescents: A Systematic Review of Population-Based Studies." *Developmental Medicine and Child Neurology* 52, no. 12 (2010): 1088–1097. doi:10.1111/j.1469-8749.2010.03793.x.

Adams, J. N., and Marilyn Deegan. "Bald's *Leechbook* and the *Physica Plinii*." *Anglo-Saxon England* 21 (1992): 87–114.

Aikin, J. M. "Etiology and Treatment of Migraine." *Journal of the American Medical Association* 39, no. 9 (1902): 485–487.

Allan, William. "The Inheritance of Migraine." *Archives of Internal Medicine* 42, no. 4 (1928): 590–599. doi:10.1001/archinte.1928.00130210138013.

———. "The Sex Ratio in Migraine." *Archives of Neurology and Psychiatry* 27, no. 6 (1932): 1436–1440. doi:10.1001/archneurpsyc.1932.02230180165010.

Alvarez, Walter. *How to Live with Your Migraine (Sick) Headaches*. Chicago: Wilcox & Follett, 1952.

———. "The Migrainous Personality and Constitution." *American Journal of the Medical Sciences* 213, no. 1 (January 1947): 1–8.

American Headache Society. "AHS Meeting Release CGRP." American Headache Society, 7 June 2017. https://americanheadachesociety.org/ahs-meeting-release-cgrp/.

Aminoff, Michael J. *Brown-Sequard: An Improbable Genius Who Transformed Medicine*. Oxford: Oxford University Press, 2011.

Anderson, Warwick, and Ian R. Mackay. *Intolerant Bodies: A Short History of Autoimmunity*. Baltimore: Johns Hopkins University Press, 2014.

Anon. "Editorial: Migraine Clinics." *British Medical Journal* (10 August 1974): 376. doi:10.1136/bmj.3.5927.376.

Anon. "St. Hildegard." *Proceedings of the Royal Society of Medicine, History of Medicine Section* (1913): vii.

Anthony, Michael, and James W. Lance. "The Role of Serotonin in Migraine." Pp. 107–123 in *Modern Topics in Migraine*, ed. J. Pearce. London: Heinemann Medical, 1975.

Anttila, Verneri, Maija Wessman, Mikko Kallela, and Aarno Palotie. "Genetics of Migraine." In "Neurogenetics, Part II," ed. Daniel H. Geschwind, Henry L. Paulson, and Christine Klein. Special issue, *Handbook of Clinical Neurology*, 3rd ser., 148 (2018): 493–503.

Arikha, Noga. *Passions and Tempers: A History of the Humours*. New York: Harper Perennial, 2007.

Arrizabalaga, Jon. "Problematising Retrospective Diagnosis in the History of Disease." *Asclepio* 54, no. 1 (2002): 51–70. doi:10.3989/asclepio.2002.v54.i1.135.

Atkinson, E. Miles. "Nasal Headaches." *British Medical Journal* (13 August 1927): 264–266.

Auld, Alexander Gunn. *Asthma, Hay Fever, Migraine, and Other Clinical Studies*. London: H. K. Lewis, 1936.

Baird, Joseph L., and Radd K. Ehrman. *The Letters of Hildegard of Bingen*, vol. 1. Oxford: Oxford University Press, 1994.

Banham, Debby. "Dun, Oxa, and Pliny the Great Physician: Attribution and Authority in Old English Medical Texts." *Social History of Medicine* 24, no. 1 (2011): 57–73.

Barker, Hannah. "Medical Advertising and Trust in Late Georgian England." *Urban History* 36, no. 3 (2009): 379–398.

Bendelow, Gillian. *Pain and Gender*. New York: Prentice Hall, 2000.

Bending, Lucy. *The Representation of Bodily Pain in Late Nineteenth-Century English Culture*. Oxford: Oxford University Press, 2000.

Benjamin, Marina. "Medicine, Morality, and the Politics of Berkeley's Tar-Water." Pp. 165–193 in *The Medical Enlightenment of the Eighteenth Century*, ed. Andrew Cunningham and Roger French. Cambridge: Cambridge University Press, 1990.

Bigal, M. E., R. B. Lipton, P. Winner, M. L. Reed, S. Diamond, and W. F. Stewart. "Migraine in Adolescents: Association with Socioeconomic Status and Family History." *Neurology* 69, no. 1 (July 2007): 16–25. doi:10.1212/01.wnl.0000265212.90735.64.

Bildhauer, Bettina. "Medieval European Conceptions of Blood: Truth and Human Integrity." *Journal of the Royal Anthropological Institute*, n.s., 19 (May 2013), S57–S76. doi:10.1111/1467-9655.12016.

Biro, David. *The Language of Pain: Finding Words, Compassion, and Relief*. New York: W. W. Norton, 2010.

Blau, Joseph Norman. *The Headache and Migraine Handbook*. London: Corgi, 1986.

———. "Migraine Pathogenesis: The Neural Hypothesis Reexamined." *Journal of Neurology, Neuropsychiatry, and Psychiatry* 47 (1984): 437–442.

———. "Problems and Paradoxes in Migraine." *Hemicrania* 2, no. 1 (1970), 6–7.

———. "Somesthetic Aura: The Experience of *Alice in Wonderland*." *The Lancet* 352, no. 9127 (15 August 1998): 582.

Bliss, Michael. *Harvey Cushing: A Life in Surgery*. Oxford: Oxford University Press, 2005.

Booth, Martin. *Cannabis: A History*. London: Doubleday, 2003.

Borsook, David, Arne May, Peter J. Goadsby, and Richard Hargreaves. "Can Imaging Change Migraine Treatment Paradigms?" Pp. 371–273 in *The Migraine Brain: Imaging Structure and Function*, ed. David Borsook, Arne May, Peter J. Goadsby, and Richard Hargreaves. Oxford: Oxford University Press, 2012.

Bourke, Joanna. *The Story of Pain: From Prayer to Painkillers*. Oxford: Oxford University Press, 2014.

Boyd, Kenneth M. "Disease, Illness, Sickness, Health, Healing, and Wholeness: Exploring Some Elusive Concepts." *Journal of Medical Ethics: Medical Humanities* 26, no. 9 (2000): 9–17.

Brain, W. Russell. *Diseases of the Nervous System*. Oxford: Oxford University Press, 1933.

Bramwell, Edwin. "Discussion on Migraine." *British Medical Journal* (30 October 1926): 765–775. doi:10.1136/bmj.2.3434.765.

Bray, George W. *Recent Advances in Allergy*. London: J. & A. Churchill, 1931.

Breuninger, Scott. "A Panacea for the Nation: Berkeley's Tar-Water and Irish Domestic Development." *Études irelandaises* 34, no. 2 (2009): 29–42. doi:10.4000/etudesirlandaises.2618.

Brockbank, William. "Sovereign Remedies: A Critical Depreciation of the 17th-Century London Pharmacopoeia." *Medical History* 8, no. 1 (1964): 1–14.

Brumberg, Joan Jacobs. *Fasting Girls: The Emergence of Anorexia Nervosa as a Modern Disease*. Cambridge, MA: Harvard University Press, 1988.

Brunton, Thomas Lauder. *Hallucinations and Allied Mental Phenomena*, reprinted from *Journal of Mental Science* (April 1902). London: Adlard & Son, 1910. WL.

Buck, R. A. "Woman's Milk in Anglo-Saxon and Later Medieval Medical Texts." *Neophilologus* 96 (2012): 467–485.

Burch, Rebecca C., Stephen Loder, Elizabeth Loder, and Todd A. Smitherman. "The Prevalence and Burden of Migraine and Severe Headache in the United States: Updated Statistics from Government Health Surveillance Studies." *Headache: The Journal of Head and Face Pain* 55, no. 1 (January 2015): 21–34. doi:10.1111/head.12482.

Burke, David. "Professor James Lance, Neurologist." Interview, 2010. Australian Academy of Science. https://www.science.org.au/learning/general-audience/history/interviews-australian-scientists/professor-james-lance-neurologist/.

Bury, Michael. "Chronic Illness as Biographical Disruption." *Sociology of Health and Illness* 4, no. 2 (July 1982): 167–182.

Buse, Dawn C., Elizabeth W. Loder, Jennifer A. Gorman, Walter F. Stewart, Michael L. Reed, Kristina M. Fanning, Daniel Serrano, and Richard B. Lipton. "Sex Differences in the Prevalence, Symptoms, and Associated Features of Migraine, Probable Migraine, and Other Severe Headache: Results of the American Migraine Prevalence and Prevention (AMPP) Study." *Headache: The Journal of Head and Face Pain* 53, no. 8 (September 2013): 1278–1299. doi:10.1111/head.12150.

Bynum, Caroline W. *Holy Feast and Holy Fast: The Significance of Food to Medieval Women*. Berkeley: University of California Press, 1987.

Bynum, William F. "Cullen and the Study of Fevers in Britain, 1760–1820." *Medical History*, Suppl. 1 (1981): 135–147.

———. "The Nervous Patient in Eighteenth- and Nineteenth-Century Britain: The Psychiatric Origins of British Neurology." Pp. 89–102 in *The Anatomy of Madness: Essays in the History of Psychiatry*, vol. 1, ed. William F. Bynum, Roy Porter, and Michael Shepherd. London: Tavistock, 1985.

Cady, Roger K., Jeanette K. Wendt, John R. Kirchner, Joseph D. Sargent, John F. Rothrock, and Harold Skaggs. "Treatment of Acute Migraine with Subcutaneous Sumatriptan." *JAMA* 265, no. 21 (1991): 2831–2835. doi:10.1001/jama.1991.03460210077033.

Cameron, Michael L. *Anglo-Saxon Medicine*. Cambridge: Cambridge University Press, 1993.

———. "Bald's *Leechbook*: Its Sources and Their Use in Its Compilation." *Anglo-Saxon England* 12 (1983): 153–182. doi:10.1017/S0263675100003392.

Canning, Kathleen. "The Body as Method? Reflections on the Place of the Body in Gender History." *Gender and History* 11, no. 3 (1999): 499–513. doi:10.1111/1468-0424.00159.

Cardinal, Roger. "Outsider Art and the Autistic Creator." *Philosophical Transactions of the Royal Society B* 364, no. 1522 (2009): 1459–1466. doi:10.1098/rstb.2008.0325.

Carel, Havi. *Illness: The Cry of the Flesh*. Stocksfield, UK: Acumen, 2008.

Carlebach, Elisheva. *Palaces of Time: Jewish Calendar and Culture in Early Modern Europe*. Cambridge, MA: Harvard University Press, 2011.

Carrington, Charles. *Rudyard Kipling: His Life and Work*. London: Macmillan, 1955.

Casper, Stephen T. *The Neurologists: A History of a Medical Specialty in Modern Britain, c. 1789–2000*. Manchester, UK: Manchester University Press, 2014.

Castle, Terry. "Eros and Liberty at the English Masquerade, 1710–1790." *Eighteenth-Century Studies* 17, no. 2 (1983): 156–176.

Caviness, Madeline. *Art in the Medieval West and Its Audience*. Aldershot, UK: Ashgate, 2001.

———. "Artist: 'To See, Hear, and Know All at Once.'" Pp. 110–124 in *Voice of the Living Light: Hildegard of Bingen and Her World*, ed. Barbara Newman. Berkeley: University of California Press, 1998.

———. "Hildegard as Designer of Illustrations." Pp. 29–62 in *Hildegard of Bingen: The Context of Her Thought and Art*, ed. Charles Burnett and Peter Dronke. London: Warburg Institute, 1998.

Charleston, Larry, and James Francis Burke. "Do Racial/Ethnic Disparities Exist in Recommended Migraine Treatments in US Ambulatory Care?" *Cephalalgia: An International Journal of Headache* 38, no. 5 (April 2018): 876–882.

Charmaz, Kathy, *Good Days, Bad Days: The Self in Chronic Illness and Time*. New Brunswick, NJ: Rutgers University Press, 1997.

Chemist and Druggist. *Pharmaceutical Formulas*. London: Chemist & Druggist, 1904.

Church, Roy A., and E. M. Tansey. *Burroughs Wellcome & Co.: Knowledge, Trust, Profit, and the Transformation of the British Pharmaceutical Industry, 1880–1940*. Lancaster, UK: Crucible, 2007. WL.

Clarke, C. A. "Gowers' Mixture." *The Practitioner* 180 (February 1958): 215–216.

Clower, William T., and Stanley Finger. "Discovering Trepanation: The Contribution of Paul Broca." *Neurosurgery* 49, no. 6 (2001): 1417–1425. doi:10.1097/00006123-200112000-00021.

Cody, Lisa Forman. "'No Cure No Money,' or the Invisible Hand of Quackery: The Language of Commerce, Credit, and Cash in Eighteenth-Century British Medical Advertisements." *Studies in Eighteenth-Century Culture* 28 (1999): 103–130.

Cohen, Esther. *The Modulated Scream: Pain in Late Medieval Culture*. Chicago: University of Chicago Press, 2010.

Cohen, Esther, Leona Toker, Manuela Consonni, and Otniel E. Dror, eds. *Knowledge and Pain*. Amsterdam: Rodopi, 2012.

Cohen, Michèle. *Fashioning Masculinity: National Identity and Language in the Eighteenth Century*. London: Routledge, 1996.

Coleborne, Catharine. *Madness in the Family*. Basingstoke, UK: Palgrave Macmillan, 2010.

Conlee, John, ed. "William Dunbar: Poems, Public and Private." In *William Dunbar: The Complete Works*. Kalamazoo, MI: Medieval Institute Publications, 2004. http://d.lib.rochester.edu/teams/text/conlee-dunbar-complete-works-poems-public-and-private/.

Cooper, Rachel. "Disease." *Studies in History and Philosophy of Science, Part C: Studies in History and Philosophy of Biological and Biomedical Sciences* 33, no. 2 (2002): 263–282.

Cooter, Roger. "The Life of a Disease?" *The Lancet* 375, no. 9709 (9–15 January 2010): 111–112.

Cornwell, Jocelyn. *Hard-Earned Lives: Accounts of Health and Illness from East London*. London: Tavistock, 1984.

Crawford, Sally. "The Nadir of Western Medicine? Texts, Contexts, and Practice in Anglo-Saxon England." Pp. 41–51 in *Bodies of Knowledge: Cultural Interpretations of Illness and Medicine in Medieval Europe*, ed. Sally Crawford and Christina Lee. Studies in Early Medicine 1. Oxford: BAR, 2010.

Critchley, Macdonald. "Discarded Theories in the Past 50 Years." Pp. 241–261 in *Migraine: Clinical, Therapeutic, Conceptual, and Research Aspects*, ed. Joseph N. Blau. London: Chapman & Hall: 1987.

———. "Migraine: General Remarks." *Proceedings of the Royal Society of Medicine* 55 (March 1962): 165–167.

———. "Towards a Definition." *Migraine News* 1 (June 1967): 1–2.

Critchley, Macdonald, and Fergus R. Ferguson. "Migraine." *The Lancet* 221, no. 5708 (21 January 1933): 123–126.

———. "Migraine." *The Lancet* 221, no. 5709 (28 January 1933): 182–187.

Crookshank, F. G. *Migraine and Other Common Neuroses*. London: Kegan Paul, 1925.

Cumings, John N. "Speculation Not the Way to a Cure." *Migraine News* 13 (December 1970): 1, 4.

Cunningham, Andrew. "Identifying Disease in the Past: Cutting the Gordian Knot." *Asclepio* 54, no. 1 (2002): 13–34. doi:10.3989/asclepio.2002.v54.i1.133.

Curth, Louise Hill. *English Almanacs, Astrology, and Popular Medicine: 1550–1700*. Manchester, UK: Manchester University Press, 2007.

Daston, Lorraine, and Peter Galison. *Objectivity*. New York: Zone Books, 2010.

Dawson, Warren R. *A Leechbook or Collection of Medical Recipes of the Fifteenth Century*. London: Macmillan, 1934.

Deegan, Marilyn. "A Critical Edition of MS B.L. Royal 12. D. xvii: Bald's Leechbook," 2 vols. PhD dissertation: University of Manchester, 1988.

Demaitre, Luke. *Medieval Medicine: The Art of Healing from Head to Toe*. Santa Barbara, CA: Praeger, 2013.

Diamond, Seymour, and Mary A. Franklin, *Headache through the Ages*. Caddo, OK: Professional Communications, 2005.

Didion, Joan. "In Bed" (1968). Pp. 168–172 in *The White Album*. New York: Farrar, Strauss, & Giroux, 1979.

DiMeo, Michelle, and Sara Pennell, eds. *Reading and Writing Recipe Books, 1550–1800*. Manchester, UK: University of Manchester Press, 2013.

Dronke, Peter. "Hildegard of Bingen." Pp. 144–201 in *Women Writers of the Middle Ages*. Cambridge: Cambridge University Press, 1984.

Duden, Barbara. *The Woman beneath the Skin: A Doctor's Patients in Eighteenth-Century Germany*. Cambridge, MA: Harvard University Press, 1998.

Eadie, Mervyn J. "Ergot of Rye—the First Specific for Migraine." *Journal of Clinical Neuroscience* 11, no. 1 (2004): 4–7.

———. *Headache through the Centuries*. Oxford: Oxford University Press, 2012.

———. "Hubert Airy, Contemporary Men of Science, and the Migraine Aura." *Journal of the Royal College of Physicians Edinburgh* 39, no. 3 (2009): 263–267. https://espace.library.uq.edu.au/view/UQ:316146/.

Eamon, William. "How to Read a Book of Secrets." Pp. 23–44 in *Secrets and Knowledge in Medicine and Science, 1500–1800*, ed. Elaine Yuen Tien Leong and Alisha Michelle Rankin. Farnham, Surrey, UK: Ashgate, 2011.

Earles, Melvin P. "The Introduction of Hydrocyanic Acid into Medicine." *Medical History* 11, no. 3 (1967): 305–312.

Edvinsson, Lars. "CGRP Receptor Antagonists and Antibodies against CGRP and Its Receptor in Migraine Treatment." *British Journal of Clinical Pharmacology* 80, no. 2 (2015): 193–199. doi:10.1111/bcp.12618.

———. "The Trigeminovascular Pathway: Role of CGRP and CGRP Receptors in Migraine." *Headache: The Journal of Head and Face Pain* 57 (May 2017): 47–55.

Elliott, R. H. "Migraine and Mysticism." *Postgraduate Medical Journal* 8, no. 86 (1932): 449–459.

Entract, J. P. "'Chlorodyne' Browne." *London Hospital Gazette* 73, no. 4 (1970): 7–11, 17. RAMC/750, WL and in BL.

Epstein, Steven. *Inclusion: The Politics of Difference in Medical Research*. Chicago: University of Chicago Press, 2007.

Evans, Jennifer. "'Gentle Purges Corrected with Hot Spices, Whether They Work or Not, Do Vehemently Provoke Venery': Menstrual Provocation and Procreation in Early Modern England." *Social History of Medicine* 25, no. 1 (2012): 2–19.

Fabbri, Christiane Nockels. "Treating Medieval Plague: The Wonderful Virtues of Theriac." *Early Science and Medicine* 12 (2007): 247–283.

Fee, Elizabeth, and Theodore M. Brown. "Using Medical History to Shape a Profession: The Ideals of William Osler and Henry E. Sigerist." Pp. 139–164 in *Locating Medical History: The Stories and Their Meanings*, ed. Frank Huisman and John Harley Warner. Baltimore: Johns Hopkins University Press, 2004.

Fee, Elizabeth, and Daniel M. Fox. *AIDS: The Burdens of History*. Berkeley: University of California Press, 1988.

Ferrari, M. D. and J. Haan. "Migraine Aura, Illusory Vertical Splitting, and Picasso." *Cephalalgia: An International Journal of Headache* 20, no. 8 (October 2000): 686. doi:10.1111/j.1468-2982 .2000.00113.x.

Field, Catherine. "'Many Hands Hands': Writing the Self in Women's Recipe Books." Pp. 49–63 in *Genre and Women's Life Writing in Early Modern England*, ed. Michelle M. Dowd and Julie A. Eckerle. Aldershot, UK: Ashgate, 2016.

Fissell, Mary. "The Marketplace of Print." Pp. 108–132 in *Medicine and the Market in England and its Colonies, c. 1450–c. 1850*, ed. Mark Jenner and Patrick Wallis. Basingstoke, UK: Palgrave Macmillan: 2007.

Flanagan, Sabina. *Hildegard of Bingen: A Visionary Life*, 2nd ed. London: Routledge, 1998.

Foster, J. B. "General Aspects of Management." Pp. 138–144 in *Modern Topics in Migraine*, ed. John Pearce. London: Heinemann Medical, 1975.

Foxhall, Katherine. "Digital Narratives: Four 'Hits' in the History of Migraine." Pp. 512–528 in *The Routledge History of Disease*, ed. Mark Jackson. London: Routledge, 2017.

Frank, Arthur. "The Rhetoric of Self-Change: Illness Experience as Narrative." *Sociological Quarterly* 34, no. 1 (1993): 39–52.

Furdell, Elizabeth Lane. "Boorde, Andrew (c. 1490–1549)." *Oxford Dictionary of National Biography*. Oxford: Oxford University Press, 2004; online ed., January 2008.

Ganidagli, Suleyman, Mustafa Cengiz, Sahin Aksoy, and Ayhan Verit. "Approach to Painful Disorders by Şerefeddin Sabuncuoğlu in the Fifteenth Century Ottoman Period." *Anesthesiology* 100, no. 1 (2004): 165–169. http://anesthesiology.pubs.asahq.org.

Gavrus, Delia. "'Making Bad Boys Good': Brain Surgery and the Juvenile Court in Progressive Era America." Pp.71–99 in *Technological Change in Modern Surgery: Historical Perspectives on Innovation*, ed. Thomas Schlich and Christopher Crenner. Rochester, NY: University of Rochester Press, 2017.

Getz, Faye M. *Medicine in the English Middle Ages*. Princeton, NJ: Princeton University Press, 1998.

Ghalioungui, Paul. *The Ebers Papyrus: A New English Translation, Commentaries, and Glossaries*. Cairo: Academy of Scientific Research and Technology, 1987.

Gil-Sotres, Pedro. "Derivation and Revulsion: The Theory and Practice of Medieval Phlebotomy." Pp. 110–155 in *Practical Medicine from Salerno to the Black Death*, ed. Luis García Ballester, Roger French, Jon Arrizabalaga, and Andrew Cunningham, Cambridge: Cambridge University Press, 1994.

Glasier, Angie. "A Stunning Look at Life with Migraine through Art." Migraine Again, 16 July 2017. https://migraineagain.com/life-with-migraine-through-art/.

Glass, S. J., H. R. Catchpole, and Betsy McKennion. "Migraine and Ovarian Deficiency." *Endocrinology* 20, no. 3 (1936): 333–338. doi:10.1210/endo-20-3-333.

Glaze, Florence Eliza. "Medical Writer: 'Behold the Human Creature.'" Pp. 125–148 in *Voice of the Living Light: Hildegard of Bingen and Her World*, ed. Barbara Newman. Berkeley: University of California Press, 1998.

Goadsby, Peter J. "The Vascular Theory of Migraine—a Great Story Wrecked by the Facts." *Brain* 132, pt. 1 (January 2009): 6–7. doi:10.1093/brain/awn321.

Goadsby, Peter J., Uwe Reuter, Yngve Hallström, Gregor Broessner, Jo H. Bonner, Feng Zhang, Sandhya Sapra, Hernan Picard, Daniel D. Mikol, and Robert A. Lenz. "A Controlled Trial of Erenumab for Episodic Migraine." *New England Journal of Medicine* 377, no. 22 (2017): 2123–2132. doi:10.1056/NEJMoa1705848.

Goldberg, Daniel S. "Pain without Lesion: Debate among American Neurologists, 1850–1900." *19: Interdisciplinary Studies in the Long Nineteenth Century* 15 (6 December 2012). https://19.bbk.ac.uk/articles/10.16995/ntn.629/.

Goltman, Alfred M. "The Mechanism of Migraine." *Journal of Allergy* 7, no. 4 (May 1936): 351–355.

Goodman, Louis S. and Alfred Gilman. *The Pharmacological Basis of Therapeutics*, 3rd ed. New York: Macmillan, 1965.

Gormley, Padhraig, Bendik S. Winsvold, Dale R. Nyholt, Mikko Kallela, Daniel I. Chasman, and Aarno Palotie. "Migraine Genetics: From Genome-Wide Association Studies to Translational Insights." *Genome Medicine* 8, no. 1 (2016): 86. doi:10.1186/s13073-016-0346-4.

Gorsky, Martin. "Sources and Resources into the Dark Domain: The UK Web Archive as a Source for the Contemporary History of Public Health." *Social History of Medicine* 28, no. 3 (2015): 596–616. doi:10.1093/shm/hkv028.

Gowers, W. R. *The Border-Land of Epilepsy*. London: Churchill, 1907.

Graham, John R. *Treatment of Migraine*. Boston: Little, Brown, 1956.

Graham, John R., and Harold G. Wolff. "Mechanism of Migraine Headache and Action of Ergotamine Tartrate." *Archives of Neurology and Psychiatry* 39, no. 4 (1938): 737–763. doi:10.1001/archneurpsyc.1938.02270040093005.

Green, Gerald, *The Last Angry Man*. New York: Charles Scribner, 1955.

Green, Monica. "Constantine the African." Pp. 145–147 in *Medieval Science, Technology, and Medicine: An Encyclopedia*, ed. Thomas F. Glick, Steven J. Livesey, and Faith Wallis. New York: Routledge, 2005.

———, ed. *A Cultural History of the Human Body in the Middle Ages*. Oxford: Berg, 2010.

———. "In Search of an 'Authentic' Women's Medicine: The Strange Fates of Trota of Salerno and Hildegard of Bingen." *Dynamis* 19 (1999): 25–54.

———. "Medical Books." Pp. 277–292 in *The European Book in the Twelfth Century*, ed. Erik Kwakkel and Rodney M. Thomson. Cambridge: Cambridge University Press, 2018.

Haan, Joost, and Michel D. Ferrari. "Picasso's Migraine: Illusory Cubist Splitting or Illusion?" *Cephalalgia: An International Journal of Headache* 31, no. 9 (May 2011): 1057–1060. doi:10.1177/0333102411406752.

Hachinski, V. C., J. Porchawka, and J. C. Steele. "Visual Symptoms in the Migraine Syndrome." *Neurology* 23, no. 6 (June 1973): 570–579. doi:10.1212/WNL.23.6.570.

Haig, Alexander. *Uric Acid as a Factor in the Causation of Disease*, 5th ed. London: J. & A. Churchill, 1900.

Ham, Chris, and K. G. M. M. Alberti. "The Medical Profession, the Public, and the Government." *British Medical Journal* (6 April 2002): 838–842. doi:10.1136/bmj.324.7341.838.

Hampshire, Edward, and Valerie Johnson. "The Digital World and the Future of Historical Research." *Twentieth Century British History* 20, no. 3 (2009): 396–414. doi:10.1093/tcbh /hwp036.

Hanington, Edda. "Migraine: A Platelet Disorder." *The Lancet* 318, no. 8249 (3 October 1981): 720–723.

———. "Preliminary Report on Tyramine Headache." *British Medical Journal* (27 May 1967): 550–551. PubMed, PMCID: PMC1842472.

Hanington, Edda, and A. Murray Harper, "The Role of Tyramine in the Aetiology of Migraine, and Related Studies on the Cerebral and Extracerebral Circulations." *Headache: The Journal of Head and Face Pain* 8, no. 3 (October 1968): 84–97. doi:10.1111/j.1526-4610.1968.hed0803084.x.

Hansen, Bert. *Picturing Medical Progress from Pasteur to Polio.* New Brunswick, NJ: Rutgers University Press, 2009.

Hansen, Jakob Møller, Anne Werner Hauge, Jes Olesen, and Messoud Ashina. "Calcitonin Gene-Related Peptide Triggers Migraine-Like Attacks in Patients with Migraine with Aura." *Cephalalgia: An International Journal of Headache* 30, no. 10 (October 2010): 1179–1186. doi:10.1177/0333102410368444.

Harrison, Mark. "From Medical Astrology to Medical Astronomy: Sol-Lunar and Planetary Theories of Disease in British Medicine, c. 1700–1850." *British Journal for the History of Science* 33, no. 1 (2000): 25–48. doi:10.1017/S0007087499003854.

Hartsock, C. L., and F. J. McGurl. "Allergy as a Factor in Headache." *Medical Clinics of North America* 22, no. 2 (March 1938): 325–331.

Hay, Kenneth Michael. "Migraine." *The Physician* 1 (1984): 579–582.

———. "The Treatment of Pain Trigger Areas in Migraine." *Journal of the Royal College of General Practitioners* 26, no. 166 (1976): 372–376. Europe PMC and PubMed, PMCID: PMC2158206.

Headache Classification Subcommittee of the International Headache Society (IHS). *The International Classification of Headache Disorders*, 2nd ed. *Cephalalgia: An International Journal of Headache* 24, Suppl. 1 (2004): 1–160.

———. *The International Classification of Headache Disorders*, 3rd ed. *Cephalalgia: An International Journal of Headache* 38, no. 1 (2018): 1–211. doi:10.1177/0333102417738202.

Hembry, Phyllis. *The English Spa, 1560–1815: A Social History.* London: Athlone Press, 1990.

Henryk-Gutt, Rita, and W. Linford Rees. "Psychological Aspects of Migraine." *Journal of Psychosomatic Research* 17, no. 2 (1973): 141–153. doi:10.1016/0022-3999(73)90015-9.

Herzberg, David. *Happy Pills in America: From Miltown to Prozac.* Baltimore: Johns Hopkins University Press, 2009.

Heyck, H. "Pathogenesis of Migraine." Pp. 1–28 in *Research and Clinical Studies in Headache: An International Review*, vol. 2, ed. Arnold P. Friedman. Basel: S. Karger, 1969.

Hitchcock, Tim. "Confronting the Digital: Or How Academic History Writing Lost the Plot." *Cultural and Social History* 10, no. 1 (2013): 9–23. doi:10.2752/147800413X13515292098070.

Hoffman, Kelly M., Sophie Trawalter, Jordan R. Axt, and M. Norman Oliver. "Racial Bias in Pain Assessment and Treatment Recommendations, and False Beliefs about Biological Differences between Blacks and Whites." *PNAS* 113, no. 16 (2016), 4296–4301.

Hogan, Susan. *Healing Arts: The History of Art Therapy.* London: Jessica Kingsley, 2001.

Horden, Peregrine. "What's Wrong with Early Medieval Medicine?" *Social History of Medicine* 24, no. 1 (2011): 5–25. doi:10.1093/shm/hkp052.

Humphrey, Patrick P. A. "The Discovery and Development of the Triptans, a Major Breakthrough." *Headache: The Journal of Head and Face Pain* 48, no. 5 (May 2008): 685–687. doi: 10.1111/j.1526-4610.2008.01097.x.

———. "The Discovery of Sumatriptan and a New Class of Drug for the Acute Treatment of

Migraine." Pp. 310 in *The Triptans: Novel Drugs for Migraine*, ed. Patrick Humphrey, Michel Ferrari, and Jes Olesen. Oxford: Oxford University Press, 2001.

——. "5-Hydroxytryptamine and the Pathophysiology of Migraine." *Journal of Neurology* 238, Suppl. 1 (1991): S38–S44.

Humphrey, Patrick P. A., and Peter J. Goadsby. "The Mode of Action of Sumatriptan Is Vascular? A Debate." *Cephalalgia: An International Journal of Headache* 14, no. 6 (December 1994): 401–410. doi:10.1046/j.1468-2982.1994.1406401.x.

Hurst, A. F. "Migraine and Its Treatment." *British Medical Journal* (12 July 1924), 60–61. doi: 10.1136/bmj.2.3315.60.

Jackson, Mark. *Allergy: The History of a Modern Malady*. London: Reaktion Books, 2007.

——. *Asthma: The Biography*. Oxford: Oxford University Press, 2009.

——. *The Borderland of Imbecility: Medicine, Society, and the Fabrication of the Feeble Mind in Late Victorian and Edwardian England*. Manchester, UK: Manchester University Press, 2000.

——. "Perspectives on the History of Disease." Pp. 1–18 in *The Routledge History of Disease*, ed. Mark Jackson. London: Routledge, 2017.

Jacyna, L. Stephen, and Stephen T. Casper, *The Neurological Patient in History*. Rochester, NY: University of Rochester Press, 2012.

Johnson, E. S., N. P. Kadam, D. M. Hylands, and P. J. Hylands, "Efficacy of Feverfew as Prophylactic Treatment of Migraine." *British Medical Journal* (31 August 1985): 569–573.

Johnson, Pamela Hansford. "The Consumer's End." In "Report of a Symposium on Migraine." *Journal of the College of General Practitioners*, Suppl. 4 (November 1963): 3–4.

Jordanova, Ludmilla, "Beth Fisher." Collaboration with Contemporary Artists, January 2010. http://www.ludmillajordanova.com/collaboration.htm.

——. "The Body of the Artist." Pp. 43–46 in *Self Portrait: Renaissance to Contemporary*, ed. Anthony Bond and Joanna Woodall. London: National Portrait Gallery & Art Gallery of New South Wales, 2005.

——. "Historical Vision in a Digital Age." *Cultural and Social History* 11, no. 3 (2014): 343–348. doi:10.2752/147800414X13983595303237.

——. *The Look of the Past: Visual and Material Evidence in Historical Practice*. Cambridge: Cambridge University Press, 2012.

——. "The Social Construction of Medical Knowledge." *Social History of Medicine* 7, no. 3 (1995): 361–381. doi:10.1093/shm/8.3.361.

Kamen, Paula. *All in My Head*. Cambridge, MA: Da Capo Press, 2005.

Karwautz, A., C. Wöber-Bingöl, and C. Wöber. "Freud and Migraine: The Beginning of a Psychodynamically Oriented View of Headache a Hundred Years Ago." *Cephalalgia: An International Journal of Headache* 16, no. 1 (February 1996): 22–26. doi:10.1046/j.1468-2982.1996.1601022.x.

Kassell, Lauren. "Casebooks in Early Modern England: Medicine, Astrology, and Written Records." *Bulletin of the History of Medicine* 88, no. 4 (2014): 595–625. doi:10.1353/bhm.2014.0066.

——. *Medicine and Magic in Elizabethan London: Simon Forman, Astrologer, Alchemist, and Physician*. Oxford: Oxford University Press, 2005.

——. "Paper Technologies, Digital Technologies: Working with Early Modern Medical Records." Pp. 120–1356 in *Edinburgh Companion to the Critical Medical Humanities*, ed. Anne Whitehead and Angela Woods. Edinburgh: Edinburgh University Press, 2016.

Keen, Elizabeth. *The Journey of a Book: Bartholomew the Englishman and the Properties of Things*. Canberra: Australian National University E Press, 2007. http://press.anu.edu.au/publications/journey-book/.

Kelly, Fran. "Experience 'Maison Migraine.'" Fran Hunt: (Fran Kelly) Prop Maker, 13 June 2016. https://frankelly.net/2016/06/13/experience-maison-migraine/.

Kelly, James. "'Drinking the Waters': Balneotherapeutic Medicine in Ireland, 1660–1850." *Studia Hibernica* 35 (2008/9): 99–146.

Kempner, Joanna. "Invisible People with Invisible Pain: A Commentary on 'Even My Sister Says I'm Acting Like a Crazy to Get a Check'; Race, Gender, and Moral Boundary Work in Women's Claims of Disabling Chronic Pain." *Social Science and Medicine* 189 (2017): 1–3. doi:10.1016/j.socscimed.2017.06.009.

———. *Not Tonight: Migraine and the Politics of Gender and Health.* Chicago: University of Chicago Press, 2014.

Kettenmann, Andrea. *Frida Kahlo, 1907–1954: Pain and Passion.* Cologne: Taschen, 1992.

Key, Felix M., Muslihudeen A. Abdul-Aziz, Roger Mundry, Benjamin M. Peter, Aarthi Sekar, Mauro D'Amato, Megan Y. Dennis, Joshua M. Schmidt, Aida M. Andrés, and Takashi Gojobori. "Human Local Adaptation of the TRPM8 Cold Receptor along a Latitudinal Cline." *PLoS Genetics* 14, no. 5 (May 2018): e1007298. doi:10.1371/journal.pgen.1007298.

Koehler, P. J. and P. C. Tfelt-Hansen, "History of Methysergide in Migraine." *Cephalalgia: An International Journal of Headache* 28 (2008): 1126–1135. doi:10.1111/j.1468–2982.2008.01648.x.

Koehler, P. J. and T. W. M. van de Wiel, "Aretaeus on Migraine and Headache." *Journal of the History of the Neurosciences* 10, no. 3 (2001): 253–261, 256. doi:10.1076/jhin.10.3.253.9089.

Lance, James W., and Jes Olesen. "Preface." In "The Classification and Diagnostic Criteria for Headache Disorders, Cranial Neuralgias, and Facial Pain." *Cephalalgia: An International Journal of Headache* 8, no. 7, Suppl. (July 1988): 9. http://journals.sagepub.com/toc/cepa/8/7_suppl.

Langham, Mike, and Colin Wells. *A History of the Baths at Buxton.* Leek, Staffordshire, UK: Churnet Valley Books, 1997.

Lardreau, Esther. "A Curiosity in the History of Sciences: The Words 'Megrim' and 'Migraine.'" *Journal of the History of the Neurosciences: Basic and Clinical Perspectives* 21, no. 1 (2012): 31–40. doi:10.1080/0964704X.2011.57638.

———. *La migraine, biographie d'une malade.* Paris: Les Belles Lettres, 2014.

Lardreau-Cotelle, Esther. "Migraine." BIU Santé, January 2008. http://www.biusante.parisdescartes.fr/histoire/medica/migraine-en.php.

Lashley, Karl Spencer. "Patterns of Cerebral Integration Indicated by the Scotomas of Migraine." *Archives of Neurology and Psychiatry*, 46, no. 2 (August 1941): 331–339.

Lassen, L. H., P. A. Haderslev, V. B. Jacobsen, Helle Klingenberg Iversen, B. Sperling, and J. Olesen. "CGRP May Play a Causative Role in Migraine." *Cephalalgia: An International Journal of Headache* 22, no. 1 (February 2002): 54–61.

Latour, Bruno. "How to Be Iconophilic in Art, Science, and Religion." Pp. 418–440 in *Picturing Science Producing Art*, ed. Carrie Jones and Peter Galison. London: Routledge, 2008.

———. "On the Partial Existence of Existing and Nonexisting Objects." Pp. 247–269 in *Biographies of Scientific Objects*, ed. Lorraine Daston. Chicago: University of Chicago Press, 2000.

Lawlor, Clark. *From Melancholia to Prozac.* Oxford: Oxford University Press, 2012.

Leão, Aristides. "Spreading Depression of Activity in the Cerebral Cortex." PhD dissertation, Harvard University, 1943.

Leder, Drew. *The Absent Body.* Chicago: University of Chicago Press, 1990.

LeJacq, Seth Stein. "Medical Recipes, Storytelling, and Surgery in Early Modern England." *Social History of Medicine* 26. no. 3 (2013): 451–468. doi:10.1093/shm/hkt006.

Leonardi, Matilde, and Colin Mathers, "Global Burden of Migraine in the Year 2000: Summary of Methods and Data Sources. " World Health Organization, Global Burden of Disease Working Paper, 2000. http://www.who.int/healthinfo/statistics/bod_migraine.pdf.

Leong, Elaine. "Collecting Knowledge for the Family: Recipes, Gender, and Practical Knowledge in the Early Modern English Household." *Centaurus* 55 (2013): 81–103. doi:10.1111/1600-0498.12019.

———. "'Herbals She Peruseth': Reading Medicine in Early Modern England." *Renaissance Studies* 28, no. 4 (2014): 556–578. doi:10.1111/rest.12079.

———. "Just Who Is This Johanna St. John?!?" The Recipes Project, 23 April 2013. https://recipes.hypotheses.org/1180/.

———. "Making Medicines in the Early Modern Household." *Bulletin of the History of Medicine* 82, no. 1 (2008): 145–168. doi:10.1353/bhm.2008.0042.

Lev, Efrayim, and Zohar Amar. *Practical Materia Medica of the Medieval Eastern Mediterranean According to the Cairo Genizah*. Leiden: Brill, 2008.

Levene, J. R. "Sir G. B. Airy, F.R.S (1801–1892) and the Symptomatology of Migraine." *Notes and Records of the Royal Society of London* 30, no. 1 (1975): 15–23.

Levine, Philippa, and Alison Bashford, eds. *The Oxford Handbook of the History of Eugenics*. Oxford: Oxford University Press, 2010.

Levy, Andrew. *A Brain Wider than the Sky*. New York: Simon & Schuster, 2009.

Lipton, Richard B, Sandra W. Hamelsky, and Walter F. Stewart. "Headache: Epidemiology and Impact." Pp. 45–62 in *Wolff's Headache and Other Head Pain*, 8th ed., ed. Stephen D. Silberstein, Richard B. Lipton, and David W. Dodick. New York: Oxford University Press, 2008.

Loder, Stephen, Huma U. Sheikh, and Elizabeth Loder. "The Prevalence, Burden, and Treatment of Severe, Frequent, and Migraine Headaches in US Minority Populations: Statistics from National Health Survey Studies." *Headache: The Journal of Head and Face Pain* 55, no. 2 (February 2015), 214–228. doi:10.1111/head.12506.

Lomas, D., and R. Howell. "Medical Imagery in the Art of Frida Kahlo." *British Medical Journal* (23 December 1989): 1584–1587. doi:10.1136/bmj.299.6715.1584.

Long, Brian. "An Eleventh-Century WebMD: The *Viaticum* of Constantine the African." Constantine Africanus, 22 May 2018. https://constantinusafricanus.com. Accessed 13 July 2018.

Lorch, Marjorie. "Language and Memory Disorder in the Case of Jonathan Swift: Considerations on Retrospective Diagnosis." *Brain* 129 (2006): 3127–3137.

Loughran, Tracey. "Shell-Shock and Psychological Medicine in First World War Britain." *Social History of Medicine* 22, no. 1 (2009): 79–95. doi:10.1093/shm/hkn093.

Löwy, Ilana. "Biotherapies of Chronic Disease in the Inter-War Period: From Witte's Peptone to *Penicillium* Extract." *Studies in History and Philosophy of Biological and Biomedical Sciences* 36, no. 4 (2005): 675–695. doi:10.1016/j.shpsc.2005.09.002.

Lu, Gwei-Djen, and Joseph Needham, *Celestial Lancets: A History and Rationale of Acupuncture and Moxa*. London: Routledge, 2002.

MacDonald, Michael. *Mystical Bedlam: Madness, Anxiety, and Healing in Seventeenth-Century England*. Cambridge: Cambridge University Press, 1981.

MacGregor, [E.] Anne. "Menstrual Migraine: The Role of Oestregen." MD dissertation, University of London, 2008. http://discovery.ucl.ac.uk/1444395/1/U591698.pdf.

MacGregor, E. Anne, Jason D. Rosenberg, and Tobias Kurth, "Sex-Related Differences in Epidemiological and Clinic-Based Headache Studies." *Headache: The Journal of Head and Face Pain* 51, no. 6 (June 2011): 843–859.

Maniyar, Farooq H., and Peter J. Goadsby. "Migraine—Some Theories and Controversies." Pp. 19–28 in *The Migraine Brain: Imaging Structure and Function*, ed. David Borsook, Arne May, Peter J. Goadsby, and Richard Hargreaves. Oxford: Oxford University Press, 2012.

Margoshes, Pamela. "Don't Say My Migraines Are All in My Head." *Washington Post*, 27 August 1986. https://www.washingtonpost.com/archive/lifestyle/wellness/1986/08/27/dont-say-my-migraines-are-all-in-my-head/7485b1c7-3ae4-4e9a-b0aa-135afca12093/.

Martelletti, Paolo. "The Application of CGRP(r) Monoclonal Antibodies in Migraine Spectrum: Needs and Priorities." *BioDrugs* 31, no. 6 (2017): 483–485.

Martin, Emily. "Blood and the Brain." *Journal of the Royal Anthropological Institute*, n.s., 19 (2013): S172–S184. doi:10.1111/1467-9655.12022.

Mathew, Ninan T., Eva Stubits, and Mool P. Nigam. "Transformation of Episodic Migraine into Daily Headache: Analysis of Factors." *Headache: The Journal of Head and Face Pain* 22. no. 2 (March 1982): 66–68. doi:10.1111/j.1526-4610.1982.hed2202066.x.

Mayer, Anna K. "When Things Don't Talk: Knowledge and Belief in the Inter-War Humanism of Charles Singer." *British Journal for the History of Science* 38, no. 3 (2005): 325–347.

McGough, Laura J. "Syphilis in History: A Response to Two Articles." *Clinical Infectious Diseases* 41 (2005): 573–574.

Micale, Mark. *Hysterical Men: The Hidden History of Male Nervous Illness.* Cambridge, MA: Harvard University Press, 2008.

Migraine Action. "A Brief History of Migraine Action." Migraine Action. http://www.migraine.org.uk/information/factsheets/history-of-migraine-action/.

Migraine Trust. "Diagnosis and Management." Facts and Figures. https://www.migrainetrust.org/about-migraine/migraine-what-is-it/facts-figures/.

———. "Feverfew." In "Treatments," Living with Migraine. https://www.migrainetrust.org/living-with-migraine/treatments/feverfew/.

Milner, Peter. "Note on a Possible Correspondence between the Scotomas of Migraine and Spreading Depression of Leão." *Electroencephalography and Clinical Neurophysiology* 10, no. 4, Suppl. (November 1958):705–710.

Moffat, William M. "Treatment of Menstrual Migraine." *Journal of the American Medical Association* 108, no. 8 (20 February 1937): 612–615.

Moisse, Katie, Mikaela Conley, and ABC News Medical Unit. "Grammy Reporter Serene Branson Suffered Complex Migraine, Not Stroke, Doctor Says." ABC News, 17 February 2011.

Moore, Martin D. "Reorganising Chronic Disease Management: Diabetes and Bureaucratic Technologies in Post-War British General Practice." Pp. 420–438 in *The Routledge History of Disease,* ed. Mark Jackson. London: Routledge, Taylor, & Francis Group, 2017.

Moscoso, Javier. *Pain: A Cultural History,* trans. Sarah Thomas and Paul House. Basingstoke, UK: Palgrave Macmillan, 2012.

Moskowitz, Michael A. "Holes in the Leaky Migraine Blood-Brain Barrier Hypothesis?" *Brain* 140, no. 6 (2017): 1537–1539. doi:10.1093/brain/awx099.

Mukherjee, Siddhartha. *The Emperor of All Maladies.* London: Fourth Estate, 2011.

Murray, T. Jock. *Multiple Sclerosis: The History of a Disease.* New York: Demos, 2005.

Musselman, Elizabeth Green. *Nervous Conditions: Science and the Body Politic in Early Industrial Britain.* Albany: State University of New York Press, 2006.

National Institutes of Health. "Estimates of Funding for Various Research, Condition, and Disease Categories (RCDC)." Research Portfolio Online Reporting Tools (RePORT), 3 July 2017. https://report.nih.gov/categorical_spending.aspx.

National Health Service. "Botox Gets Nod for Migraine." NHS Choices, 11 May 2012. https://www.nhs.uk/news/medication/botox-gets-nod-for-migraine/.

National Health Service England. "Clinical Commissioning Policy: Occipital Nerve Stimulation for Adults with Intractable Chronic Migraines and Medically Refractory Chronic Cluster Headaches." NHS England, July 2015. https://www.england.nhs.uk/commissioning/wp-content/uploads/sites/12/2015/07/d08-p-c.pdf.

Newman, Barbara. "Hildegard of Bingen: Visions and Validation." *Church History* 54, no. 2 (June 1985): 163–175.

———. "'Sibyl of the Rhine': Hildegard's Life and Times." Pp. 1–29 in *Voice of the Living Light: Hildegard of Bingen and Her World,* ed. Barbara Newman. Berkeley: University of California Press, 1998.

———. "Three-Part Invention: The *Vita S. Hildegardis* and Mystical Hagiography." Pp. 189–210 in *Hildegard of Bingen: The Context of Her Thought and Art,* ed. Charles Burnett. London: Warburg Institute, 1998.

———, ed. *Voice of the Living Light: Hildegard of Bingen and Her World*. Berkeley: University of California Press, 1998.

Nuttall, Jenni. "On His Heid-Ake: A Medieval Migraine." Stylisticienne: Her Newe Poetrye, 14 February 2015. http://stylisticienne.com/medieval-migraine/.

Olesen, J., I. Lekander, P. Andlin-Sobocki, and B. Jönsson. "Funding of Headache Research in Europe." *Cephalalgia: An International Journal of Headache* 27, no. 9 (September 2007): 995–999. doi:10.1111/j.1468-2982.2007.01397.x.

Olesen, J., P. Tfelt-Hansen, L. Henriksen, and B. Larsen. "The Common Migraine Attack May Not Be Initiated by Cerebral Ischaemia." *The Lancet* 318, no. 8244 (29 August 1981): 438–449. doi:10.1016/S0140-6736(81)90774-1.

O'Neal, Rebecca. "A Love of 'Words as Words': Metaphor, Analogy and the Brain in the Work of Thomas Willis." PhD dissertation, Queen Mary University of London, 2017.

Oppenheim, Janet. *Shattered Nerves: Doctors, Patients, and Depression in Victorian England*. Oxford: Oxford University Press, 1991.

Osborn, Sally A. "The Role of Domestic Knowledge in an Era of Professionalisation: Eighteenth-Century Manuscript Medical Recipe Collections." PhD dissertation, University of Roehampton, 2016.

Osler, William. *The Evolution of Modern Medicine: A Series of Lectures Delivered at Yale University on the Silliman Foundation in April, 1913*. New Haven, CT: Yale University Press, 1922.

Overy, C., and E. M. Tansey, eds. *Migraine: Diagnosis, Treatment, and Understanding, c. 1960–2010*. Wellcome Witnesses to Contemporary Medicine 49. London: Queen Mary, University of London, 2014.

Owen, Gilbert Roy. "The Famous Case of Lady Anne Conway." *Annals of Medical History* 9 (1937): 567–571.

Pardee, Irving H. "Pituitary Headaches and Their Cure." *Archives of Internal Medicine* 23, no. 2 (1919): 174–184. WL.

Parry, T. Wilson. "Neolithic Man and the Penetration of the Living Human Skull." *The Lancet* 218, no. 5651 (19 December 1931): 1388–1390.

Pearce, J. M. "Historical Aspects of Migraine." *Journal of Neurology, Neurosurgery, and Psychiatry* 49, no. 10 (1986): 1097–1103. doi:10.1136/jnnp.49.10.1097.

Peitzman, Steven J. *Dropsy, Dialysis, Transplant; A Short History of Failing Kidneys*. Baltimore: Johns Hopkins University Press, 2007.

Peterlin, B. Lee, Saurabh Gupta, Thomas N. Ward, and Anne MacGregor. "Sex Matters: Evaluating Sex and Gender in Migraine and Headache Research." *Headache: The Journal of Head and Face Pain* 51, no. 6 (June 2011): 839–842. doi:10.1111/j.1526-4610.2011.01900.x.

Pilloud, Séverine, and Micheline Louis-Courvoisier. "The Intimate Experience of the Body in the Eighteenth Century: Between Interiority and Exteriority." *Medical History* 47, no. 4 (2003): 451–472. doi:10.1017/S0025727300057343.

Podoll, Klaus. "Further Competitions Inspired by the Migraine Art Concept." Migraine Aura Foundation, 13 November 2004. http://www.migraine-aura.com/content/e24966/e25413/e25452/index_en.html. Migraine Aura Foundation website accessed 22 February 2018; URL no longer valid.

Podoll, Klaus, and Derek Robinson. "Lewis Carroll's Migraine Experiences." *The Lancet* 353, no. 9161 (17 April 1999): 1366. doi:10.1016/S0140-6736(05)74368-3.

———. *Migraine Art: The Migraine Experience from Within*. Berkeley, CA: North Atlantic Books, 2008.

———. "Migraine Experiences as Artistic Inspiration in a Contemporary Artist." *Journal of the Royal Society of Medicine* 93, no. 5 (May 2000): 263–265. doi:10.1177/014107680009300515.

Porter, Roy, *Health for Sale: Quackery in England*. Manchester, UK: Manchester University Press, 1989.

———. "The Patient's View: Doing Medical History from Below." *Theory and Society* 14, no. 2 (1985): 175–198.

Pressman, Jack D. *Last Resort: Psychosurgery and the Limits of Medicine*. Cambridge: Cambridge University Press, 1998.

Puledda, Robert Messina, and Peter J. Goadsby. "An Update on Migraine: Current Understanding and Future Directions." *Journal of Neurology* 264, no. 9 (2017): 2031–2039.

Rachford, Benjamin Knox. *Neurotic Disorders of Childhood*. New York: E. B. Treat, 1905.

Rankin, Alisha. *Panaceia's Daughters: Noblewomen as Healers in Early Modern Germany*. Chicago: University of Chicago Press, 2013.

Rapoport, Allan, and John Edmeads. "Migraine: The Evolution of Our Knowledge." *Archives of Neurology* 57, no. 8 (2000): 1221–1223.

Rasmussen, Birthe Krogh. "Epidemiology of Headache." *Cephalalgia: An International Journal of Headache* 15, no. 1 (February 1995): 44–67. doi:10.1046/j.1468-2982.1995.1501045.x.

Rawcliffe, Carole. *Medicine and Society in Later Medieval England*. Stroud, Gloucestershire, UK: Alan Sutton, 1995.

Rawson, Malcolm D., and L. A. Liversedge, "The Clinical Pharmacology of Migraine." Pp. 145–156 in *Modern Topics in Migraine*, ed. John Pearce. London: Heinemann Medical, 1975.

Raz, Mical. *The Lobotomy Letters: The Making of American Psychosurgery*. Rochester, NY: University of Rochester Press, 2013.

Regush, Nicholas. "Migrainekiller." *Mother Jones* (September/October 1995): 26–31, 70. Google Books.

Richardson, William "Topcliffe, Richard (1531–1604)." *Oxford Dictionary of National Biography*. Oxford: Oxford University Press, 2004; online ed., January 2008. doi:10.1093/ref:odnb/27550.

Risse, Guenter B., and John Harley Warner, "Reconstructing Clinical Activities: Patient Records in Medical History." *Social History of Medicine* 5, no. 2 (1992): 183–205. doi:10.1093/shm /5.2.183.

Robbins, Nathaniel M., and James L. Bernat. "Minority Representation in Migraine Treatment Trials." *Headache: The Journal of Head and Face Pain* 57, no. 3 (27 January 2017): 525–533.

Robinson, Richard. "News from the American Headache Society Annual Meeting: Positive Trial Results for Anti-Migraine Drugs Targeting CGRP Could 'Change the Way Neurologists Practice,' Experts Say." *Neurology Today* 17, no. 13 (6 July 2017): 31–32. doi:10.1097/01 .NT.0000521716.95578.

Rocca, Julius. "Galen and the Uses of Trepanation." Pp. 253–271 in *Trepanation: History, Discovery, Theory*, ed. Robert Arnott, Stanley Finger, and Christopher Upham Murray Smith. Amsterdam: Swets & Zeitlinger, 2003.

Rose, F. Clifford. "The History of Migraine from Mesopotamian to Medieval Times." *Cephalalgia: An International Journal of Headache* 15, no. 15 (October 1995): 1–3. doi:10.1111/j.1468 -2982.1995.tb00040.x.

———. "An Overview from Neolithic Times to Broca." Pp. 347–363 in *Trepanation: History, Discovery, Theory*, ed. Robert Arnott, Stanley Finger, and Christopher Upham Murray Smith. Lisse, Netherlands: Swets & Zeitlinger, 2003.

Rosenberg, Charles. "What Is Disease? In Memory of Owsei Temkin." *Bulletin of the History of Medicine* 77, no. 3 (2003): 491–505. doi:10.1353/bhm.2003.0139.

Rosenberg, Charles, and Janet Golden. *Framing Disease: Studies in Cultural History*. New Brunswick, NJ: Rutgers University Press, 1992.

Rydzewski, Wladyslaw. "Serotonin (5-HT) in Migraine: Levels in Whole Blood in and between Attacks." *Headache: The Journal of Head and Face Pain* 16, no. 1 (March 1976): 16–19. doi: 10.1111/j.1526-4610.1976.hed1601016.x.

Sacks, Oliver. *Hallucinations*. London: Picador, 2012.

———. *Migraine*. New York: Vintage Books, 1992.

———. *Migraine: Understanding the Common Disorder*. London: Pan Books, 1985.

Sanders-Bush, Elaine. *The Serotonin Receptors*. Clifton, NJ: Humana Press, 1988.

Scarry, Elaine. *The Body in Pain: The Making and Unmaking of the World*. Oxford: Oxford University Press, 1987.

Schimmel, Paul. *Sigmund Freud's Discovery of Psychoanalysis: Conquistador and Thinker*. Hove, East Sussex, UK: Routledge, 2014.

Schuster, David G. "Neurasthenic Nation: The Medicalization of Modernity in the United States (1869–1920)." PhD dissertation, University of California, Santa Barbara, 2006.

Schwartz, Michael. "Is Migraine an Allergic Disease?" *Journal of Allergy* 23, no. 5 (1952): 426–428. doi:10.1016/0021-8707(52)90006-3.

Scott, Ann, Mervyn Eadie, and Andrew Lees. *William Richard Gowers, 1845–1915: Exploring the Victorian Brain*. Oxford: Oxford University Press, 2012.

Sengoopta, Chandak. "A Mob of Incoherent Symptoms: Neurasthenia in British Medical Discourse, 1860–1920." Pp. 97–115 in *Cultures of Neurasthenia: From Beard to the First World War*, ed. Roy Porter and Marijke Gijswijt-Hofstra. Amsterdam: Rodopi, 2011.

———. *The Most Secret Quintessence of Life: Sex, Glands, and Hormones*. Chicago: University of Chicago Press, 2006.

Seymour, Michael. *Bartholomaeus Anglicus and his Encyclopedia*. Aldershot, UK: Ashgate, 1992.

———, ed. *On the Properties of Things: John Trevisa's Translation of Bartholomaeus Anglicus De Proprietatibus Rerum; A Critical Text*, 3 vols. Oxford, Clarendon Press, 1975–1988.

Sharratt, Mary. "Were Hildegard's Visions Caused by Migraine?" "Christianity," Feminism & Religion, 8 July 2015. https://feminismandreligion.com/2015/07/08/were-hildegards-visions-caused-by-migraines/.

Shaw, Jane. *Miracles in Enlightenment England*. New Haven, CT: Yale University Press, 2006.

Shuttleworth, Sally. *The Mind of the Child: Child Development in Literature, Science, and Medicine, 1840–1900*. Oxford: Oxford University Press, 2010.

Sicuteri, Federigo. "Prophylactic and Therapeutic Properties of 1-Methyl-Lysergic Acid Butanolamide in Migraine." *International Archives of Allergy and Immunology* 15, no. 4–5 (1959): 300–307.

Sicuteri, Federigo, A. Testi, and B. Anselmi. "Biochemical Investigations in Headache: Increase in the Hydroxyindoleacetic Acid Excretion during Migraine Attacks." *International Archives of Allergy and Immunology* 19, no. 1 (1961): 55–58.

Silberstein, Stephen D., David W. Dodick, Marcelo E. Bigal, Paul P. Yeung, Peter J. Goadsby, Tricia Blankenbiller, Melissa Grozinski-Wolff, Ronghua Yang, Yuju Ma, and Ernesto Aycardi. "Fremanezumab for the Preventive Treatment of Chronic Migraine." *New England Journal of Medicine* 377, no. 22 (2017): 2113–2122. doi:10.1056/NEJMoa1709038.

Silberstein, S[tephen] D., J. Olesen, M.-G. Bousser, H.-C. Diener, D. Dodick, M. First, P. J. Goadsby, H. Göbel, M. J. A. Lainez, J. W. Lance, et al. "The *International Classification of Headache Disorders*, 2nd ed. (ICHD-II)—Revision of Criteria for 8.2 'Medication-Overuse Headache.'" *Cephalalgia: An International Journal of Headache* 25, no. 6 (June 2005): 460–465. doi:10.1111/j.1468-2982.2005.00878.x.

Silvas, Anna, ed. and trans. *Jutta and Hildegard: The Biographical Sources*. University Park: Pennsylvania State University Press, 1999.

Singer, Charles. *From Magic to Science*. New York: Dover, 1958.

———. "Science." Pp. 106–148 in *Mediaeval Contributions to Modern Civilization*, ed. F. J. C. Hearnshaw. London: George G. Harrap, 1921.

———. "The Scientific Views and Visions of Saint Hildegard (1098–1180)." Pp. 1–55 in *Studies in the History and Method of Science*, vol. 1, ed. Charles Singer. Oxford: Clarendon Press, 1917.

Singh, Inder, Inderjit Singh, and Devinder Singh. "Progesterone in the Treatment of Migraine." *The Lancet* 249, no. 6457 (31 May 1947): 745–747. doi:10.1016/S0140-6736(47)91493-1.

Skwire, Sarah E. "Women, Writers, Sufferers: Anne Conway and An Collins." *Literature and Medicine* 18, no. 1 (1999): 1–23. doi:10.1353/lm.1999.0010.

Slack, Paul. "Mirrors of Health and Treasures of Poor Men: The Uses of the Vernacular Medical Literature of Tudor England." Pp. 237–274 in *Health, Medicine, and Mortality in the Sixteenth Century*, ed. Charles Webster. Cambridge: Cambridge University Press, 1979.

Slight, David. "Migraine." *Canadian Medical Association Journal* 35, no. 3 (September 1936): 268–273. Europe PMC and PubMed, PMCID: PMC1561861.

Smith, Alan G. R. *Servant of the Cecils: The Life of Sir Michael Hickes, 1543–1612.* London: Cape, 1977.

Smith, Lisa W. "'An Account of an Unaccountable Distemper': The Experience of Pain in Early Eighteenth-Century England and France." *Eighteenth-Century Studies* 41, no. 4 (2008): 459–480. doi:10.1353/ecs.0.0015.

———. "Imagining Women's Fertility before Technology." *Journal of the Medical Humanities* 31, no. 1 (2010): 69–79. doi:10.1007/s10912-009-9097-1.

———. "Women's Health Care in England and France (1650–1775)." PhD thesis, University of Essex, 2002.

Smith, Matthew. *Another Person's Poison: A History of Food Allergy.* New York: Columbia University Press, 2015.

Smith, Timothy. "Some Insurance Companies May Be Placing Unfair Restrictions on Access to New Migraine Prevention Treatments." National Headache Foundation, 5 July 2018. https://headaches.org/2018/07/05/.

Smith, Wesley D. *Hippocrates*, vol. 7. Cambridge, MA: Harvard University Press, 1994.

Snyder, Laura J. *The Philosophical Breakfast Club.* New York: Broadway, 2011.

Solomon, S., S. Diamond, N. Mathew, and E. Loder. "American Headache through the Decades: 1950–2008." *Headache: The Journal of Head and Face Pain* 48, no. 5 (May 2008): 671–677. doi:10.1111/j.1526-4610.2008.01120.x.

Staines, Richard. "Novartis/Amgen's migraine drug hits market at lower than expected price." *Pharmaforum*, 18 May 2018. https://pharmaphorum.com/news/novartis-amgens-aimovig-hits-market-at-lower-than-expected-price/.

Stein, Claudia. "'Getting' the Pox: Reflections by an Historian on How to Write the History of Early Modern Disease." *Nordic Journal of Science and Technology Studies* 2, no. 1 (2014): 53–60. https://www.ntnu.no/ojs/index.php/njsts/article/view/2137/2062/.

Steiner, Timothy J., Lars J. Stovner, and Gretchen L. Birbeck. "Migraine: The Seventh Disabler." *Journal of Headache and Pain* 14, no. 1 (2013): 1. doi:10.1186/1129-2377-14-1.

Steiner, Timothy J., Lars J. Stovner, and Theo Vos. "GBD 2015: Migraine Is the Third Cause of Disability in Under 50s." *Journal of Headache and Pain* 17, no. 1 (2016): 104–107. doi:10.1186/s10194-016-0699-5.

Stewart, H. C. "Ergometrine for Migraine." *British Medical Journal* (24 November 1945): 745. doi:10.1136/bmj.2.4429.745.

Stewart, Walter F., Richard B. Lipton, and Joshua Liberman. "Variation in Migraine Prevalence by Race." *Neurology* 47, no. 1 (1 July 1996): 52–59.

Stone, Marvin J. "Samuel Wilks: The 'Grand Old Man' of British Medicine." *Proceedings of Baylor University Medical Center* 23, no. 3 (July 2010): 263–265. Europe PMC and PubMed, PMCID: PMC2900981.

Sutherland, E. Harvey. *Migraine Clinic: A Seven-Year Survey of Preventive Treatment.* London: Saint Catherine Press, 1957.

Sweet, Victoria. *Rooted in the Earth, Rooted in the Sky: Hildegard of Bingen and Premodern Medicine.* New York: Routledge, 2006.

Symonds, C. P. "Discussion on Migraine." *Proceedings of the Royal Society of Medicine* 20, no. 7 (May 1927): 1097–1110. PubMed, PMCID: PMC2100823. https://www.ncbi.nlm.nih.gov/pmc/issues/154855/.

Taavitsainen, Irma. "Transferring Classical Discourse Conventions into the Vernacular." Pp. 37–72 in *Medical and Scientific Writing in Late Medieval English*, ed. Irma Taavitsainen and Päivi Pahta. Cambridge: Cambridge University Press, 2004.

Talley, Colin L. *A History of Multiple Sclerosis*. Westport, CT: Praeger, 2008.

Tekle Haimanot, Redda. "Burden of Headache in Africa." *Journal of Headache and Pain* 4, no. 1 (2003): S47–S54.

Tfelt-Hansen, P[eer C.]. "History of Headache Research in Denmark." *Cephalalgia: An International Journal of Headache* 21, no. 7 (September 2001): 748–752. doi:10.1111/j.1468-2982.2001 .00242.x.

Tfelt-Hansen, Peer C., and Peter J. Koehler. "History of Use of Ergotamine and Dihydroergotamine in Migraine from 1906 Onward." *Cephalalgia: An International Journal of Headache* 28, no. 8 (August 2008): 877–886. doi:10.1111/j.1468-2982.2008.01578.x.

———. "One Hundred Years of Migraine Research: Major Clinical and Scientific Observations from 1910–2010." *Headache: The Journal of Head and Face Pain* 51, no. 5 (May 2011): 752–788. doi:10.1111/j.1526-4610.2011.01892.x.

Thomson, Mathew. "Neurasthenia in Britain: An Overview." Pp. 77–95 in *Cultures of Neurasthenia: From Beard to the First World War*, ed. Roy Porter and Marijke Gijswijt-Hofstra. Amsterdam: Rodopi, 2011.

———. *Psychological Subjects: Identity, Culture, and Health in Twentieth-Century Britain*. Oxford: Oxford University Press, 2006.

Thomson, William A. R. *Spas That Heal*. London: Adam & Charles Black, 1978.

Throop, Priscilla, trans. *Causes and Cures of Hildegard of Bingen*, 2nd ed. Charlotte, VT: MedievalMS, 2008.

Torres-Ferrús, M., M. Quintana, J. Fernandez-Morales, J. Alvarez-Sabin, and P. Pozo-Rosich. "When Does Chronic Migraine Strike? A Clinical Comparison of Migraine according to the Headache Days Suffered per Month." *Cephalalgia: An International Journal of Headache* 37, no. 2 (February 2017): 104–113.

Travitsky, Betty, and Anne Lake Prescott. *Seventeenth-Century English Recipe Books: Cooking, Physic, and Chirurgery in the Works of W. M. and Queen Henrietta Maria, and of Mary Tillinghast*. Aldershot, UK: Ashgate, 2008.

Tredgold, Alfred Frank. "II. The Feeble-Minded—a Social Danger." *Eugenics Review* 1, no. 2 (July 1909): 97–104.

Triptan Cardiovascular Safety Expert Panel. "Consensus Statement: Cardiovascular Safety Profile of Triptans (5-HT$_{1B/1D}$ Agonists) in the Acute Treatment of Migraine." *Headache: The Journal of Head and Face Pain* 44, no. 5 (May 2004): 414–425. doi:10.1111/j.1526-4610.2004 .04078.x.

Turner, David M. "Disability and Crime in Eighteenth-Century England." *Cultural and Social History* 9, no. 1 (2012): 47–64. doi:10.2752/147800412X13191165982953.

Twarog, Betty M., and Irvine H. Page. "Serotonin Content of Some Mammalian Tissues and Urine and a Method for Its Determination." *American Journal of Physiology-Legacy Content* 175, no. 1 (September 1953): 157–161.

Underwood, Emily. "FDA Just Approved the First Drug to Prevent Migraines: Here's the Story of Its Discovery—and Its Limitations." *Science Magazine*, 18 May 2018.

Urbach, Erich, and Philip M. Gottlieb. *Allergy*, 2nd ed. London: Heinemann, 1946.

Van Arsdall, Anne. *Medieval Herbal Remedies: The Old English Herbarium and Anglo-Saxon Medicine*. New York: Routledge, 2002.

Vaughan, Warren T. "Allergic Migraine." *Journal of the American Medical Association* 88, no. 18 (1927), 1383–1386. WL.

———. *Allergy and Applied Immunology*. London: Henry Kimpton, 1934.

Vick, Randy M., and Kathy Sexton-Radek. "Art and Migraine: Researching the Relationship between Artmaking and Pain Experience." *Art Therapy* 22, no. 4 (2005): 193–204. doi:10.1080 /07421656.2009.10129371.

Voigts, Linda Ehrsam. "Fifteenth-Century English Banns Advertising the Services of an Itinerant Doctor." Pp. 245–278 in *Between Text and Patient: The Medical Enterprise*, ed. Florence Eliza Glaze and Brian K. Nance. Florence: SISMEL—Edizioni del Galluzzo, 2011.

Voigts, Linda E[hrsam], and Michael R. McVaugh. *A Latin Technical Phlebotomy and Its Middle English Translation*. Philadelphia: American Philosophical Society, 1984.

Volger, B. K., M. H. Pittler, and E. Ernst. "Feverfew as a Preventive Treatment for Migraine: A Systematic Review." *Cephalalgia: An International Journal of Headache* 18, no. 10 (December 1998): 704–708.

Wailoo, Keith. *Pain: A Political History*. Baltimore: Johns Hopkins University Press, 2014.

Wainscott, Gillian, F. M. Sullivan, G. N. Volans, and Marcia Wilkinson. "The Outcome of Pregnancy in Women Suffering from Migraine." *Postgraduate Medical Journal* 54, no. 628 (February 1978): 98–102. doi:10.1002/pnp.137.

Walker, Vera. "The Place of Allergy." In "Report of a Symposium on Migraine." *Journal of the College of General Practitioners*, Suppl. 4 (November 1963): 21–25.

Wallis, Faith. *Medieval Medicine: A Reader*. Toronto: University of Toronto Press, 2010.

Wallis, Patrick. "Consumption, Retailing, and Medicine in Early Modern London." *Economic History Review* 61, no. 1 (2008): 26–53.

Walsham, Alexandra. "Holywell: Contesting Sacred Space in Post-Reformation Wales." Pp. 211–236 in *Sacred Space in Early Modern Europe*, ed. Will Coster and Andrew Spicer. Cambridge: Cambridge University Press, 2005.

———. *The Reformation of the Landscape: Religion, Identity, and Memory in Early Modern Britain and Ireland*. Oxford: Oxford University Press, 2011.

Waters, W. E. "Controlled Clinical Trial of Ergotamine Tartrate." *British Medical Journal* (9 May 1970): 325–327. doi:10.1136/bmj.2.5705.325.

Waters, W. E., and P. J. O'Connor. "Prevalence of Migraine." *Journal of Neurology, Neurosurgery, and Psychiatry* 38 (1975): 613–616.

Wear, Andrew. *Knowledge and Practice in English Medicine, 1550–1680*. Cambridge: Cambridge University Press, 2000.

Weatherall, Mark W. "The Migraine Theories of Liveing and Latham: A Reappraisal." *Brain* 135, no. 8 (2012): 2560–2568. doi:10.1093/brain/aws020.

Weisz, George. *Chronic Disease in the Twentieth Century: A History*. Baltimore, Johns Hopkins University Press, 2014.

Weller, Toni. *History in the Digital Age*. London: Routledge, 2013.

Whitaker-Azmitia, Patricia Mack. "The Discovery of Serotonin and Its Role in Neuroscience." *Neuropsychopharmacology* 21, no. 2 (August 1999), 2S–8S. doi:10.1016/S0893-133X(99)00031-7.

Wickersheimer, Ernest. "Textes médicaux chartrains des IXe, Xe, et XIe siècles." Pp. 164–176 in *Science, Medicine, and History: Essays on the Evolution of Scientific Thought and Medical Practice Written in Honour of Charles Singer*, ed. E. Ashworth Underwood. London: Oxford University Press, 1953.

Wigley, Samuel. "The Best 80s Sci-Film Posters." BFI: Film Forever, 29 October 2014. http:// www.bfi.org.uk/news-opinion/news-bfi/features/best-80s-sci-fi-film-posters/.

Wilkinson, Marcia. "Are Classical and Common Migraine Different Entities?" *Headache: The Journal of Head and Face Pain* 25, no. 4 (June 1985): 211–212. doi:10.1111/j.1526-4610.1985.hed 2504211.x.

———. "Clonidine for Migraine." *The Lancet* 294, no. 7617 (23 August 1969): 430. https://doi.org /10.1016/S0140-6736(69)90131-7.

———. "Migraine—Treatment of Acute Attack." *British Medical Journal* (26 June 1971): 754–755.

Wilkinson, Marcia, and Hansruedi Isler. "The Pioneer Woman's View of Migraine: Elizabeth

Garrett Anderson's Thesis 'Sur la migraine.'" *Cephalalgia: An International Journal of Headache* 19, no. 1 (January 1999), 3–15. doi:10.1111/j.1468-2982.1999.1901003.x.

Wilkinson, Marcia, and Jane Woodrow. "Migraine and Weather." *Headache: The Journal of Head and Face Pain* 19, no. 7 (November 1979): 375–378. doi:10.1111/j.1526-4610.1979.hed 1907375.x.

Williams, Kevin. *Read All About It! A History of the British Newspaper.* Abingdon, UK: Routledge, 2009.

Wilper, Andrew, Steffie Woolhandler, David Himmelstein, and Rachel Nardin. "Impact of Insurance Status on Migraine Care in the United States: A Population-Based Study." *Neurology* 74, no. 15 (2010): 1178–1183.

Wilson, Adrian. "On the History of Disease Concepts: The Case of Pleurisy." *History of Science* 38, no. 3 (2000): 271–319. doi:10.1177/007327530003800302.

Wilson, Peter. "National Migraine Art Competition." *Migraine Newsletter* 3 (August 1980): 11.

Withey, Alun. " 'Persons That Live Remote from London': Apothecaries and the Medical Marketplace in Seventeenth- and Eighteenth-Century Wales." *Bulletin of the History of Medicine* 85 (2011): 222–247.

Woldeamanuel, Yohannes W., and Robert P. Cowan. "Migraine Affects 1 in 10 People Worldwide Featuring Recent Rise: A Systematic Review and Meta-analysis of Community-Based Studies Involving 6 Million Participants." *Journal of the Neurological Sciences* 372 (2017): 307–315. doi:10.1016/j.jns.2016.11.071.

Wolff, Harold G. *Headache and Other Head Pain.* Oxford: Oxford University Press, 1948.

Woolf, Virginia. "On Being Ill" (1930). *The Moment, and Other Essays,* published 1947. http://gutenberg.net.au/ebooks15/1500221h.html#ch3/.

World Health Organization. "Headache Disorders." Updated 8 April 2016. http://www.who.int/mediacentre/factsheets/fs277/en/.

———. "WHO Model List of Essential Medicines, 20th List, March 2017, amended August 2017." Reprint of text on the WHO Medicines website. http://www.who.int/medicines/publications/essentialmedicines/20th_EML2017_FINAL_amendedAug2017.pdf?ua=1/.

Wright, C. E., ed. *Bald's Leechbook: British Museum Royal Manuscript 12 D.xvii.* Copenhagen: Rosenkilde & Bagger, 1955.

Wrobel Goldberg, Stephanie, and Stephen David Silberstein. "Targeting CGRP: A New Era for Migraine Treatment." *CNS Drugs* 29 (2015): 443–452.

Yearl, Katherine Keblinge. "The Time of Bloodletting." PhD dissertation, Yale University, 2005.

Yeh, Ju-Fen. "Monoclonal Antibodies for Chronic Pain: A Practical Review of Mechanisms and Clinical Applications." *Molecular Pain* 13 (2017): 1–14. doi:10.1177/1744806917740233.

Young, William B. "De-stigmatizing Migraine—with Words." *Headache: The Journal of Head and Face Pain* 58, no. 2 (15 November 2017): 319–321. doi:10.1111/head.13209.

Ziegler, Dewey K. "The Headache Symptom: How Many Entities?" *Archives of Neurology* 42, no. 3 (1985): 273–274. doi:10.1001/archneur.1985.04060030091014.

Zilkha, K. J. "Clinics." *Migraine News* 1 (June 1967): 3.

Zimmer, Carl. *Soul Made Flesh: The Discovery of the Brain—and How It Changed the World.* London: Arrow Books, 2005.

Page numbers in italics refer to figures.

acupuncture, 28, 37, 221n21
Adler, Alfred, 165
advertising, 34–35, 70–75, 170–173; and patient art, 191–192; testimonials in, 74, 76–78
Africa, 213–214
Aikin, J. M., 159
Airy, George Biddell, 117, 124
Airy, Hubert, 1, 111–112, 117–122, 124–125, 133, 192, 202; authority of his images, 9, 13, 19, 112, 125, 132, 140, 142, 217; reproduction of his images, 121–122, 124–125
alcohol, 72, 97, 180–181; avoidance of, 58, 201
alcoholism, 101, 174
Allbutt, Thomas Clifford, 96, 125, 127
allergy, 14, 144, 155, 157, 159–161, 167, 189; desensitization therapies, 160, 175–176, 187; theory of migraine, 16, 158, 182
alternative medicine, 75, 147
Alvarez, Walter, 165–166, 190
American Ad Hoc Committee on Classification of Headache, 179–180
American Headache Society, 211–212
amyl nitrite, 96, 97, 108, 175
anaphylaxis, 151, 160, 234n10
Andral, Gabriel, 113
animal parts, 54–55, 70. *See also* earthworms
Anstie, Francis, 97, 125
Anthony, Michael, 177
antidepressants, 176, 206
antifebrine, 107, 108
antipyrin, 106, 107, 108, 126
apoplexy, 29, 51, 52, 62, 71, 72, 117, 127
apothecaries, 60, 69–70, 72
Aretaeus of Cappadocia, 27–28
arsenic, 97, 108
art therapy, 20, 190–191
asthma, 15, 122–123, 129, 152, 160, 212
astrology, 66–69, 71, 83; and phlebotomy, 39–41
astronomy, 117–118
asylums, lunatic, 96–98, 99, 128; Sussex County, 96–98, 108; West Riding, 96, 127
aura: in art, 1–2, 13, 21, 140–141, 146–147, 150, 192–193, 199, 204, 206, 208–209; causes of, 120, 124, 180; centrality of, in modern migraine categories, 19, 132–133, 144, 153–154, 183; and CGRP, 211; and cortical spreading depression, 180; diagnostic primacy of, 9, 144, 153–154, 217; diagrams of, 1, 110–111, 117, 140; duration of, 5, 201; in *Epidemics*, 27; epileptic, 138; fortification spectrum, 1, 113–115, 118, 120, 126, 135, 143; gendered experience of, 7; hemiopsy, 88, 116–117, 120; and Hildegard of Bingen, 145–147; ocular spectra, 114–116, 119; scintillating scotoma, 1, 118, 135, 141–142, 192; sensory symptoms of, 6, 180; zigzag, 6, 88, 103, 110, 116, 138, 140, 185, 192

Bacon, Francis, 80, 113
Bald's *Leechbook*, 18, 22–27, 35, 38
Barrough, Philip, 48–49, 58, 69–70
Bartholomaeus Anglicus, 30–32, 35
Bath, 62, 65
Beard, George, 126–128
Beck, Mr., 110–112, 133
belladonna, 98, 107, 108
Berkeley, George, 75
bilious headache, 81, 90, 92, 94, 122, 124, 217
biliousness, 84, 90–92, 94–95, 183
Blagden, Sir Charles, 81–83
Blau, Joseph N. (Nat), 150, 175, 180, 192, 202
blood, 3, 12, 31, 35–41, 76; circulation of, 48, 180; cleansing of, 66, 71; deficiency and surplus of, 92–93; humoral, 26, 28, 48, 149; supply to the brain, 91, 92
blood-brain barrier, 5, 12, 212
bloodletting. *See* phlebotomy
blood platelets, 12, 177–178
Blount, Thomas, 62
bodily constitution, 91, 108, 116–117, 130; in humoral theory, 25, 27; inherited, 164, 190; in phlebotomy, 35; society's corruption of, 84–85
Boehringer Ingelheim, 184
Boorde, Andrew, 47–48, 57
Borumborad, Dr. Achmet, 76–78
botox, 213
Brain, Walter Russell, 157
Bray, George, 160

breastfeeding, 31, 92–93, 102, 130, 222n37
Brewster, David, 117, 188
British Migraine Association, 20, 184, 186, 189
British Ophthalmological Society, 110–111
Broca, Paul, 139
Brunton, Thomas Lauder, 136, 138, 142
Buchan, William, 92, 116, 130
Bullein, William, 39, 50
Burleigh, Lord, 61
Burroughs Wellcome, 170
Bury, Michael, 102
Butter, Jean, 191–192
Buxton, 61–66
Buzzard, Thomas, 105

caffeine, 98, 108, 127, 131, 170, 174
calcium channel blockers, 176
calomel, 102, 107, 126
cannabis, 96–98, 108, 127, 131
Carroll, Lewis, 150
Cartwright, Thomas, 50
Cave, Jane, 74
cephalalgia, 27
cephelaea, 27, 30
CGRP blocking antibodies, 12, 211–212; gepants, 212
Cheyne, George, 84
children, 7, 25, 88, 128–130, 156, 163, 189; age of onset in, 7, 160; artworks by, 190, 199, 200; personality of, 166; symptoms in, 129; treatments for, 72, 126, 205
Chinese medicine, 28
chlorodyne, 105
chocolate, 72, 91, 160, 161
chronic daily headache, 4
chronic illness, 14–15, 62, 77–78, 187, 196; as biographical disruption, 102
chronic migraine, 148, 208, 211, 213, 216; and long-term medication, 11, 212, 215; and socioeconomic status, 7
civilization, migraine as result of, 90, 139
classic (or classical) migraine, 6, 158, 180–181, 192
classification, 6, 27–8, 81, 89, 90–93, 122, 179–181; debates about, 92–93, 152–153, 157–158, 162; and drug response, 182; standardization of, 6, 181, 216
class status. *See* socioeconomic status
Clendinning, John, 97

clinical trials, 158, 169, 173–174, 180–181; inadequate representation in, 183, 214
clinics, 182, 186, 187–189; City of London, 175, 180–181, 192; Copenhagen Acute Headache Clinic, 189; Putney, 175–176, 186–187
clonidine, 189, 191
Clouston, Thomas, 97, 125
Clowes, William, 38
cluster headache, 4, 181
coffee, 72, 91, 98, 127, 131
Cogan, Thomas, 52
Collins, Thomas, 49
common migraine, 6, 180–181, 216
comorbidity, 61, 68, 77
Constantine the African, 30, 31
Conway, Anne, 136, 137, 147–149, 150, 153–154, 156
Copland, William, 50, 52
Corlyon, Mrs., 18, 42–46, 53–55, 57–58
correspondence, 12, 19, 61–62, 78–83, 87, 117–119
cortical spreading depression, 180
creativity, 150–151, 190–191, 195, 208–209, 239n27
criminal trials, 93–95
Critchley, Macdonald, 151, 157, 160, 162, 168, 182, 187
Cromwell, Thomas, 63
Crookshank, Francis Graham, 164–165
Cullen, William, 79–80, 84, 90, 106, 227n87
Culpeper, Nicholas, 50, 53
Cumings, John, 178
cure: absence of, 11, 15, 97–98, 176, 182, 212; claims of, 22, 28, 34, 46, 57, 65–66, 71–78, 126
Curran, Don, 177
Curtis, Thomas, 81–83
Cushing, Harvey, 148, 155–156

Darwin, Charles, 13, 150
de Sauvages, Boissier, 81
diagnosis, 9, 15, 152, 158; aura as requirement for, 9, 144, 153–154, 217; difficulties of, 147–148, 151–152, 234n68; instructions for, 48; modern frameworks for, 179–181; to placate patients, 153. *See also* retrospective diagnosis
Didion, Joan, 189–190, 204
diet: and blood platelets, 178, 188–189; faulty, 84–85, 91, 168, 188; management of, 206; and nervous disease, 62; as self-help, 75, 105; as treatment, 91, 93, 102, 103, 107, 123, 126, 131
digitalis, 97, 107, 175
digitization, 17, 209–210

Dioscorides, 26, 50, 55
disability, 5, 14, 78, 214–215
discrimination, 7
disease concepts, 15–16
doctor-patient relationships, 12–13, 158, 79, 81–82,
    130; in art, 185, 194–195; effect of multiple
    theories on, 163; and gender, 9; and gendered
    marketing, 171–173; and patient personality,
    167–168
Dodoens, Rembert, 50, 70
domestic medicine, 43
Doré, Gustav, 140, 142
Dr. Stephen's water, 54
drugs: abortive, 11, 15, 178–179, 208; in artworks,
    206, 207; and blood-brain barrier, 5, 12; and end
    of psychological framework, 168–169, 176; to
    induce attack, 126; by injection, 169–170, 171,
    174–175, 177, 213; migraine-specific, 169–170, 176,
    211–212; physiological mechanisms of, 169–170,
    174–175, 177–178; response and classification,
    182; side effects of, 11, 97, 107, 170–171, 174, 176,
    179, 207, 212
Dublin, 76–78
du Bois-Reymond, Emile, 125
Dunbar, William, 4, 33–34, 35

Eadie, Mervyn, 16, 132
earthworms, 11, 43, 54–57
Ebers papyrus, 27
Elizabeth I (Queen), 61
Elliott, R. H., 143–144, 151
Elyot, Thomas, 46
emigranea, 4, 24, 29–31, 41, 145
emotions: as cause, 67, 87, 95, 123, 127, 133; effect of
    migraine on, 207, 215; in humoral system, 25;
    migraine as *pique*, 80; and personality, 166–167;
    repression of, 164–165; as symptoms, 5, 123
endocrinology, 5–6, 16, 144, 151, 158, 161–163
"English Spaw," the, 66
epilepsy, 5, 9, 82, 101; and degenerate heredity, 128,
    129, 190; eugenic views of, 163–164; as functional
    nervous disorder, 122–123, 128; at National
    Hospital, 99–100; and "nerve-storm theory,"
    125–126, 127, 152; relationship to migraine, 4,
    62, 95, 100, 122, 125, 132–133; and social class,
    128; treatment of, 29, 66, 71, 97, 106–107, 156;
    trepanning for, 139–140
ergometrine, 170

ergotamine, 20, 168–176, 187; as "dirty" drug, 174;
    effects on pain, 169–170; side effects of, 170, 174,
    207
ergotin, 131
ergotism, 174
ergot of rye, 97, 108, 169, 173–174
E. T. the Extra-Terrestrial, 203
eugenics, 129, 163–164, 235n30
eyestrain, 152

Ferguson, Fergus, 157, 162–163
Ferrier, David, 99
feverfew, 54, 205
fibromyalgia, 14
Food and Drug Administration (FDA), 212
foods, 84–85, 90, 204; avoidance of "smoky" foods,
    57–58, 199; sensitivity to, 155, 160, 161; tyramine
    in, 178
Fordyce, John, 83
Forman, Simon, 66–67
Fothergill, John, 84–85, 91, 113, 122
Frederica, Duchess of York, 87
French culture, influence of, 85–87
Freud, Sigmund, 165
Friedman, Arnold P., 179

Galen, 3–4, 23–24, 32, 138; on bloodletting, 35, 39,
    41; theory of migraine, 25, 30, 41; on trepanation,
    138
Garrett Anderson, Elizabeth, 130, 188
gender, 3, 8, 9–11, 14, 17, 133, 192–193; differing
    experiences of men and women, 6–7, 123–124,
    127, 218; emergence of assumptions about, 19,
    62, 89, 108; in marketing, 171–173; in nineteenth
    century, 92–93, 124, 130; and personality
    theories, 167–168; prevalence ratio, 6–7, 67,
    130–131, 181, 218; and social class, 129–130,
    133–134; and stereotypes of national character,
    86–87
genetics, 5, 12, 203, 213–214, 215–216
Gerard, John, 57
Glaxo, 179, 188, 208
global burden, 5, 9, 213–215
Goadsby, Peter, 182–183, 212
Goltman, Alfred, 155–157, 160
gout, 34, 40, 46, 63, 90, 116, 125–126, 152
Gowers, William, 1; on diagrams of aura, 110–112,
    133; on migraine and nervous disease, 131–132,

Gowers, William (*continued*)
133–134, 157; at the National Hospital, 99, 103, 106–107, 108
Gowers' Mixture, 107, 108, 175
Graham, John R., 1, 167–170, 174, 178; blind men and elephant parable, 158–159; and classification, 179
Grant, Ulysses S., 150
Green, Gerald, 189
Greene, Richard, 97–98
Guillemeau, Jacques, 39
Gyer, Nicholas, 39

Haig, Alexander, 126, 133, 160
half headache, 22–23, 25, 26–27, 34; logic of, 29
Halford, Sir Henry, 87
Hall, Marshall, 91
Hanington, Edda, 177–178, 183
Harvey, William, 138, 148
headache, 3–4; characteristics of, 5–6, 48, 88, 131, 152; classical division into three types of, 27–28, 46, 92; and diagnosis of migraine, 131, 152, 158; hot or cold causes of, 25–26, 31–32, 41, 49, 66; internal or external causes of, 30, 46, 167; migraine as *more than* a, 9, 35, 84, 218; one-sided, 4, 23, 28, 29, 34, 38, 80, 102–103, 113; "open head" as cause of, 42–43, 46; and "smoky" foods, 57–58
headache disorders, 9, 19, 94, 214–215
Heberden, William, 113
hemicrania, 3, 4, 8, 23–41, 68, 80, 148; changing meaning of, 19, 82; descriptions of, 3, 47–48; humoral causes of, 25–26, 41, 90
hemicranick, 62
herbal remedies, 11, 22–24, 29, 32–33, 43–46, 49–60; as evidence of chronic migraine, 58–60; kitchen ingredients in, 22, 27, 43, 49, 52, 57–58; regional adaptations of, 53, 59–60; therapeutic action of, 52
herbals, printed, 50, 52–53, 57
herbs, 22, 26, 43; betony, 49, 53; chamomile, 49–50, 53, 54; daisy, 57; dill, 49; houseleek, 49, 56, 58; laurel, 22, 33, 59, 106; nettle, 22, 26–27; pellitory, 26, 50, 52–53, 54; qualities of, 26–27, 49–54, 56, 59; rosemary, 29, 43, 49–54, 59; sage, 50, 52–54, 57; spikenard, 32–33, 83; stavesacre, 53; valerian, 32, 79, 83, 108, 131; vervain, 49–50, 53

heredity, 3, 8, 19, 96, 128–129, 148, 162, 202; and allergy, 160; in artworks, 202; and degeneration, 129, 163–165, 217; of nervous disorders, 90, 96, 101, 124, 190
Herschel, Sir John, 114–120, 124
heterocrania, 28
Hickes, Sir Michael, 61
Hildegard of Bingen, 29, 140–147, 149–150, 153–154; diagnosis of, 135–137, 217; her illness, 29, 145; medieval historians on, 145–147, 149; on migraine treatment, 29; as patron saint, 136, 147
Hinterberger, Anthony, 177
Hippocratic corpus, 25, 27, 138
histamine, 175, 176
hives. *See* nettle rash
hormones, 161–162, 178; pure and synthetic extracts, 162–163; therapies, 175–176, 187
House of Commons debate, 186–187
human genome, 216
humoral theory, 3, 8, 24, 25–26, 28–31, 40–41, 62; rejection of, 125–26
humors, 16, 24–31, 35–40, 44, 46–49, 57, 68–69, 147, 217
Humphrey, Patrick, 178–179, 188
hypothalamus, 5
hysteria, 4, 19, 62, 81, 93, 127, 128, 130; as female disorder, 93, 94–96
hysterical migraine, 81, 93, 95–96

identity, 62, 86, 185
images, 2–3, 13, 18; for bloodletting, 37, 39–40; as diagnostic authority, 133, 135, 140–142; in Migril marketing, 171–173; retrospective diagnosis using, 135, 138, 141–147; as scientific evidence, 9, 111–112, 121–122, 169–170, 191–192. *See also* Migraine Art Competitions
Imitrex. *See* sumatriptan
inflammation, 5, 12, 48, 131, 152, 161
insanity, 95–96, 129, 132, 164
intelligence: and children, 133, 163, 166; and excess study, 84, 91, 116–117, 164; migraine as disease of, 86, 126, 128, 130, 142–143, 149, 165
International Classification of Headache Disorders (*ICHD*), 6, 181, 213, 215, 216, 242nn25–26
International Headache Society, 181
internet, 209–210
irritation, nervous, 9, 91, 124, 149, 151–152, 211

Jackson, John Hughlings, 88, 96, 99–100, 125
Johnson, Pamela Hansford, 186
Jones, John, 66–67
Jung, Carl, 165

Kahlo, Frida, 195
Kamen, Paula, 9, 37, 75
Kempner, Joanna, xiii, 9–10, 96, 216
Kipling, Rudyard, 4, 150
Klebs, Arnold, 141

Labarraque, Henri, 91
Lance, James, 177
Langham, William, 54
Lardreau, Esther, 81, 86
Latham, Peter W., 124–125, 131, 157
Leão, Aristides, 180
leech, itinerant, 18, 34–35, 113
leeches, 38, 74, 79, 228n11
Lees, F. Arnold, 95
legitimacy, 9–10, 87, 127, 153, 165, 176, 187, 216; and
    creativity, 195
lesion, 100, 125
Levy, Andrew, 13, 124, 139, 149–151, 193
Leyton, Neville, 175, 186–187
life, effect of migraine on, 6, 59, 78, 89, 94–95,
    102–106, 167–168; in art, 184, 194–207; in
    marketing, 171–73
life events, effect of, 68, 90, 102, 106
lifestyle, 8, 62, 84, 90, 168, 208
Lifting the Burden's Global Campaign Against
    Headache, 214
literature, 80, 150, 186
Liveing, Edward, 4, 112, 122–127, 148; ongoing
    influence of, 132–134, 144, 157, 160–161; *On
    Megrim*, 19, 122–124
lobotomy, 11, 156, 190
Lucas-Championnière, Just, 139

MacGregor, Anne, 7, 181, 182
magic, 29, 143
Mary, Queen of Scots, 65
masquerade balls, 85–87
Mead, Richard, 83
Mease, James, 91
medical imaging, 13, 182, 216
medical knowledge: divergence of lay and
    professional, 94–95, 108; exchange between
    manuscript and print, 49–50, 60; international
    exchange of, 81–82, 83, 126–128, 159, 180–181,
    189; lay, 33–35, 43–45, 58–60, 94–95, 101–103;
    moments of change in, 14, 57, 62, 133, 168–170,
    176, 179–183, 185, 212; professional, 22–23, 25,
    37, 69–70, 102, 119, 122, 131–134, 158; twentieth-
    century fragmentation of, 157–168; and use of
    history, 136, 142, 154
medical marketplace, 18, 62, 72–75, 78–79
medical texts: early printed, 4, 17, 31–32, 39–41,
    46–50, 52, 56–57; head-to-toe arrangement of,
    24–25, 30, 46; as stores of knowledge, 45, 69–70;
    translation of, 4, 24, 30–33, 35, 39, 50, 80, 148,
    181
medication overuse headache, 215
megrim: and blood deficiency, 93; changing
    meaning of, 4, 8, 19, 95, 217; and dizziness,
    80–81; early modern ideas about, 39–41, 47–48;
    in the head, 44, 68, 77, 80; in horses, 80–81;
    nineteenth-century revival of, 122; preference
    for French term over, 131; spellings of, 4, 53–54,
    57–58
men, 7, 27, 123–125, 127, 131, 167, 217–218; accounts
    of migraine by, 33–34, 61–62, 68–69, 76–77,
    81–83, 93–4, 102, 103–104; art by, 191–193, 205;
    effects of war on, 164–165; marketing aimed at,
    170–173; scientific authority of, 110–112, 114–122,
    133–134, 143
menopause, 103, 104, 129
menstrual migraine, 158, 163
menstruation, 3, 16, 6–7, 37, 96, 100, 130–131, 152,
    183; disorders of, 93, 153, 159; hormones and, 162
Mental Deficiency Act (1913), 164
mental illness, 14, 15, 51, 95–96, 171, 177; creative
    responses to, 191; and hereditary diathesis, 129,
    132, 164; in institutions, 96; treatments for, 71, 97,
    156
metaphors, 2, 196–198; arrows, 8, 34, 194, 195, 205;
    burning, 18, 30, 196, 199; companion, 4, 199, 204;
    computer, 1, 5; gendered, 9, 87; hammers, 30,
    196, 199; historical specificity of, 103; of holding
    down, 197, 198; monsters, 196; nails, 193, 195;
    for pain, 8, 30, 196–198; people-like, 196, 197;
    piercing, 30, 196; telephone, 197; television, 201;
    tools, 196, 200; vise, 8, 147; of weight, 196
methysergide, 176, 177

Michaelangelo, 203

migraine: as acute and chronic, 12, 14–15, 18, 44, 58; biochemical processes in, 12, 177–180, 215; as chronic, 61–62, 67–69, 94–95, 103–106; French meaning of, 80, 82–83; as moral failure, 10, 85, 86–87, 165, 189–190, 216; as multiple disorders, 180–181; theories of, 9, 12, 16, 19–20, 23, 108, 151–153, 159, 176

Migraine Action, 184, 209, 238n4

Migraine Art Competitions, xiv, 2, 13, 20–21, 184–185, 191–210, 217; children's entries, 185, 199, 202; driving, 201–202; everyday life, 184, *185*, 204–208; isolation, 197, *198*; pain, 193–210; social life, 199, 205–206; winners of, 192–193

migraine lunatique, 82

migraine personality, 20, 86, 124, 157, 165–168, 189–190

migraineur, xiii, 185, 189–190

migraine with aura (MA), 6, 158, 180–183

migraine without aura (MO) 6, 180–183

Migril, 170–175, 194

modernity, 84, 126–127, 128, 168, 171–173, 201

monoclonal antibodies. *See* CGRP blocking antibodies

moon, 40, 82–83

morphine, 105, 107, 126

motherhood, 89, 92–93, 96, 123, 130, 205

Moulton, Thomas, 50

Moysey, Abel, 81

Murphy, Patrick J., 92–93

Napier, Richard, 66–69

National Health Service (NHS), 187, 213

National Hospital for the Paralysed and Epileptic, xiii, 88–90, 98–109, 110, 125, 128, 175

nerve-storm, 123–125, 130, 131, 151, 157, 159, 161, 165

nervous disorders, 90, 96, 116–117, 160; ability to change into each other, 125, 127, 132; effect of world wars on research into, 144, 164–165; functional, 108, 122, 144; and luxurious living, 62, 84; migraine as, 84–85, 95, 132, 135

nettle rash, 88, 108

neurasthenia, 100, 126–128, 130, 133

neurology, 2, 12, 15–16, 158, 175, 179–183; approach to migraine's history, 16–17, 148–150, 137, 143–145, 154; in clinics, 187–188; foundations of, 99, 148, 218, 229n25; and identity, 190; and migraine as "symphony," 180; neurotic diathesis, 126, 129;

racial theories in, 213–214; and vascular theories, 144, 180, 188

nitroglycerine, 107, 131, 175

objectivity, 14, 108, 110, 112, 120, 191, 218

occipital nerve stimulation, 213

ocular migraine, 81

ocular theory, 116, 151, 182

Old Bailey, 93–95

Olesen, Jes, 174, 180–182, 189

opioids, 11, 174

opium, 76, 97, 106, 114, 126

Osler, William, 139–140, 141

outsider art, 190–191

Owen, Gilbert Roy, 147

pain, 7–10, 14–15; artistic representations of, 21, 193–210; in children, 7, 129; chronic, 77–78; in classical definitions, 3–4, 19, 25, 27–28; denial of, 19–20, 112, 115, 117, 124; discrimination, 7; effect of drugs on, 105, 131, 169–170, 179; effect of serotonin on, 177; and gender, 5–7, 171–173; intensity of, 23–24, 34, 68–69, 102–107, 139; language of, 103, 240n42; location of, 30–31, 46–47, 89, 100, 122, 148, 195; medieval, 24, 29, 30–31, 33–34; quality of, 48–49, 56, 67–69, 70, 84, 103, 113, 122, 131, 155; severity of, 30, 34, 48, 81, 103–104, 113, 193–199, 217; shape of, 47–48; from windiness, 30, 48, 70

pain relief, 8, 20, 32, 79, 149; cannabis for, 98; fantasies of, 139; pharmacological, 105, 107, 131, 169–172; politics of, 187–188, 212–213; promises of, 70–71, 77–78

paralysis, 96, 99

Paré, Ambroise, 48, 80

Parry, Caleb Hillier, 91, 113

Partridge, John, 49

patients, 9–13; advocacy, 20, 185, 188; casenotes, 12, 67–69, 88–90, 99–107; compliance with treatment, 58, 95, 174; confidentiality, 17; information for, 41, 47, 57, 170–171; in institutions, 19, 88–90, 99–107; and patienthood, 12–13, 19, 191; personality of, 165–168, 176; reliability of, 9, 14, 101, 119, 124, 191; and therapeutic experimentation, 89, 106–107, 155–156, 169–170, 177, 180–181, 182, 188–189. *See also* doctor-patient relationships

Pechey, John, 53

pharmaceutical industry, 185, 187

pharmaceutical research, 178–181, 182–183, 186–191, 211–212; funding for, 9, 182

pharmacology, 96–98, 105–108

phenacetin, 106, 107, 108

phlebotomy, 12, 28, 35–41, 44, 68, 70, 74, 83, 91, 149; almanacs, 39–40; astrological considerations in, 39–41; derivative and revulsive, 38–39; instructions for, 31, 35–40; patient care in, 37; scars of, 14

photography, 120

Picasso, Pablo, 150

pituitary gland, 144, 147, 162

Pliny the Elder, 25, 30, 32

poetry, 33–34, 39, 74

potassium bromide, 97, 105, 106, 107, 108, 128, 130, 152

Potter, Samuel, 108

poverty, 76–78, 99, 130, 133, 168. *See also* socioeconomic status

pregnancy, 163, 174, 189

prevalence, 5, 17, 181, 213–215; in children, 7, 186; of chronic migraine, 7, 11; gender ratio, 6–7, 67, 130–131, 181, 218

Prior, Thomas, 76

prophylaxis, 38, 131, 163, 175–176, 211–212

proprietary medicines, 70–74, 105, 107

psychiatry, 96–98, 129, 156, 158, 165, 170, 176, 182

psychoanalysis, 164–165

psychological theories of migraine, 16, 144, 164–168, 182, 190; criticism of, 168, 176, 186

quackery, 67, 75, 85–86, 149, 217

Queen Square, 88, 98–99, 108–109. *See also* National Hospital for the Paralysed and Epileptic

quinine, 97, 102, 106

race and ethnicity, 7, 17, 139, 213–214, 215

Rachford, Benjamin, 130

Raskin, Neil, 176

recipe collections, manuscript, 11–12, 42, 44–45, 49–50

Regimen Sanitatis Salerni, 39

religion, 29, 61–65, 78, 140–141, 145–147, 195

retrospective diagnosis, 14–16, 135–137, 141–144, 147–151, 153–154

rheum, 4, 48–49, 52–54, 65, 70

rheumatism, 160

rheumatoid arthritis, 102, 212

Robinson, Derek, 150, 191–192, 207

Royal Society of London, 81, 119–120, 121

Royal Society of Medicine, 141, 152–153

Sābūr ibn Sahl, 32

Sacks, Oliver, 144–145, 190, 196

Salmon, William, 71–2

Sandoz Chemical Company, 169–170

sciatica, 61

sedatives, 11, 29, 83, 174, 175–176, 187

self-experimentation, 83, 106, 126

self-medication, 74–75, 77, 105, 106, 165

Semmes, Raphael Eustace, 155–156

serotonin, 12, 176–179

Shaw, Miss, recipe collection, 50

sick headache, 19, 89, 101, 113, 124–125, 158, 206, 217; and blood, 91–2, 93; distinct from migraine, 122, 152; emergence of term, 4, 81, 90; and errors of diet, 84–85, 93; and gender, 130; as lay knowledge, 91–95; and neurasthenia, 127

Singer, Charles, 135, 141–146, 153

sinuses, 81, 91, 152–153, 162

sleep, 31, 147, 175

socioeconomic status, 7, 17, 88–90, 92, 108, 123–124, 130, 217; and access to drugs, 212–213. *See also* poverty

Speed, John, 63–64

spices, 22, 32, 43, 49; cumin, 27, 43, 48, 59, 68; imported, 49, 50, 59; mustard, 22, 26–27, 33, 43, 49, 50, 52, 58; nutmeg, 32–33, 43

Staker, John, 81

stigma, xiii, 99, 127, 196, 216

stimulants, 97, 98, 174

St. John, Johanna, 54

stomach: disturbance of, 19, 30, 77; in Galenic thought, 3, 25, 81–83, 90–91, 103, 104, 113, 116; medicine for, 48, 54, 66, 79; in migraine art, 194, 196, 206; sympathy with nerves of the head, 84

sumatriptan, 178–179, 182, 208

surgery, 11, 20, 23, 155–156, 175

Symonds, C. P., 152

Symonds, John Addington, 122

symptoms, 3–4, 5–6, 34, 42, 113; in art, 193–196, 199, 204, 206; auditory, 30, 103, 122, 138; clusters of, 68; dizziness, 8, 28, 76, 80–81, 100, 127, 217; firsthand accounts of, 89, 99–107, 113, 118, 189; gastric, 4, 81, 117; nausea, 4, 5, 28, 90, 112, 153, 155, 170–171, 174, 176, 178–189; phonophobia, 147,

symptoms (*continued*)
180; photophobia, 5, 28, 30, 34, 147, 180;
postdrome, 103, 180; prodrome, 103, 180;
sensory, 34, 41, 100, 118, 131, 152, 196–197

Talbot, Alathea, 42, 44, 45, 225n56
tea, 90, 98, 126, 127, 131, 188
tension-type headache, 181, 214
terminology, xiii–xiv; changes in, 3–4, 19, 80–81,
82, 94–96; influence of French ideas about, 4,
82–83, 122
tetanus, 96
theriac, 29, 91
Thomson, Francis, 18, 61–63
Thompson, Theophilus, 91
Tissot, Samuel Auguste David, 84, 113, 122–123
Todd, John, 150
Topcliffe, Richard, 61, 65
Townsend, family recipe collection, 53
toxins, 151, 152, 159, 182
tranquilizers, 171, 175, 187
transcutaneous electrical nerve stimulation, 37
treatments, 11–12; access to, 7, 99, 212–213; behavioral, 167–168; cost of, 34, 70, 72, 212–213; drinks
and gargles, 22, 43; efficacy of, 31, 59, 77–78, 95,
106, 152, 157, 169–170, 180, 208; electrical, 105, 131;
experimental, 13, 96–98, 107, 188; inadequacies
of, 74–75, 105, 151, 174–176, 188, 206, 210; nard
oil, 32–33; for an open head, 42–43, 45; patient
compliance with, 95, 174; pills, 1, 71–75, 171–172,
204, 207; plasters and caps, 13, 32, 43, 49–50,
55–59, 68, 70, 91; purgative, 28, 49, 57, 68; and
undertreatment, 9, 215; warming, 32, 52
Tredgold, Alfred, 163–164
trepanation, 136, 137–140, 141
trigeminovascular system, 4, 12, 182, 211
trigger factors, 11, 103, 158, 204
triptans, 181, 182, 208, 237n93
Trotter, Thomas, 90
Twarog, Betty Mack, 177
tyramine, 177–178, 188–189

Urbach, Erich, 161, 163–64
uric acid theory, 126, 159
urine analysis, 34

vapors: ascent of, 25, 48–49, 80; as nervous
disorder, 62, 76, 84; therapeutic action of, 52

vascular theories, 5, 12, 124, 144, 149, 216; compat-
ibility with personality theories, 169; demise of,
180, 182–183; influence on classification, 179–180;
rise to prominence of, 157–158, 166, 176
vasoconstriction, 12, 170, 176–178
vasodilation, 9; drug effects on 107, 169–170, 175,
178, 211; pain due to, 5, 124, 138, 157–158
vasomotor theory, 125, 129, 131
Vaughan, Warren T., 160
vein man diagrams, 13, 35–40
vertigo, 4, 8, 51, 62, 68, 71–72, 80–81, 107, 116
Vicary, Thomas, 52
vomiting: in art, 194, 199, 207; caused by serotonin
fluctuations, 178; in childhood, 129; as drug side
effect, 174; as relief, 113; as symptom, 5, 27, 48–49,
103–106, 155, 158, 178; as treatment, 79, 83, 91
von Hilden, Wilhelm Fabry, 138

Walker, Vera, 161, 174
waters: for bathing, 18, 61–66, 82, 149; chemical
properties of, 64, 65–66, 75–76; to drink, 46, 54,
75–76, 85, 149, 159; herbal, 31, 33; hot to put feet
in, 38–39
weather, 39, 79, 158, 189
Wilkinson, Marcia, 175, 180–181, 188, 192
Wilks, Samuel, 106, 128, 130
Willis, Thomas, 99, 122, 138, 147–148
Wilson, Peter, 186
Woakes, Edward, 169
Wolff, Harold, 166–169, 178, 179
Wollaston, William Hyde, 115
women, 3, 5–7; artists, 184–185, 194–198, 201–209;
and clinical trials, 183, 214; and functional
disorders, 127–128; as healers, 24, 45–47, 54, 149;
and humoral theory, 26; as inpatients, 99–102,
103, 104–107, 130; knowledge networks, 45;
marginalization of, 3, 108; as "martyrs," 89, 93,
130; and personality theories, 165–168, 174;
portrayed as sufferers, 3, 16, 86–87, 92–93, 95,
108, 165–168, 171; pressures of domestic life on,
123, 130, 133, 204–205, 208; relationships with
do[...] oductive
di[...]
Woo[...]
work[...] –131,
158[...] 62,
77[...]
Worl[...] 4